KU-102-170

WITHDRAWN

LIVERPOOL JMU LIBRARY

3 1111 00739 9437

Schools & Health

Our Nation's Investment

Diane Allensworth, Elaine Lawson, Lois Nicholson, and James Wyche,
Editors

Committee on Comprehensive School Health Programs in Grades K–12

Division of Health Sciences Policy

INSTITUTE OF MEDICINE

NATIONAL ACADEMY PRESS
Washington, D.C. 1997

National Academy Press • 2101 Constitution Avenue, NW • Washington, DC 20418

NOTICE: The project that is the subject of this report was approved by the Governing Board of the National Research Council, whose members are drawn from the Councils of the National Academy of Sciences, the National Academy of Engineering, and the Institute of Medicine. The members of the committee responsible for this report were chosen for their special competences and with regard for appropriate balance.

The report has been reviewed by a group other than the authors according to procedures approved by a Report Review Committee consisting of members of the National Academy of Sciences, the National Academy of Engineering, and the Institute of Medicine.

The Institute of Medicine was chartered in 1970 by the National Academy of Sciences to enlist distinguished members of the appropriate professions in the examination of policy matters pertaining to the health of the public. In this, the Institute acts under both the Academy's 1863 congressional charter responsibility to be an adviser to the federal government and its own initiative in identifying issues of medical care, research, and education. Dr. Kenneth I. Shine is president of the Institute of Medicine.

Additional copies of this report are available for sale from the National Academy Press, Lock Box 285, 2101 Constitution Avenue, N.W., Washington, DC 20055.

Call (800) 624-6242 or (202) 334-3313 (in the Washington metropolitan area), or visit the NAP on-line bookstore at **http://www.nap.edu/nap/bookstore**.

Call (202) 334-2352 for more information on the other activities of the Institute of Medicine, or visit the IOM home page at **http://www.nas.edu/iom**.

Library of Congress Cataloging-in-Publication Data

Schools and health : our nation's investment / Committee on
    Comprehensive School Health Programs in Grades K-12, Division of
    Health Sciences Policy, Institute of Medicine ; Diane Allensworth
    ... [et al.], editors.
        p. cm.
    Includes bibliographical references and index.
    ISBN 0-309-05435-4
    1. School health services—United States. 2. School health
services—United States—Planning. 3. Health education—United
States. I. Allensworth, Diane DeMuth. II. Institute of Medicine
(U.S.). Committee on Comprehensive School Health Programs.
  LB3409.U5S33 1997
  371.7'1'0973—dc21   97-21177

Copyright 1997 by the National Academy of Sciences. All rights reserved.

Printed in the United States of America.

The serpent has been a symbol of long life, healing, and knowledge among almost all cultures and religions since the beginning of recorded history. The image adopted as a logotype by the Institute of Medicine is based on a relief carving from ancient Greece, now held by the Staatliche Museen in Berlin.

COMMITTEE ON COMPREHENSIVE SCHOOL HEALTH PROGRAMS IN GRADES K–12

DIANE D. ALLENSWORTH (*Cochair*), Executive Director, American School Health Association, Kent, Ohio

JAMES H. WYCHE (*Cochair*), Associate Provost, Brown University

BEVERLY J. BRADLEY, Certified Health Education Specialist, San Diego City Schools, California

DOROTHY R. CALDWELL, Director, Child Nutrition Programs, Arkansas Department of Education, Little Rock

JOY G. DRYFOOS, Independent Researcher, Hastings-on-Hudson, New York

STEVE A. FREEDMAN, Director, Institute for Child Health Policy, Gainesville, Florida

LA BARBARA GRAGG, Superintendent of Schools, Pontiac, Michigan (retired); Palm City, Florida

JUDITH B. IGOE, Associate Professor and Director, School Health Programs, School of Nursing, University of Colorado, Denver

ELAINE L. LARSON,* Dean, School of Nursing, Georgetown University

JOSEPH D. McINERNEY, Director, Biological Sciences Curriculum Study, Colorado Springs, Colorado

PHILIP R. NADER, Professor and Director, Child and Family Health Studies, Community Pediatrics DIvision, University of California, San Diego

ELENA O. NIGHTINGALE,*† Scholar in Residence, Board on Children and Families, National Academy of Sciences, Washington, D.C.

GUY S. PARCEL, Director, Center for Health Promotion Research and Development, the University of Texas Health Sciences Center, Houston

KEN RESNICOW, Associate Professor, Department of Behavioral Sciences and Health Education, Rollins School of Public Health, Emory University

AARON SHIRLEY,* Director, Jackson Hinds Comprehensive Health Center, Jackson, Mississippi

BECKY J. SMITH, Executive Director, Association for the Advancement of Health Education, Reston, Virginia

LENORE K. ZEDOSKY, Director, Office of Healthy Schools, West Virginia Department of Education, Charleston

---

*Institute of Medicine member.

†Resigned committee September 1995 due to health reasons.

Study Staff

VALERIE P. SETLOW, Director, Division of Health Sciences Policy
LOIS NICHOLSON, Study Director (through May 1996)
ELAINE LAWSON, Research Associate
LINDA A. DEPUGH, Administrative Assistant
MARGO CULLEN, Project Assistant (through October 1996)

Preface

    In late 1994, an Institute of Medicine (IOM) committee was convened to carry out a study of comprehensive school health programs (CSHPs) in grades K–12. These programs are a new concept that combines—in an integrated, systemic manner—health education, health promotion and disease prevention, and access to health and social services at the school site. Whereas earlier generations of school health programs were predominantly concerned with stemming the threat of infectious disease, these problems have now to a large extent been ameliorated and replaced with the "new social morbidities"—injuries, violence, substance abuse, risky sexual behaviors, psychological and emotional disorders, and problems due to poverty—and many students' lack of access to reliable health information and health care. Because schools touch all families and schools are, for the most part, where the children are, CSHPs hold promise for addressing many of the health-related problems of today's children and young people.

    When a study of CSHPs was first contemplated, the IOM was well aware that many groups were already active in school health and sought to determine whether it could make a unique contribution to the field. An outside planning group was convened in 1993 to advise the Institute on the need for and feasibility of its undertaking a study of CSHPs. The planning group identified a broad set of school health issues in the areas of (1) education and curriculum, (2) health promotion and disease prevention, (3) health services, and (4) national strategies and policies that could potentially benefit from the results of an IOM study. The planning group also noted that the IOM—and its partner organization, the National Research Council—had special expertise in such relevant areas as K–12 science education, child and family policy, nutrition, health promotion and disease prevention, and health care policy. Based on the planning group's recommendations and encouragement, the Institute then began the necessary groundwork to assemble the committee and launch the full study.

The resulting 17-member Committee on Comprehensive School Health Programs in Grades K–12 represented a diversity of backgrounds, including physicians, nurses, health educators, science educators, social scientists, basic scientists, school administrators, and experts in public and child health policy. The original charge to the committee was to (1) assess the status of CSHP's, (2) examine what factors appear to predict success (or failure) of these programs; and if appropriate, (3) identify strategies for wider implementation of such programs. This charge was refined by the committee at its first meeting to better describe the scope of work to be undertaken. The revised charge states that the committee will develop a framework for (1) determining the desirable and feasible health outcomes of comprehensive school health programs; (2) examining the relationship between health outcomes and education outcomes; (3) considering what factors are necessary in the school setting to optimize these outcomes; (4) appraising existing data on the effectiveness (including cost-effectiveness) of comprehensive school health programs; and (5) if appropriate, recommending mechanisms for wider implementation of those school health programs that have proven to be effective.

At the onset of the committee's work, it became evident that a broad range of constituencies had become interested and involved in CSHPs and that a variety of opinions existed about what these programs are and what they do. The members of the committee themselves came into the study with a diverse range of backgrounds and experiences; therefore, they determined that it would be useful to establish their own working definition of the term "comprehensive school health program" to use as a guide for further work and to stimulate discussion and feedback from others in the field. In the spring of 1995, the committee developed, published, and distributed an interim statement presenting this working definition and identifying issues that the committee planned to address in its study (IOM, 1995)[1]. The definition and models for CSHPs are further discussed in Chapter 2 of this report.

---

[1]Institute of Medicine. 1995. *Defining a Comprehensive School Health Program.* Washington, D.C.: National Academy Press. Although this report is now out of print, the full text is available on line at www2.nap.edu/readingroom.

The committee met four times during the course of the study. At its first meeting, representatives from various federal agencies presented their programs and priorities in the area of school health. The committee expresses its special thanks to the following agency representatives from the U.S. Department of Health and Human Services, Public Health Service: Linda Johnston, Health Resources and Services Administration, Maternal and Child Health Bureau; Jane Martin, Bureau of Primary Health Care, Health Resources and Services Administration; William Harlan, Office of the Assistant Secretary for Health, Department of Health and Human Services, and Office of Health Promotion and Disease Prevention, National Institutes of Health; Evelyn Kappeler, Office of Population Affairs, and Peter Cortese, Division of Adolescent and School Health, Program Development and Services Branch, Centers for Disease Control and Prevention; and Connie Garner, U.S. Department of Education, Federal Interagency Coordinating Council, Office of the Undersecretary.

A public workshop was convened in conjunction with the first meeting to examine selected elements of a CSHP in depth. The committee appreciates the contributions of the following workshop speakers: Tom O'Rourke, Ph.D., M.P.H., professor, Department of Community Health, University of Illinois, for his review of new directions in health education; Mary Jackson, B.S.N., M.Ed., nurse consultant, Bureau of Women and Children, Texas Department of Health, for her analysis of the relationship of health education to the core curriculum; Eulalia Muschik, M.S., R.D., supervisor of food services, Carroll County (Maryland) Public Schools, for her examination of nutrition education and food services; Karla Shepard-Rubinger, M.S., The Conservation Company, and John Santelli, M.D., M.P.H., medical epidemiologist, Baltimore City Health Department, and adjunct assistant professor of Maternal and Child Health, Johns Hopkins School of Hygiene and Public Health, for their presentations about school-affiliated clinics and service delivery; and Genie L. Wessel, R.N., M.S., project director, Making the Grade Program, Maryland Governor's Office, for her presentation on approaches for integrating school health programs.

Because research and evaluation are major challenges for CSHPs, a subcommittee on research and evaluation was appointed after the first meeting to examine issues in this area. At the second meeting, the subcommittee reported its findings on the status and results of current research to the full committee and outlined the most difficult problems and obstacles in conducting research on these multifaceted programs. As a result of the full committee discussion, a paper by Mary Ann Pentz, Ph.D., was commissioned, which stresses that schools are just one part of a broader community system and describes various evaluation studies on school–community programs and interactions. (See Appendix A.)

Also at the second meeting, one day was devoted to a discussion of financing school health programs and services. The committee thanks the following speakers for their presentations on the topic: Harriette Fox, M.S., of Fox Health Policy Consultants; Susan L. Lordi, administrative project director, School Health Programs, Los Angeles County Office of Education; and Ruth Rich, Ed.D., director of Drug, Alcohol, and Tobacco Education Programs, Los Angeles Unified School District.

The third committee meeting examined school-affiliated services. The committee appreciates the views expressed by the following speakers at that meeting: Phyllis L. Gingiss, Dr. P.H., associate dean of research, College of Education, University of Houston, for her presentation on the education and training of school health personnel; Deborah Klein Walker, Ed.M., Ed.D., assistant commissioner, Bureau of Family and Community Health, Massachusetts Department of Public Health, for her overview of school-affiliated services; and Thomas W. Payzant, Ed.D., assistant secretary for elementary and secondary education, U.S. Department of Education, for his analysis of school-affiliated services from the educator or administrator's point of view. The committee also thanks the following individuals for their participation in a panel discussion on school-affiliated services: Kevin Dwyer, M.A., NCSP, assistant executive director, National Association of School Psychologists; Isadora Hare, ACSW, LCSW, National Association of Social Workers; Olga Wright, representing the National Association of School Nurses, from the Alexandria (Virginia) City Public Schools; and Judith Ladd, representing the American School Counselor Association, from Prince William County (Virginia) Public Schools.

At the fourth and final meeting, the committee met in working session to finalize the report and its recommendations.

Thus, in the final analysis, the committee has responded to its charge throughout the chapters of this report. The committee's response to the first element of the charge, to develop a framework for determining the desirable and feasible health outcomes (including mental, emotional, and social health) of CSHPs, can be found in Chapters 3 and 4. The second element, to examine the relationship between health outcomes and education outcomes, is addressed in Chapter 1, in which the committee found that dropouts are more likely to have costly medical problems, and Chapter 2. The third element, to consider what factors are necessary in the school setting to optimize these outcomes, is addressed in Chapters 3 and 4. The fourth element, to appraise existing data on effectiveness (including cost-effectiveness) of comprehensive school health programs and identify possible additional strategies for evaluation of the effectiveness of these programs, is discussed in Chapter 6. The fifth and final element, to recommend mechanisms for wider implementation of those health programs that have proven to be effective, is discussed extensively in Chapter 5.

This important report would not have been possible without the excellent staff work at the Institute of Medicine. The committee thanks Valerie P. Setlow, Ph.D., Director of the Division of Health Sciences Policy, for her revisions to the text, constant enthusiasm, encouragement, and guidance during the study and throughout the report review process. Thanks also are due to Study Director Lois Nicholson, M.S., who provided staff leadership during the course of the study by weaving together the separate contributions of individual committee members to develop the original draft of this report. The committee also thanks Research Associate Elaine Lawson, M.S., for developing the study concept at its inception, and for her efforts in gathering and organizing information, working with committee members in writing their contributions, and helping to develop the response to review. Appreciation is extended to Project Assistant Margo Cullen for her excellent administrative support in making meeting and travel arrangements, and facilitating communication among committee members and staff. Sincere thanks go to Linda DePugh, Administrative Assistant, for making editorial corrections to the entire report and for producing the tables and figures and the camera ready manuscript for publication. Thanks also go to Claudia Carl for her patience and guidance in shepherding the report through the review process; and Mike Edington for getting the report to the press in rapid and good condition and for finding Florence Pollion, who edited the report. Finally, we thank the sponsors, NIH, CDC, HRSA, and the Department for Education for their support and vision about the need for this report. We are greatly appreciative of their confidence throughout this process. The cochairs thank all the committee members for their extraordinary spirit of teamwork and dedication. Working with such a distinguished and dedicated group has been a wonderful experience; all of us have learned from each other and are richer for the opportunity.

Diane Allensworth, *Cochair*
James Wyche, *Cochair*

Support for this project was provided by the Centers for Disease Control and Prevention (Division of Adolescent and School Health), the Health Resources and Services Administration (Bureau of Primary Care and Maternal and Child Health Bureau), the National Institutes of Health (Office of Disease Prevention, Office of the Director, National Cancer Institute, National Institute of Environmental Health Sciences, National Institute for Drug Abuse, National Institute for Dental Research, National Center for Research Resources, and National Institute of Arthritis and Musculoskeletal and Skin Diseases), the U.S. Department of Education, and the U.S. Department of Health and Human Services, Public Health Service (Office of the Assistant Secretary and Office of Population Affairs). Support for dissemination of this report was provided by the Kaiser Family Foundation and the Centers for Disease Control and Prevention (Division of Adolescent and School Health). This support does not constitute an endorsement by the U.S. Department of Health and Human Services or the U.S. Department of Education of the views expressed in the report.

Contents

EXECUTIVE SUMMARY   1
    Background, 1
    Findings, Conclusions, and Recommendations, 3
    Moving School Health Programs into the Future, 14

1   INTRODUCTION   16
    Background of the Study, 16
    The Current Context for School Health Programs, 18
    The Comprehensive School Health Program, 28
    Major Issues and Questions Considered by the Committee, 29
    Organization of the Remainder of This Report, 29

2   EVOLUTION OF SCHOOL HEALTH PROGRAMS   33
    Historical Overview, 33
    The Comprehensive School Health Program, 50
    Summary, 76

3   EDUCATION   81
    The Role of Physical Education in Comprehensive School
      Health Programs, 81
    The Role of Health Education in Comprehensive
      School Health Programs, 99
    Summary of Findings and Conclusions, 139
    Recommendations, 140

4   SCHOOL HEALTH SERVICES   153
      Introduction, 153
      Overview of Basic School Services, 161
      Extended Services, 181
      Research on School Health Services, 186
      Matching Level of Services to Needs, 199
      Confidentiality of Students' Health and Education Records, 204
      Financing of School Health Services, 206
      First Steps for a Community in Establishing School Services, 216
      Summary of Findings and Conclusions, 225
      Recommendations, 226

5   BUILDING THE INFRASTRUCTURE FOR
      COMPREHENSIVE SCHOOL HEALTH PROGRAMS   237
      The National Infrastructure, 238
      The State and Local Infrastructure, 246
      Summary of Findings and Conclusions, 261
      Recommendations, 261

6   CHALLENGES IN SCHOOL HEALTH RESEARCH
      AND EVALUATION   271
      Overview of Research and Evaluation, 271
      Methodological Challenges, 276
      Challenges and Future Directions for School Health
        Education Research, 280
      Summary of Findings and Conclusions, 288
      Recommendations, 289

7   THE PATH TO THE FUTURE   296
      The Unique Position of the School, 296
      Moving School Health Programs into the Future, 297
      An Investment in the Future, 299
      Concluding Remarks, 301

APPENDIXES
A   THE SCHOOL–COMMUNITY INTERFACE IN
      COMPREHENSIVE SCHOOL HEALTH EDUCATION   305
B   GUIDELINES FOR COMPREHENSIVE SCHOOL
      HEALTH PROGRAMS   337
C   MODELS OF HEALTH BEHAVIOR CHANGE USED
      IN HEALTH EDUCATION PROGRAMS   356
D   NEW APPROACHES TO THE ORGANIZATION OF
      HEALTH AND SOCIAL SERVICES IN SCHOOLS   365

E   GUIDELINES FOR ADOLESCENT PREVENTIVE SERVICES   416
F   FEDERAL FUNDING STREAMS FOR COMPREHENSIVE
     SCHOOL HEALTH PROGRAMS   430
G-1 A VISION OF INTEGRATED SERVICES FOR CHILDREN
     AND FAMILIES   443
G-2 THE WEST VIRGINIA EXPERIENCE:
     AN INFRASTRUCTURE MODEL   456
G-3 CONNECTICUT SCHOOL HEALTH SERVICES MODELS   463

ACRONYMS AND ABBREVIATIONS   474

INDEX   478

Executive Summary

BACKGROUND

Schools have been the site for health programming in the United States since the early colonial period. When public education became compulsory in the mid-nineteenth century, the strategic role that schools could play in promoting and protecting health became recognized; schools soon became the front line in the fight against infectious disease and the hub for providing a wide range of health and social services for children and families.

As times changed, school health programs have changed to keep pace with the changing needs of children and adolescents. The Centers for Disease Control and Prevention (CDC) has noted that six categories of behavior are responsible for 70 percent of adolescent mortality and morbidity: unintentional and intentional injuries, drug and alcohol abuse, sexually transmitted diseases and unintended pregnancies, diseases associated with tobacco use, illnesses resulting from inadequate physical activity, and health problems due to inadequate dietary patterns. A significant segment of our nation's youth is at risk for dropping out of school as a consequence of a broad range of health and behavioral problems; further, many children do not have access to basic preventive and primary care.

The concept of a comprehensive school health program (CSHP) was proposed in the 1980s to address many of the health-related[1] problems of

---

[1]The committee uses the term "health" in its broadest sense. Health is more than simply the absence of disease; health involves optimal physical, mental, social, and emotional functioning and well-being.

today's children and young people. CSHPs are intended to take advantage of the pivotal position of schools in reaching children and families by combining—in an integrated, systemic manner—health education, health promotion and disease prevention, and access to health-related services at the school site. CSHPs may be a promising way both to improve health and educational outcomes for students and to reduce overall health care costs by emphasizing prevention and easy access to care.

The original charge to the committee was to: (1) assess the status of CSHPs; (2) examine what factors appear to predict success (or failure) of these programs; and if appropriate, (3) identify strategies for wider implementation of such programs. This charge was refined by the committee at its first meeting to better describe the scope of work to be undertaken. The revised charge states that the committee will develop a framework for (1) determining the desirable and feasible health outcomes of CSHPs; (2) examining the relationship between health outcomes and education outcomes; (3) considering what factors are necessary in the school setting to optimize these outcomes; (4) appraising existing data on the effectiveness (including the cost-effectiveness) of CSHPs; and (5) if appropriate, recommending mechanisms for wider implementation of those school health programs that have proven to be effective.

Early in the course of the study, the committee established its own working definition of a CSHP as follows:

> A comprehensive school health program is an integrated set of planned, sequential, school-affiliated strategies, activities, and services designed to promote the optimal physical, emotional, social, and educational development of students. The program involves and is supportive of families and is determined by the local community, based on community needs, resources, standards, and requirements. It is coordinated by a multidisciplinary team and accountable to the community for program quality and effectiveness.

In developing this definition, the committee examined a variety of models and definitions of school health programs. However, whatever the program model, the committee found that there are three critical areas that should be considered in designing a CSHP.

The first critical area is the **school environment,** which includes (1) the *physical environment*, involving proper building design, lighting, ventilation, safety, cleanliness, freedom from environmental hazards that foster infection and handicaps, safe transportation policies, and having emergency plans in place; (2) the *policy and administrative environment*, consisting of policies to promote health and reduce stress, and regulations ensuring an environment free from tobacco, drugs, weapons, and violence; (3) the *psychosocial environment*, including a supportive and nurturing atmosphere, a cooperative academic setting, respect for individual differences, and involvement of families; and (4) *health promotion for staff*, in order that staff members can become positive role models and increase their commitment to student health.

The second critical area is **education,** which consists of *physical education,* which teaches the knowledge and skills necessary for lifelong physical fitness; *health education*, which addresses the physical, mental, emotional, and social dimensions of health; and *other curricular areas*, which promote healthful behavior and an awareness of health issues as part of their core instruction.

The third critical area is **services**, which includes *health services*, that depend on the needs and preferences of the community and services for students with disabilities and special health care needs; *counseling, psychological, and social services*, which promote academic success and address the emotional and mental health needs of students; and *nutrition and foodservices*, which provide nutritious meals, nutrition education, and a nutrition-promoting school environment.

Three of the most common models examined include the following:

• **The Three-Component Model**: This is the traditional model for CSHPs. According to this model, the three essential components of a school health program are health education, health services, and a healthful environment.

• **The Eight-Component Model**: According to this model, the eight essential components of a CSHP are health education, physical education, health services, nutrition services, health promotion for school staff, counseling and psychological services, a healthy school environment, and parent and community involvement.

• **Full-Service Schools**: In addition to quality education, these combine a wide range of health services, mental health services, and family welfare and social services for students and their families.

The committee determined that the most frequently encountered models and definitions for school health programs had much in common and that no single model was best. CSHPs must be locally tailored—with the involvement of all critical stakeholders—to meet each community's needs, resources, perspectives, and standards.

FINDINGS, CONCLUSIONS, AND RECOMMENDATIONS

The committee examined four topics of school health in depth: education, services, infrastructure, and research and evaluation. The principal findings, conclusions, and recommendations pertaining to each area are presented in the remainder of this section.

Education

Findings and Conclusions

The status of the two curricular components of a CSHP—physical education and health education—is sometimes questioned because they were not originally mentioned in the National Education Goals as "core subjects" in which students should demonstrate competence. However, with each updated report, the National Education Goals panel has added language emphasizing the importance of physical education and health education, affirming that these two subjects should be an integral part of the school curriculum.

Physical Education   Research has confirmed a direct relationship between a physically active life-style and improved long-term health status. Therefore, the new generation of physical education programs is shifting emphasis from competitive sports to physical activity and fitness. Three recent documents—the National Standards for Physical Education, the School Health Policies and Programs Study[2] (SHPPS), and the CDC's Guidelines for School and Community Health Programs to Promote Physical Activity Among Youth—emphasize the new priorities and recommendations in physical education and collectively provide a sound basis for developing quality physical education programs in the future. The committee supports these recommendations.

Health Education   The traditional health education curriculum has been based on 10 conceptual areas identified by the School Health Education Study of the 1960s: community health, consumer health, environmental health, family life, mental and emotional health, injury prevention and safety, nutrition, personal health, prevention and control of disease, and substance use and abuse. Recently, CDC recommended that the six major contributors to adolescent mortality and morbidity mentioned earlier be priority areas of emphasis for health education because these problems are based in behaviors that can be prevented or changed. The overarching goal of the recently released National Health Education Standards is the development of health literacy—the capacity to obtain, interpret, and understand basic health information and services and the competence to use such information and services to enhance health.

---

[2]The School Health Policies and Programs Study was conducted in 1994 by the Centers for Disease Control and Prevention to examine policies and programs across multiple components of school health programs at the state, district, school, and classroom levels.

Research conducted since 1970 has shown that specific health education curricula are effective, for example, those focused on categorical problems such as tobacco avoidance. Studies have shown that in order for health education to produce behavior change, effective strategies, considerable instructional time, and well-prepared teachers are required. Students' behavioral decisions are also heavily influenced by environmental variables—peers, family, schools, community, and the media. A recent cost–benefit analysis shows that school health education is cost-effective, and several recent national surveys indicate that parents and students overwhelmingly consider health education to be very important and useful.

Despite the potential effectiveness and favorable perception of health education, SHPPS found a considerable gap between what health educators consider to be desired practice and actual current practice. Typically, only one semester of health education is required at the middle or junior high level and one semester at the high school level, and the attention given to certain priority topics falls considerably short of recommended goals. Although most teachers of health education have not majored in the field, there is not an overwhelming demand for staff development. This lack of demand may be due to a lack of awareness on the part of teachers and administrators of the potential and complexities of health education or the fact that teachers with majors in other fields prefer to teach in those fields and see no value in improving their skills in health education.

Recommendations

The committee believes that three recently released documents—the National Action Plan for Comprehensive School Health Education, the National Health Education Standards, and the SHPPS report—collectively provide comprehensive recommendations and a strong framework to move health education forward in the future. Beyond this, however, several aspects of health education merit further emphasis and discussion.

The committee believes that the period prior to high school is the most crucial for shaping attitudes and behaviors. By the time students reach high school, many are already engaging in risky behaviors or may at least have formed accepting attitudes toward these behaviors.

The committee recommends that all students receive sequential, age-appropriate health education every year during the elementary and middle or junior high grades.

At all grade levels, instruction should focus on achieving the performance indicators outlined in the National Health Education Standards. Early years might focus on such topics as nutrition and safety, but beginning at the late elementary or early middle school grades, instruction should shift focus to an intensive, age-appropriate emphasis on the CDC priority behaviors and should be provided by teachers who understand early adolescents and are especially prepared to deal with these sensitive and difficult topics.

The committee recommends that a one-semester health education course at the secondary level immediately become a minimum requirement for high school graduation. Instruction should follow the National Health Education Standards, use effective up-to-date curricula, be provided by qualified health education teachers interested in teaching the subject, and emphasize the six priority behavioral areas identified by the CDC.

According to SHPPS, 83.9 percent of all senior high schools already require at least one semester of health education, and within this 83.9 percent, the CDC topics are frequently emphasized. Thus, such an immediate requirement is not unrealistic. Additional courses or electives in health education at the high school level would be preferable to a single semester.

The committee debated how to reconcile the call for students to receive health education every year, from kindergarten through the twelfth grade, with the reality of the crowded curriculum at the secondary level and decided that the critical issue should be whether high school students achieve the performance indicators described in the National Health Education Standards, not the amount of "seat time." Thus, the committee recommends that the "seat time" be a minimum of at least one semester, but that student health knowledge and understanding be assessed at the end of this course. If a community finds its young people falling short on this assessment, the existing course must be improved or additional courses instituted. The committee believes that some form of health education must occur every year at the secondary level but that some of this education can take place through alternative approaches, such as "booster" sessions, health modules in other courses, field trips, assemblies, school-wide campaigns, after-school peer discussion groups, and one-on-one or small group counseling for students with identified needs.

Effective elementary health education is the foundation for the future critical middle school years, and well-prepared elementary teachers are the key for providing this education.

The committee recommends that all elementary teachers receive

substantive preparation in health education content and methodology during their preservice college training. This preparation should give elementary generalist teachers strategies for infusing health instruction into the curriculum and prepare upper elementary teachers to lay the groundwork for the intensive middle or junior high health education program.

Services

Findings and Conclusions

Although the scope of school health services varies from one school district to another, many common elements exist throughout the country. Most schools provide screenings, monitor student immunization status, and administer first aid and medication. Schools are also required to provide a wide range of health services for students with disabilities and special health care needs.

There is agreement among virtually all school districts that a core set of services is needed in schools, but the topic currently generating a great deal of discussion is the role of the school in providing access to "extended services" that go beyond traditional basic services, such as primary care, social, and family services. The committee believes that extended services should not be the sole—or even the major—responsibility of the schools; instead, the school should be considered by other community agencies and providers as a partner and a potentially effective site for provision of needed services—services that will ultimately advance the primary academic mission of the school.

Although the demands and complexity of basic school services have increased, these services are often supervised by education-based administrators who have no clinical preparation in the delivery of health services. Thus, it is important to develop closer links between the school and community health systems and to encourage greater involvement of community health care professionals in the planning and implementation of basic services. School-based health centers (SBHCs) and other extended services are a relatively new phenomenon, and research in this area is in its early stages. Studies have shown that SBHCs provide access to care for needy students and increase students' health knowledge significantly. However, it has been difficult to measure the impact of SBHCs on students' health status or high-risk behavior, such as sexual activity or drug use. This is consistent, however, with other interventions to reduce high-risk behavior—increased knowledge has little effect unless the environment and perceived norms are changed. The committee believes that access, utilization, and possibly a reduction in absenteeism may be more appropriate **measures of outcomes of effectiveness** of SBHCs than change in health status or high-risk behavior.

Recommendations

> **School health services should be formally planned, and the quality of services should be continuously monitored as an integral part of the community public health and primary care systems.**

In the planning process, school health services should be considered an integral part of the overall community public health and primary care system. The range of services actually provided at the school site must be determined locally, based on community characteristics and needs. Special concerns should be emphasized about two areas of services that a significant proportion of students need—mental health or psychological counseling and school foodservice. The committee believes that mental health and psychological services are essential in enabling many students to achieve academically; these should be considered mainstream, not optional, services. The committee also believes that the school foodservice should serve as a learning laboratory for developing healthful eating habits and should not be driven by profit-making or forced to compete with other food options in school that may undermine nutrition goals.

Many questions remain unanswered about school services, particularly questions regarding the relative advantages, disadvantages, quality, and effectiveness of providing extended services at the school rather than at other sites in the community. Thus, the committee recommends the following:

> **Research should be conducted on school-based services, particularly on the organization, management, efficacy, and cost-effectiveness of extended services.**

Additionally, the committee found that there is no current consistent school health data collection process among and between schools. Accurate data collection protocols and standards would greatly facilitate school health research of all kinds.

So that the privacy of families and adolescents be maintained, the committee recommends the following:

> **Confidentiality of health records should be given high priority by the school. Confidential health records of students should be handled and shared in the school setting in a manner that is**

consistent with the manner in which health records are handled in nonschool health care settings in the state.

The lack of a consistent and adequate funding base has been a barrier to establishing school health services. Thus, the committee recommends the following:

Established sources of funding for school health services should continue from both public health and education funds, and new approaches must be developed.

Strategies that have shown promise and should be explored further include billing Medicaid for services to eligible students, developing school-based insurance groupings, forming alliances with managed care organizations and other providers, instituting special taxes, and placing surcharges or special premiums on existing insurance policies.

The CSHP Infrastructure

Findings and Conclusions

Many parts of the infrastructure—the basic framework of policies, resources, organizational structures, and communication channels—needed to support CSHPs already exist or are emerging. However, these parts are often fragmented and uncoordinated, and resources are typically transient or limited to specific categorical activities. Leadership and coordination at all levels—national, state, local—will be crucial for programs to become established and grow.

Recommendations

At the national level, the federal Interagency Committee on School Health (ICSH) was established in 1994 to improve coordination among federal agencies, identify national needs and strategies, and serve as a national focal point for school health. The National Coordinating Committee on School Health (NCCSH), which works closely with the ICSH, brings together federal departments with approximately 40 national nongovernmental organizations to provide national leadership in school health.

The committee recommends that the mission of the federal Interagency Committee on School Health be revitalized so that the ICSH fulfills its potential to provide national leadership

and to carry out critical new national initiatives in school health. In addition, the committee recommends that the National Coordinating Committee on School Health serve as an official advisory body to the ICSH and that individual NCCSH organizations mobilize their memberships to promote the development of a CSHP infrastructure at the state and local levels. The committee also recommends that the membership of the NCCSH be expanded to include representatives from managed care organizations, indemnity insurers, and others who will be key to resolving financial issues of CSHPs.

The responsibilities of the national leadership should include coordinating programs and funding streams, providing technical assistance to states, and advancing the CSHP research agenda.

At the state level, the infrastructure can be anchored by a structure similar to the ICSH–NCCSH arrangement at the national level.

The committee recommends that an official state interagency coordinating council for school health be established in each state to integrate health education, physical education, health services, physical and social environment policies and practices, mental health, and other related efforts for children and families. Further, an advisory committee of representatives from relevant public and private sector agencies, including representatives from managed care organizations and indemnity insurers, should be added.

The state coordinating council should coordinate state programs and funding streams, propose appropriate state policies and legislation, and provide assistance to local districts. Establishing a regional "school health extension service," modeled after the Agricultural Extension Service offers a particularly promising approach for providing technical assistance.

To anchor the infrastructure at the community or district level, the committee recommends the following:

A formal organization with broad representation—a coordinating council for school health—should be established in every school district.

Among its duties, the district coordinating council should involve the community in conducting a needs and resource assessment, developing plans and policies, coordinating programs and resources, and providing assistance to individual schools. Communities must be prepared to confront barriers in building their CSHP infrastructure, including time and resource constraints, turf battles, indifference, or controversy over sensitive aspects of programs. An effective method for mobilizing support has been to enlist parents and other community leaders as program advocates. Compromise on small issues may be essential for the sake of advancing the larger program.

At the school level:

The committee recommends that, at the school level, individual schools should establish a school health committee and appoint a school health coordinator to oversee the school health program.

Under this leadership, schools should address the major issues facing students and/or the components of the CSHP, develop policies, coordinate activities and resources, and seek the active involvement of students and families in designing and implementing programs.

In order to implement quality comprehensive school health programs, the training and utilization of competent, properly prepared personnel should be expanded.

Specific personnel needs are described in the full report. In general, an interdisciplinary approach is needed in the preservice and inservice preparation of CSHP professionals to enable them to communicate and collaborate with each other. Educators in all disciplines—particularly administrators—need preparation in order to understand the philosophy and potential of CSHPs.

Research and Evaluation

Findings and Conclusions

Research and evaluation of CSHPs can be divided into three categories: basic research, outcome evaluation, and process evaluation. Basic research involves inquiry into the fundamental determinants of behavior as well as mechanisms of behavior change. A primary function of basic research is to inform the development of interventions that can then be tested in outcome evaluation trials. Outcome evaluation involves the empirical examination of interventions on targeted outcomes, based on the randomized clinical trial approach with experimental and control groups. Process evaluation determines whether a proven intervention was properly implemented and examines factors that may have contributed to the intervention's success or failure. Basic research and outcome evaluation are typically conducted by professionals from university or other research centers and are largely beyond the capacity of local education agencies. The committee believes that process evaluation is the appropriate level of evaluation in local programs.

Research and evaluation are particularly challenging for CSHPs. Since these programs comprise multiple interactive components, it is often difficult to attribute observed effects to specific components or to separate program effects from those of the family or community. Determining what outcomes are realistic and measuring outcomes in students is often problematic, especially when outcomes involve sensitive matters such as drug use or sexual behavior. Furthermore, since CSHPs are unique to a particular setting, the results of even the most rigorous evaluations may not be generalizable to other situations.

Interventions associated with the separate, individual components of CSHPs—health education, health services, and nutrition services—should be developed and tested using rigorous methods involving experimental and control groups. However, such an approach is likely to be difficult—and possibly not feasible—for studying entire comprehensive programs or determining the differential effects of individual components and combinations of components.

A fundamental issue involves determining what outcomes are appropriate and reasonable to expect from CSHPs. The committee recognizes that, although influencing health behavior and health status is an ultimate goal of a CSHP, such end points involve factors beyond the control of the school. The committee believes that the reasonable outcomes on which a CSHP should be judged are equipping students with the knowledge, attitudes, and skills necessary for healthful behavior; providing a health-promoting environment; and ensuring access to high-quality services.[3] Other outcomes—improved cardiovascular fitness or a reduction in absenteeism, drug abuse, or teen pregnancies, for example—may also be considered, but the committee believes that such measures must be interpreted with caution, since they are influenced by factors beyond the control of the school. In particular, null or negative measures for these outcomes should not necessarily lead to declaring the CSHP a failure; rather, they may imply that other sources of influence oppose and outweigh that

---

[3]This is consistent with the view that for the local school, the desired level of evaluation is process evaluation. If the school is providing health curricula and services that have been shown through basic research and outcome evaluation to produce positive health outcomes, the committee suggests that the crucial question at the school level should be whether the interventions are implemented properly.

of the CSHP or that the financial investment in the CSHP is so limited that returns are minimal.

Recommendations

In order for CSHPs to accomplish the desired goal of influencing behavior, the committee recommends the following:

An active research agenda on comprehensive school health programs should be pursued to fill critical knowledge gaps; increased emphasis should be placed on basic research and outcome evaluation and on the dissemination of these research and outcome findings.

Research is needed about the effectiveness of specific intervention strategies such as skills training, normative education, or peer education; the effectiveness of specific intervention messages such as abstinence versus harm reduction; and the required intensity and duration of health services and health education programming. Evidence suggests that common underlying factors may be responsible for the clustering of health-compromising behaviors and that interventions may be more effective if they address these underlying factors in addition to intervening to change risk behaviors. Additional research is needed to understand the etiology of problem behavior clusters and to develop optimal problem behavior interventions. And finally, since the acquisition of health-related social skills—such as negotiation, decisionmaking, and refusal skills—is a desired end point of CSHPs, basic research is needed to develop valid measures of social skills that can then be used as proxy measures of program effectiveness. Diffusion-related research is critical to ensure that efforts of research and development lead to improved practice and a greater utilization of effective methods and programs. Therefore, high priority should be given to studying how programs are adopted, implemented, and institutionalized. The feasibility and effectiveness of techniques of integrating concepts of health into science and other school subjects should also be examined.

Since the overall effects of comprehensive school health programs are not yet known and outcome evaluations of such complex systems pose significant challenges, the committee recommends the following:

A major research effort should be launched to establish model comprehensive programs and to develop approaches for their study.

Specific outcomes of overall programs should be examined, including education (improved achievement, attendance, and graduation rates), personal health (resistance to "new social morbidities," improved biological measures), mental health (less depression, stress, and violence), improved functionality, health systems (more students with a medical home; reduction in use of emergency rooms or hospitals), self-sufficiency (pursuit of higher education or job), and future health literacy and health status. Studies could examine differential impacts of programs produced by such factors as program structure, characteristics of students, and type of school and community.

A thorough understanding of the feasible and effective (including cost-effective) interventions in each separate area of a CSHP will be necessary to provide the basis for combining components to produce a comprehensive program.

The committee recommends that further study of each of the individual components of a CSHP—for example, health education, health services, counseling, nutrition, school environment—is needed.

Additional studies are needed in a number of other areas. First, more data are needed about the advantages (cost and effectiveness) and disadvantages of providing health and social services in schools compared to other community sites—or compared to not providing services anywhere—as a function of community and student characteristics. This information will require overall consensus about the criteria to use for determining the quality of school health programs. It is also important to know how best to influence change in the climate and organizational structure of school districts and individual schools in order to bring about the adoption and implementation of CSHPs. Finally, there is a need for an analysis of the optimal structure, operation, and personnel needs of CSHPs.

MOVING SCHOOL HEALTH PROGRAMS INTO THE FUTURE

Schooling is the only universal entitlement for children in the United States. The committee believes that students, as a part of this entitlement, should receive the health-related programs and services necessary for them to derive maximum benefit from their education and to enable them to become healthy, productive adults. This view appears to be broadly accepted, since the committee has found that many of the components of a CSHP already exist in many schools across the country—health education, physical education, nutrition and foodservice programs, basic school health services, counseling and psychological services, and policies addressing the quality of the school environment. The question then arises: What would it take to transform existing programs in typical communities into the vision of a comprehensive school health program?

First, although many components of a CSHP already exist widely, their implementation and quality require attention. New standards and recommendations have been released in many fields that have yet to reach the local level. Another serious deficiency is the apparent lack of involvement of critical community stakeholders in designing and supporting current programs. Perhaps the most difficult issue to resolve before existing programs can be considered "comprehensive" involves the role of the school in providing access to services typically considered the responsibility of the private sector, such as certain preventive and primary health care services. "Providing access" does not necessarily mean that services will be delivered at the school site; rather, it implies ensuring that all students are able to obtain and make use of needed services. Each community must devise appropriate strategies to ensure that all of its students have access to these basic preventive and primary care services.

Although there are divergent opinions about some categorical aspects of school health programs, the committee found a uniform belief that school health programs are important and valuable. Nonetheless, despite this uniform opinion, there is a wide gap between the conceptualization of programs and their implementation. Before school health programs can achieve their promise, concerted action will be needed to bridge this gap. Such action could include coordinating scattered activities; improving the quality and consistency of implementation; engaging the participation of crucial stakeholders; and providing an adequate, stable funding base.

Although dedication and cooperation will be required, the committee believes that the vision of a comprehensive school health program is attainable, and the situation is not so complicated that, even today, a local community could not begin to work toward this vision. The committee is not calling for schools to do more on their own; instead, it is asking communities to recognize and take advantage of the key role that schools can play in promoting and protecting the health and well-being of our nation's children and youth. An investment in the health and education of today's children and young people is the ultimate investment for the future.

1

Introduction

BACKGROUND OF THE STUDY

Times have changed, and so have school health programs. Many adults remember school health as consisting of lessons about first aid and the four food groups, with occasional visits to the school nurse for minor illnesses or injuries. While these issues have not disappeared, today's school health programs also are faced with a new array of difficult and seemingly intractable problems: the "new social morbidities"—violence, drug and alcohol abuse, acquired immunodeficiency syndrome (AIDS) and other sexually transmitted diseases (STDs), teen pregnancy, and depression; students' lack of access to reliable health information and health care; changing family structures; and increasing poverty. Traditional approaches to school health programs may no longer be sufficient to deal with these complex issues.

A new concept of school health programming—the "comprehensive school health program"—was proposed in the 1980s as a means to address many of these health-related[1] problems of our nation's children and young people. Comprehensive school health programs (CSHPs) are de-

---

[1]Throughout its study and this report, the committee uses the term "health" in its broadest sense. Health is much more than simply the absence of disease; health involves optimal physical, mental, social, and emotional functioning and well-being. The World Health Organization has defined health as "a state of complete physical, mental, and social well-being, and not merely the absence of disease or infirmity." (World Health Organization, 1996).

signed to take advantage of the pivotal position of the school in reaching children and families by combining—in an integrated, systemic manner—health education, health promotion and disease prevention, and access to health and social services at the school site. CSHPs are implemented in conjunction with other educational reforms to join together the movement toward quality education with health enhancement. CSHPs may be promising not only for improving health and educational outcomes for students but also for reducing overall health care costs by emphasizing prevention, adoption of health-enhancing behaviors, and early identification of health problems and by providing easy access to care.

The Committee on Comprehensive School Health Programs in Grades K through 12 (K–12) was convened by the Institute of Medicine (IOM) to carry out a 15-month study to develop a framework for (1) determining the desirable and feasible health outcomes (including mental, emotional, and social health) of comprehensive school health programs; (2) examining the relationship between health outcomes and education outcomes; (3) considering what factors are necessary in the school setting to optimize these outcomes; (4) appraising existing data on the effectiveness (including cost-effectiveness) of comprehensive school health programs and identifying possible additional strategies for evaluation of the effectiveness of these programs; and (5) if appropriate, recommending mechanisms for wider implementation of those school health programs that have proven to be effective. The committee found that many aspects of CSHPs are in place in numerous schools. However, a comprehensive, integrated, and synergistic program remains a concept in most school systems. The task of the committee was to examine the rationale, structure, and status of these programs and to consider whether and how the concept might become a reality.

The committee began its study with the following basic assumptions:

1. The primary goal of schools is education.
2. Education and health are linked. Educational outcomes are related to health status, and health outcomes are related to education.
3. There are certain basic health needs of children and young people. These include nurturing and support; timely and relevant health information, knowledge, and skills necessary to adopt healthful behavior; and access to health care.
4. The school has the potential to be a crucial part of the system to provide these basic health needs. Schools are where children and youth spend a significant amount of their time, and schools can reach entire families. However, the school is only part of the broader community system; the responsibility does not and should not fall only on the schools.

LIVERPOOL JOHN MOORES UNIVERSITY
LEARNING SERVICES

THE CURRENT CONTEXT FOR
SCHOOL HEALTH PROGRAMS

A variety of important reports have been released in recent years raising concern about the health, education, and social condition of many of our nation's children and young people (Carnegie Council on Adolescent Development, 1989; National Commission on Children, 1991; National Commission on the Role of the School and the Community in Improving Adolescent Health, 1990; National Research Council, 1993; Office of Technology Assessment, 1991; U.S. General Accounting Office, 1993, 1994a, 1994b). These concerns include the fact that economically, children are the poorest segment of our citizenry,[2] and infant mortality rates in some parts of the country are as high as those in many developing countries.[3] Two seminal documents recently have been released containing new recommendations for the health supervision of children and adolescents in order to address the changing problems of today. *Bright Futures: Guidelines for Health Supervision of Infants, Children, and Adolescents*[4] emphasizes that new strategies are needed to address the major economic, social, and demographic changes that have occurred in recent decades and have had a dramatic effect on the health and welfare of children (Green, 1994). These changes include a decrease in the time parents spend with children, the disintegration of families and an increase in the number of children living in single-parent households, and a rapid escalation of the numbers of children living in poverty. *Guidelines for Adolescent Preventive Services*, published by the American Medical Association, recommends that new strategies are needed to deal with health problems of adolescents, which are now predominantly behavioral rather than biomedical (Elster and Kuznets, 1994). Both reports stress the need for a more comprehensive approach that involves families and for an emphasis on prevention of problems before they become established.

The Importance of Education

Concern about students' academic performance and our national competitiveness has led to a national education reform movement and volun-

---

[2]The following poverty rates existed in 1992: children under age 18, 21.9 percent; adults 18–64, 11.7 percent; adults 65 and older, 12.9 percent (National Research Council, 1995).

[3]For example, the infant mortality rate for U.S. blacks ranks 40th when compared with other countries' overall rates; countries ranking higher include Jamaica, Costa Rica, Malaysia, and Sri Lanka (Children's Defense Fund, 1994).

[4]This document was developed by a large number of health professionals, in collaboration with consumers and experts in other fields, under the sponsorship of the Maternal and Child Health Bureau, U.S. Public Health Service.

tary national standards in core academic subjects. The relationship between academic achievement and student health status has been acknowledged by the National Education Goals, a bipartisan effort that began at a national governors' summit convened by President Bush in 1989. Among its directives, the National Education Goals call for (National Education Goals Panel, 1994) the following:

1. students to start school with the healthy minds, bodies, and mental alertness necessary for learning,
2. safe and disciplined school environments that are free of drugs and alcohol,
3. access for all students to physical education and health education to ensure that students are healthy and fit, and
4. increased parental partnerships with schools in order to promote the social, emotional, and academic growth of children.

The future of our country depends on an educated, productive workforce. The unskilled blue collar jobs of previous generations are disappearing, and schools are expected to prepare all students, not just a select few, for the demanding workplace of the future (Marshall and Tucker, 1992; Secretary's Commission on Achieving Necessary Skills, 1991). The Hudson Institute's Workforce 2000 report notes that unless workforce basic skills are improved substantially, there will be more joblessness among the least skilled, accompanied by a chronic shortage of workers with advanced skills (Johnston and Packer, 1987). However, the U.S. General Accounting Office (GAO) has suggested that the education—and thus the future—of a significant segment of our nation's children and adolescents is being threatened by a broad range of health and behavioral problems, increasing poverty, and deteriorating family and community conditions (GAO, 1993, 1994a, 1994b).

One of these GAO reports estimates that about one-third of the school-age population, or approximately 15 million children in 1992, is at risk of dropping out of school. This report cites a 1989 study that predicted male high school dropouts can expect to earn $260,000 less and pay $78,000 less in taxes during their lifetimes than male high school graduates; comparable estimates for female dropouts are $200,000 and $60,000, respectively. The report also notes that studies have shown that dropouts are more likely to be poor, have costly medical problems as a result of their economic status, and require job training. Currently, many dropouts populate U.S. prisons (GAO, 1993).

Concern about the effect of school dropouts on the nation's budget, workforce, and ability to compete globally in the future is reflected in the National Education Goal to increase the high school graduation rate to at least 90 percent by the year 2000. In 1992, the high school completion rate for people aged 19 to 20 was 84.7 percent, and for those aged 21 to 22, the rate was 86.2 percent. Although the difference between current school completion rates and the National Education Goal does not appear to be great, the graduation rate is significantly lower in many inner city and rural areas. Furthermore, the Bureau of the Census has projected that the population of academically at-risk children will continue to grow. Because these children are more likely to fail and drop out of school, the 90 percent goal may be more difficult to attain than the data indicate. To assist the growing number of school-aged children at risk of school failure, some experts have proposed comprehensive interventions that deliver a range of human services to students in schools (GAO, 1993).

The New Social Morbidities

A century ago, infectious disease and untreated physical defects put students at risk of school failure. Today, most of these problems can be addressed in whole or in part with immunizations, antibiotics, eyeglasses, and other medical treatments. Yesterday's problems, however, have been replaced by special health care needs, chronic diseases, and a new set of problems based in behavior and life-style choices, and these problems are not amenable to simple well-defined solutions. The Centers for Disease Control and Prevention (CDC) has found that the following six categories of behavior are responsible for 70 percent of the mortality and morbidity among adolescents: (1) behaviors that cause unintentional and intentional injuries, (2) drug and alcohol abuse, (3) sexual behaviors that cause sexually transmitted diseases and unintended pregnancies, (4) tobacco use, (5) inadequate physical activity, and (6) dietary patterns that cause disease (Kann et al., 1995). These problems are based in behaviors that can be prevented or changed. These behaviors usually are established during youth, persist into adulthood, are interrelated, and contribute simultaneously to poor health, education, and social outcomes.

The CDC's Youth Risk Behavior Survey of 1993 (CDC, 1995) found that 19.1 percent of all high school students rarely or never used a safety belt, 35.3 percent had ridden with a driver who had been drinking alcohol during the 30 days preceding the survey, 22.1 percent had carried a weapon during the preceding 30 days, 80.9 percent had ever consumed alcohol, 32.8 percent had ever used marijuana, and 8.6 percent had attempted suicide during the 12 months preceding the survey. Among high school seniors, 89 percent reported having used alcohol, and 39 percent of seniors reported having five or more drinks at one time in the past two weeks. In addition, 53 percent of students in grades 9–12 have had sexual intercourse, and 19 percent of them have had four or more sexual partners in their lifetime. Among twelfth graders, 68 percent have had sexual intercourse, and 27 percent of them have had four or more sexual partners in their lifetime.

In addition, health-compromising behaviors frequently tend to occur in clusters; individuals engaging in one type of high-risk behavior also tend to engage in other types of high-risk behaviors (Donovan and Jessor, 1985; Donovan et al., 1988; National Research Council, 1993; Resnicow et al., 1995). Those who smoke are also more likely drink alcohol, drive after drinking, and have unprotected sexual intercourse. Dryfoos estimated that 10 percent of adolescents are at very high risk for dropping out of school because of engaging in a variety of risky behaviors, an additional 15 percent are at high risk, and 25 percent are at moderate risk (Dryfoos, 1990).

Beyond these major risk areas, adolescents also engage in significant health-compromising practices that endanger health over the long term into adulthood. The CDC's Youth Risk Behavior Survey found that 30.5 percent of high school students smoke cigarettes, only 15.4 percent eat five or more servings of fruits and vegetables per day, and only 34.3 percent attend physical education class daily. The major causes of chronic disease and death among adults—cancer, heart disease, injury, stroke, and liver and lung disease—are influenced by health behaviors and life-styles established during childhood and youth (U.S. Department of Health and Human Services, 1991).

In 1979, the U.S. Public Health Service identified the four major factors leading to early illness or death and the extent of each contribution: heredity (20 percent), environment (20 percent), inadequate health care delivery system (10 percent), and an unhealthy lifestyle (50 percent) (U.S. Department of Health and Human Services, 1979). Studies by the U.S. Department of Health and Human Services have shown that 99 percent of health expenditures go to medical treatment and only 1 percent goes to population-wide public health prevention strategies. However, estimates predict that medical treatment can prevent only 10 percent of our nation's premature deaths, whereas population-wide public health approaches have the potential to prevent 70 percent of early deaths (U.S. Department of Health and Human Services, 1993).[5] The debate surrounding the re-form of health care delivery systems would be well advised to consider the fact that cost containment might be achieved by shifting the focus from medical care financing to an emphasis on illness and accident pre-vention.

---

[5]Approximately 20 percent of premature deaths are attributable to genetic conditions and are not preventable, at least at this time.

TABLE 1-1 Ten Most Prevalent Conditions at Time of Death in 1990

Cause	Number of Deaths
Heart disease	720,000
Cancer	505,000
Cerebrovascular disease	144,000
Unintentional injuries	92,000
Chronic lung disease	87,000
Pneumonia and influenza	80,000
Diabetes mellitus	48,000
Suicide	31,000
Chronic liver disease	26,000
HIV infection	25,000
Total	1,758,000

NOTE: HIV = human immunodeficiency virus.

SOURCE: McGinnis and Foege, 1993.

Certificates filed at the time of death generally indicate the primary pathophysiological conditions identified at the time of death; although these conditions are commonly thought of as the "causes" of death, in fact they may not be the root causes. For 1990, the 10 most prevalent conditions at time of death are shown in Table 1-1. Noting that most diseases or injuries are multifactorial in nature, McGinnis and Foege (1993) carried out an analysis to determine the relative contribution of the underlying factors that led to these most frequently reported causes of death in 1990. Their results are shown in Table 1-2. McGinnis and Foege point out that most of these underlying causes of death are based on behavior and lifestyle choices, and these avoidable underlying causes impose a substantial public health burden.

To improve the health of all age groups, the U.S. Public Health Service, in partnership with practitioners and private organizations, developed the *Healthy People 2000* initiative, a set of nearly 300 national health promotion and disease prevention objectives to be achieved by the year 2000 (U.S. Department of Health and Human Services, 1991). An examination shows that one-third of these objectives can be influenced significantly or achieved in or through the schools (McGinnis and DeGraw, 1991).

Problems Due to Poverty

As mentioned earlier, the poverty rate for children under the age of 18

TABLE 1-2 Underlying Factors Leading to Death in 1990

Underlying Factors	Number of Deaths
Tobacco	400,000
Diet/inactivity patterns	300,000
Alcohol	100,000
Infections	90,000
Toxic agents	60,000
Firearms	35,000
Sexual behavior	30,000
Motor vehicles	25,000
Drug use	20,000
Total	1,060,000

SOURCE: McGinnis and Foege, 1993.

is 21.9 percent, the highest of any age group in this country. The poverty rate varies considerably by race and ethnicity, however, with close to 40 percent of black children and 32 percent of Hispanic children living in poverty, according to 1990 figures. Between 1980 and 1990, the percentage of children living in low-income families increased and the percentage living in families with comfortable or prosperous income decreased across all racial and ethnic groups (U.S. Department of Commerce, 1993). The increasing number of poor and at-risk students requires schools to contend with more students who are potentially low achievers and who have health and other problems that interfere with learning. Even the youngest kindergartners arrive at school with backgrounds that will have a profound influence on their school experience; some are at a physical and mental disadvantage even before entering school, due to their mother's lack of prenatal care and to inadequate care and nurturing after birth.

A report of the Carnegie Task Force on Meeting the Needs of Young Children found that there are three major "protective factors" that help a child to achieve positive outcomes: perinatal factors such as full-term birth and normal birthweight, dependable caregivers whose childbearing practices are positive and appropriate, and community support. Scientists have learned that brain development that takes place before age 1 is more rapid and extensive than previously realized, with infants' earliest experiences with their parents providing the essential building blocks for intellectual competence and language comprehension. Therefore, the care and nurturing that take place even before a child reaches kindergarten play an important role in that child's future (Carnegie Task Force, 1994).

A GAO study reports that poor children have more health problems than other children, their conditions are often more severe, and they are less likely to receive regular health care. Poor children typically receive only episodic and crisis-related care, leaving preventive, chronic, and dental health needs not met. For example, of the 19 million children eligible for Medicaid's Early and Periodic Screening, Diagnostic, and Treatment Program in 1992, fewer than 7 million had been screened. More than 40 percent of poor school-aged children had no dental visits in 1989, compared with 28 percent for all children. Children from poor families (those with less than $10,000 annual income) are nearly twice as likely to be hospitalized and spend more than twice the number of days in the hospital than are children from families with annual incomes of $35,000 or more (GAO, 1994b). Poor children are also more likely to be limited in school or play activities by chronic health problems and to suffer more severe consequences than children from high-income families when afflicted by the same illness (Newacheck et al., 1995).

The new social morbidities, which are expressed as negative behaviors, also have a disproportionate impact on poor students. While school health programs attempt to address many of the social and environmental factors that influence human behavior, biomedical factors can also profoundly influence behavior and thus the effectiveness of school programs. For example, an obsessive–compulsive disorder would affect dramatically the ability of an individual to benefit from behavioral interventions. It may be that a significant share of the negative health behaviors currently ascribed primarily to social and environmental factors actually are caused by, or at least aggravated by, biomedical factors. Thus, health and education outcomes may be much less promising for a child with an undiagnosed and untreated neurological deficit—or other "hidden" biomedical disorders—growing up in social and environmental deprivation.

Schools with many children who live in poverty have higher rates of absenteeism and grade retention—or repeated grades—among their student populations. Further, these students have more health problems and inadequate nutrition. Compounding these problems is the increased mobility associated with poor and at-risk children. Changing schools frequently disrupts the child's education, making learning and achievement difficult (GAO, 1994a).

Schools with higher percentages of students in poverty are often inferior structurally, may be unsafe, and may even be harmful to children's health. It is estimated that approximately $112 billion is necessary to repair or upgrade America's facilities. Of this, $11 billion (10 percent) is needed in the next three years to comply with federal mandates that require schools to make all programs accessible to all students; to remove or correct hazardous substances, such as asbestos, lead in water or paint, materials in underground storage tanks, and radon; or to meet other requirements. Based upon a GAO study of a national sample of schools, although two-thirds of the schools reported that all buildings were in at least overall adequate condition, one-third reported that the schools needed extensive repair or replacement of one or more buildings. Fourteen million students attend classes in these buildings that have leaky roofs, unsanitary bathrooms, and inadequate plumbing that make them unsafe and harmful to children's health (GAO, 1995).

The measure of the number of students in poverty in a school is the number of students who receive free and/or reduced-price lunches. In those schools that have 70 percent or more of students receiving free or reduced-cost lunches, the proportion of schools reporting unsatisfactory environmental factors greatly exceeds those schools with less than 20 percent of students receiving such lunches. In the highest-poverty schools, 19.1 percent report unsatisfactory lighting compared to 14.3 percent of schools with lower numbers of students in poverty; 22.6 percent report inadequate indoor air quality compared to 15.8 percent of low-poverty schools; 32.8 percent report unsatisfactory acoustics compared to 24.1 percent of low-poverty schools; and 30 percent report unsatisfactory physical security compared to 19.4 percent of low-poverty schools (GAO, 1995).

It seems especially ironic that the one institution within the community that requires attendance of all students, rather than serving as a safe haven, may be a dangerous and unhealthy setting for many of our children who are most at risk. The deplorable physical state of some of these schools sends a message to students about their own self-worth and about the importance of their education, further exacerbating the downward spiral of educational and health outcomes.

Changing Family Structures

Involvement of the family is critical to a student's achievement. When schools involve families in meaningful ways to support learning, students tend to succeed not just in school but throughout life. Studies have found that the most accurate predictor of a child's success in school is the degree to which the family creates a home environment that encourages learning, has high expectations for the child's achievement, and becomes involved with the child's education. Students with supportive families are more likely to receive higher grades and test scores, have better attendance, complete more homework, have fewer placements in special education, attain higher graduation rates, and enroll more often in post-secondary education (Henderson and Berla, 1994).

Social and economic changes have reduced the support and nurturing available from the family and have increased family stress. The number of traditional two-parent families with extended family nearby for support and assistance is dwindling. According to 1990 census figures, only 14 percent of children live in such "traditional" families with fathers who work year-round and mothers who stay home, and only 3 percent of children living in two-parent families have a grandparent in the home.

In many families, parents are increasingly making the decision, often driven by economics, to have both parents work outside the home (Gordon, 1995); 15 percent of children live in two-parent families in which both parents work full-time, and another 24 percent live in two-parent families in which the father works full-time and the mother works part-time. For children living with their mothers, whether in single- or two-parent families, only 28 percent had mothers who stayed home full-time in 1990, compared to 40 percent in 1980 (U.S. Department of Commerce, 1993). Ambition to improve the family's standard of living has been frustrated because of the lack of growth in real wages. Between 1983 and 1992, the weekly earnings for full-time workers, adjusted for inflation, grew by a total of only 1 percent. In contrast, real family incomes grew an average of 4 percent per year during the 25 years of economic prosperity following the end of World War II. Particularly noteworthy are the declining earnings of young workers, which fell by 9 percent during the 1983–1992 period (Zill and Nord, 1994).

Increasing numbers of children do not live in two-parent families (U.S. Department of Commerce, 1993). The percentage of children living in a one-parent family grew from 18 percent in 1980 to 24 percent in 1990. An examination of the family situation of 1-year-olds—children with which schools will be dealing well into the twenty-first century—shows that 27 percent of them lived in families with one or no parent in 1990, compared to 21 percent in 1980. For black children, 68 percent of 1-year-olds lived in families with one or no parent in 1990, compared to 60 percent in 1980. Similar figures for Hispanic 1-year-olds are 36 percent in 1990 compared to 29 percent in 1980. More than four out of every five children living with one parent lived with their mother. It is estimated that approximately half of American children will live in a single-parent family for some period of their lives (Cohen, 1992; Kirst and Kelly, 1995).

In addition to the lack of financial progress, there is concern that time devoted to employment detracts from parents' ability to provide nurturing and supportive functions (Zill and Nord, 1994). It may be difficult for working parents to take their children to the doctor or spend time at home with a sick child (U.S. GAO, 1994b). For adults, the hours away from home required by full-time employment often do not match the hours that children spend at school. Latchkey children with time on their hands and without supervision are the result. Often the only "babysitter" is the television. The Search Institute, in its analysis of 15,000 adolescents, found that the combination of inadequate supervision of children and more than three hours of television daily was directly related to a life-style marked by more health-debilitating behaviors than was the case with youngsters who were more closely supervised (Blythe and Rochlkepartain, 1993).

With increased family stress and the decreased time and direct supervision that parents are able to give to their children, schools are increasingly asked to fill the role of surrogate or supplemental parents.

Access to Health Care

Estimating the number and percentage of children under the age of 18 with no health insurance is difficult, and different models give different figures. For example, estimates range from 8.7 million (12.6 percent) to 11.1 million (16.1 percent) uninsured children in 1993 (Lewit and Schuurmann-Baker, 1995), although a figure as high as 12 million uninsured children has been cited recently (American Medical Association Council on Scientific Affairs, 1990). Millions of other children have inadequate insurance plans that fail to cover even such basic preventive services as immunizations (National Health/Education Consortium, 1992). According to a recent GAO report, 12 million children do not get such basic preventive care as periodic physical examinations or immunizations at the proper intervals, and only about half of all elementary school children routinely receive health care. Although 7.5 children under the age of 18 require mental health services, fewer than one in eight actually receives them (GAO, 1994b). Oral health problems are significant among schoolchildren and often go untreated (National Institute of Dental Research, 1995).

Of major concern is the decline of employer-sponsored health coverage for children. Solloway and Budetti (1995) report that between 1979 and 1986, 1.26 million children lost health insurance coverage because of reductions in their parents' employer-based plans. The largest decline occurred in conventional two-parent, single wage earner families, in which coverage of children decreased by 11.7 percent between 1977 and 1987 (Solloway and Budetti, 1995). Between 1987 and 1992, another 4.5 percent of children lost their employer-based coverage. Even if dependent coverage is available, high cost-sharing requirements for premiums and large copayments or out-of-pocket expenses are major problems, especially for low- and middle-income wage earners. Further, uninsured children with chronic illnesses may be excluded because of preexisting condition, and lifetime benefit caps are an obstacle for those with insurance. In addition, young families are often the least protected and most vulnerable in an unstable job market, frequently the first fired or working in temporary jobs with no employer-based insurance coverage.

Access to health care can include concerns beyond mere financial issues. Transportation, convenience, and cultural sensitivity are also factors. In addition, parental support and encouragement, as well as understanding the importance of health care and how to approach the system, influence students' access to health care.

Even with access to health care, young people may not be receiving the attention they need. When adolescents with access to physicians are asked what they want to discuss and what they actually discuss with the physician, the percentage drops on virtually every topic from nutrition, to sex, to drug use (Marks et al., 1983). Even those adolescents with insurance and family doctors do not seek help from health care professionals for problems of greatest importance for their high-risk behaviors. In fact, doctors themselves do not feel qualified to discuss most adolescent health behaviors—only 38 percent feel they have adequate training in alcohol and drug abuse, and a mere 11 percent feel qualified to discuss depression with a youth (Beringer, 1990). Studies have shown that an initial history and physical examination for a new adolescent patient should require 30 to 45 minutes. Although 23 percent of adolescent physician visits are first encounters, half of all visits last 10 minutes or less, 30 percent last 11 to 15 minutes, and only 4 percent are 30 minutes or longer (Klein et al., 1993).

THE COMPREHENSIVE SCHOOL HEALTH PROGRAM

The comprehensive school health program is seen as a new paradigm needed to deal with the problems of today's children and families. It became clear to the IOM committee at the onset of its study that although a variety of conceptions and models exist, coordinated comprehensive programs are still essentially an unrealized ideal in most communities. The committee members themselves came into the study with a range of backgrounds and experiences, and the committee determined that it needed to establish its own working definition of the term "comprehensive school health program," which would guide further work. This definition was published and distributed in the committee's interim statement in the spring of 1995, along with additional background information and an outline of issues the committee planned to address in its study. The definition of a CSHP, as well as various program models and essential components, is further discussed in Chapter 2 of this report.

MAJOR ISSUES AND QUESTIONS
CONSIDERED BY THE COMMITTEE

As mentioned above, early in its study the committee identified a set of issues and questions to be examined. These include the following:

• There is no consensus on what the responsibilities of the school should be relative to the health of children in this country. What are schools doing now? What have they done in the past? What should our schools be doing in the future?

• What is the status of CSHPs? What are considered their essential elements, and how do programs work? How does a CSHP differ from previous models of school health programs?

• Given the problems of today's children and young people, what are the desired outcomes of CSHPs? What outcomes are feasible and measurable? What factors appear to optimize these outcomes?

• What is known about the effectiveness (including cost-effectiveness) of comprehensive school health programs and their components? What are the data gaps and possible ways of filling them?

• In this era of cost containment, what are the implications for CSHPs of reforms in the health care delivery system and possible changes in Medicaid?

• How can effective CSHPs be disseminated and replicated? What are the barriers and obstacles to wider implementation of effective programs?

ORGANIZATION OF THE REMAINDER OF THIS REPORT

Chapter 2 traces the evolution of school health programs from their early beginnings in the mid-nineteenth century to today's definition and concept of a CSHP. Chapter 3 considers the two important educational components of CSHPs, physical education and health education. Chapter 4 examines the wide range of health-related services available in the schools—including health, mental health, and nutrition or foodservices—and some of the new approaches for providing extended services to students with greatest needs. Chapter 5 considers how the infrastructure—the basic interconnected framework and support structure—for CSHPs can be built, from the national level to the local school level. Chapter 6 reviews research on CSHPs and their components, noting the limitations and methodological difficulties in carrying out research on these complex systems. Chapter 7 provides a summary of the committee's findings and concluding remarks.

Recognizing that schools are just one part of a broader community system, the committee sought to understand the nature and potential of school–community collaboration in promoting and protecting the health of students. A paper by an outside author was commissioned that examines this topic; it can be found in Appendix A. Appendixes C and D contain material written by committee members that served as background for the committee; Appendix C examines some of the theoretical models of behavior change that form the basis for health education programs, and Appendix D describes and gives examples of new approaches for providing health and related services through schools. Appendixes B, E, F, and G provide supplemental background information.

REFERENCES

American Medical Association Council on Scientific Affairs. 1990. Providing medical services through school-based health programs. *Journal of School Health* 60(3):87–91.

Blum, R.W., and Beringer, L.H. 1990. Knowledge and attitudes of health professionals toward adolescent health care. *Journal of Adolescent Health Care* 11(4):289–294.

Blythe, D.A., and Rochlkepartain, E.C. 1993. *Healthy Communities, Healthy Youth: How Communities Contribute to Positive Youth Development.* Minneapolis: Search Institute.

Carnegie Council on Adolescent Development. 1989. *Turning Points: Preparing American Youth for the 21st Century.* Washington, D.C.: Carnegie Council on Adolescent Development.

Carnegie Task Force on Meeting the Needs of Young Children. 1994. *Starting Points: Meeting the Needs of Our Youngest Children.* New York: Carnegie Corporation.

Centers for Disease Control and Prevention. 1995. CDC surveillance summaries. *Morbidity and Mortality Weekly Report* 44(SS–1), March 24.

Children's Defense Fund. 1994. P. 14 in *The State of America's Children Yearbook.* Washington, D.C.: Children's Defense Fund.

Cohen, D. 1992. Despite widespread income growth, study finds increase in child poverty. *Education Week* 11(40):24.

Donovan, J.E., and Jessor, R. 1985. Structure of problem behavior in adolescence and young adulthood. *Journal of Consulting and Clinical Psychology* 53:890–904.

Donovan, J.E., Jessor, R., and Costa, F.M. 1988. Syndrome of problem behavior in adolescence: A replication. *Journal of Consulting and Clinical Psychology* 56:762–765.

Dryfoos, J.G. 1990. *Adolescents at Risk: Prevalence and Prevention.* New York: Oxford University Press.

Elster, A.B., and Kuznets, N.J. 1994. *American Medical Association Guidelines for Adolescent Preventive Services: Recommendations and Rationale.* Baltimore: Williams and Wilkins.

Gordon, E.W. 1995. Commentary: Renewing familial and democratic commitments. In *School-Community Connections: Exploring Issues for Research and Practice,* I.C. Rigsby, M.C. Reynolds, and M.C. Wang, eds. San Francisco: Jossey-Bass.

Green, M., ed. 1994. *Bright Futures: Guidelines for Health Supervision of Infants, Children, and Adolescents.* Arlington, Va.: National Center for Education in Maternal and Child Health.

Henderson, A.T., and Berla, N., eds. 1994. *A New Generation of Evidence: The Family is Critical to Student Achievement.* Washington, D.C.: National Committee for Citizens in Education.

Johnston, W.B., and Packer, A.H. 1987. *Workforce 2000: Work and Workers for the 21st Century.* Indianapolis, Ind.: Hudson Institute.

Kann, L., Collins, J.L., Pateman, B.C., Small, M.L., Russ, J.G., and Kolbe, L.J. 1995. The School Health Policies and Programs Study (SHPPS): Rationale for a nationwide status report on school health programs. *Journal of School Health* 65(8):291–294.

Kirst, M.W., and Kelly, C. 1995. Collaboration to improve education and children's services: Politics and policy making. In *School-Community Connections: Exploring Issues for Research and Practice,* I.C. Rigsby, M.C. Reynolds, and M.C. Wang, eds. San Francisco: Jossey-Bass.

Klein, J.D., Slap, G.B., Elster, A.B., and Cohn, S.E. 1993. Adolescents and access to health care. *Bulletin of the New York Academy of Medicine* 70(3):219–235.

Lewit, E.M., and Schuurmann-Baker, L. 1995. Child indicators: Health insurance coverage. In *The Future of Children: Long-Term Outcomes of Early Childhood Programs,* R.E. Behrman, ed. Los Altos, Calif.: Center for the Future of Children, David and Lucille Packard Foundation 5(3):192-204, Winter.

Marks, A., Malizio, J., Hoch, J., Brody, R., and Fisher, M. 1983. Assessment of health needs and willingness to utilize health care resources of adolescents in a suburban population. *Journal of Pediatrics* 102(3):456–460.

Marshall, R., and Tucker, M. 1992. *Thinking for a Living: Work, Skills, and the Future of the American Economy.* New York: Basic Books.

McGinnis, J.M., and DeGraw, C. 1991. Healthy Schools 2000: Creating partnerships for the decade. *Journal of School Health* 61(7):292–297.

McGinnis, J.M., and Foege, W.H. 1993. Actual causes of death in the United States. *Journal of the American Medical Association* 270(18):2207–2212.

National Commission on Children. 1991. *Beyond Rhetoric: A New American Agenda for Children and Families.* Washington, D.C.: U.S. Government Printing Office.

National Commission on the Role of the School and the Community in Improving Adolescent Health. 1990. *Code Blue: Uniting for Healthier Youth.* Washington, D.C.: American Medical Association and the National Association of State Boards of Education.

National Education Goals Panel. 1994. *The National Education Goals Report: Building a Nation of Learners.* Washington, D.C.: U.S. Government Printing Office.

National Health/Education Consortium. 1992. *Creating Sound Minds: Health and Education Working Together.* Washington, D.C.: National Health/Education Consortium.

National Institute of Dental Research. 1995. Personal communication.

National Research Council. 1993. *Losing Generations.* Washington, D.C.: National Academy Press.

National Research Council. 1995. *Measuring Poverty: A New Approach.* Washington, D.C.: National Academy Press.

Newacheck, P.W., Hughes, D.C., English, A., Fox, H.B., Perrin, J., and Halfon, N. 1995. The effect on children of curtailing Medicaid spending. *Journal of the American Medical Association* 274(18):1468–1471.

Office of Technology Assessment, Congress of the United States. 1991. *Adolescent Health.* Washington, D.C.: U.S. Government Printing Office.

Resnicow, K., Ross, D., and Vaughan, R. 1995. The structure of problem and conventional behaviors in African American youth. *Journal of Clinical and Consulting Psychology* 63(4):594–603.

Secretary's Commission on Achieving Necessary Skills. 1991. *What Work Requires of Schools: A SCANS Report for America 2000.* Washington, D.C.: U.S. Department of Labor.

Solloway, M.R., and Budetti, P.P. 1995. *Child Health Supervision: Analytical Studies in the Financing, Delivery, and Cost-Effectiveness of Preventive and Health Promotion Services for Infants, Children, and Adolescents.* Arlington, Va.: National Center for Education in Maternal and Child Health.

U.S. Department of Commerce. 1993. *We the American Children.* Washington, D.C.: U.S. Government Printing Office.

U.S. Department of Health and Human Services, Public Health Service. 1979. *Healthy People: Surgeon General's Report on Health Promotion and Disease Prevention*. Washington, D.C.: U.S. Department of Health and Human Services.

U.S. Department of Health and Human Services, Public Health Service. 1991. *Healthy People 2000: National Health Promotion and Disease Prevention Objectives*. DHHS Publication No. (PHS) 91-50213, Washington, D.C.: U.S. Government Printing Office.

U.S. Department of Health and Human Services, Public Health Service. 1993. *The Core Function Project. Health Care Reform and Public Health: A Paper on Population-Based Core Functions*. Washington, D.C. U.S. Department of Health and Human Services.

U.S. General Accounting Office. 1993. *School-Linked Human Services: A Comprehensive Strategy for Aiding Students at Risk of School Failure*. Washington, D.C.: U.S. General Accounting Office, December.

U.S. General Accounting Office. 1994a. *School-Age Children: Poverty and Diversity Challenge Schools Nationwide*. Washington, D.C.: U.S. General Accounting Office, April.

U.S. General Accounting Office. 1994b. *Health Care: School-Based Health Centers Can Expand Access for Children*. Washington, D.C.: U.S. General Accounting Office, December.

U.S. General Accounting Office. 1995. *School Facilities: Condition of America's Schools*. Washington, D.C.: U.S. General Accounting Office, February.

World Health Organization. 1996 [Online]. Available World Wide Web (WWW) site. http //www.who.ch/programmes/inf/facts/fact126.htm [August].

Zill, N., and Nord, C.W. 1994. *Running in Place: How American Families are Faring in a Changing Economy and an Individualistic Society*. Washington, D.C.: Child Trends.

2

Evolution of School Health Programs

HISTORICAL OVERVIEW

Schools have been the focus of numerous and varied efforts to promote and secure the health of American children and young people since the colonial era. In its interim statement, the committee reviewed some of the historical aspects of school health programming to provide a context for its definition of a comprehensive school health program (CSHP) and a background for identifying issues to be examined in the committee's study. The following section extends that review. An understanding of the evolution of school health programs gives insight into how educational, political, and societal issues—as well as health issues—have influenced these programs over the years and provides lessons for the future development of school health programs.

School Health Through the Early Twentieth Century

During the colonial period, only limited attention was paid to any aspect of school health. Benjamin Franklin advocated a "healthful situation" and promoted physical exercise as one of the primary subjects in the schools that were developing during his time. Samuel Moody, headmaster of the Dummer Grammar School, which opened in 1763 as the first private boarding school, taught the value of exercise and participated in it himself. Prior to the mid-1800s, however, public education was still in a formative stage and efforts to introduce health into the schools were iso-

lated and sparse. It was not until 1840 that Rhode Island passed legislation to make education compulsory, and other states soon followed
(Means, 1975).

School health professionals often state that the "modern school health
era" began in 1850 (Pigg, 1992). In that year, the Sanitary Commission of
Massachusetts, headed by Lemuel Shattuck, produced a report that had a
significant impact on school health and has become a classic in the field of
public health. Shattuck served as a teacher in Detroit and as a member of
the school committee in Concord, Massachusetts, where he helped reor-
ganize the public school system. His background led to school programs
receiving major attention as a means to promote public health and prevent disease (Means, 1975). The report states the following:

> Every child should be taught early in life, that, to preserve his own life
> and his own health and the lives and health of others, is one of the most
> important and constantly abiding duties. By obeying certain laws or
> performing certain acts, his life and health may be preserved; by disobe-
> dience, or performing certain other acts, they will both be destroyed. By
> knowing and avoiding the causes of disease, disease itself will be avoid-
> ed, and he may enjoy health and live; by ignorance of these causes and
> exposure to them, he may contract disease, ruin his health, and die.
> Everything connected with wealth, happiness and long life depends
> upon health; and even the great duties of morals and religion are per-
> formed more acceptably in a healthy than a sickly condition.

Soon after the release of the Shattuck report, the medical and public
health sectors began to recognize the role that schools could play in controlling communicable disease with their "captive audience" of children
and young people. For example, even though a vaccine had been developed years earlier, smallpox continued to strike well into the latter half of
the nineteenth century, due to the constant influx of new immigrants and
the mobility of the population. When New York City was faced with an
outbreak of smallpox in the 1860s, no mechanism was in place to provide
free vaccinations to those who needed them, so the Board of Health turned
to the schools. Education officials agreed to permit inspection of school
children to determine whether or not they had been vaccinated, and in
1870, smallpox vaccination became a prerequisite to school attendance
(Duffy, 1974).

Although the schools of this period had the potential to confront and
control communicable disease, no doubt they also contributed to the
spread of disease. In the late 1860s and early 1870s, the New York City
Board of Health instituted a program of sanitary inspections of all public
schools twice a year. These inspections revealed a filthy environment and
excessive crowding. Modern plumbing was nonexistent, and schools were
sometimes overrun by rats. Frequently, more than 100 students occupied

a single small classroom, with two or three children sitting at the same desk. Classrooms lacked ventilation and fresh air, a problem exacerbated by using stoves for heating and gaslights for illumination. These problems continued in New York City even into the early twentieth century, and no doubt the situation was not unique to New York (Duffy, 1974).

The era of school "medical inspection" began in earnest at the end of the nineteenth century (Means, 1975). In 1894, Boston appointed 50 "medical visitors" to visit schools and examine children thought to be "ailing." By 1897, Chicago, Philadelphia, and New York had all started comparable programs, and most of the participating medical personnel provided their services without compensation. The success of these early programs developed into more formalized medical inspection. In 1899, Connecticut made examination of school children for vision problems compulsory. In 1902, New York City provided for the routine inspection of all students to detect contagious eye and skin diseases, and employed school nurses to help the students' families seek and follow through with treatment. In 1906, Massachusetts made medical inspection compulsory in all public schools, a step that ushered in broad-based programs of medical inspections in which school nurses and physicians participated. Legislative mandates became the means of ensuring medical inspections, and legislation continues to this day to be the basis for many elements of school health programs.

Around the turn of the century, the role and advantages of school nurses began to be recognized. In 1902, Lillian Wald demonstrated in New York City that nurses working in schools could reduce absenteeism due to contagious diseases by 50 percent in a matter of weeks (Lynch, 1977). For minor conditions, nurses treated students in school and instructed them in self-care. For major illnesses, nurses visited the homes of children who had been excluded from school because of illness or infection, educated parents on their child's condition, provided information on available medical and financial resources, and urged the parents to have their child treated and returned to school. School nurses began to assume a major role in the daily medical inspection of students, treatment of minor conditions, and referral of major problems to physicians. By 1911, there were 102 cities employing cadres of school nurses. In 1913, New York City alone had 176 school nurses (Means, 1975). This expansion of the role of school nurses freed physicians to spend more time in conducting medical inspections of individual students with recognized needs rather than in inspecting entire classes.

Medical inspections in the early part of the century were no doubt perfunctory and superficial. For example, in New York City in 1904, it was reported that 8,261,733 examinations were given and 515,505 students were treated by school nurses and physicians, yet the total number of medical inspectors was only 50! Another factor reducing the effectiveness of medical inspections was the Victorian attitude toward exposing the body. As late as 1914, school inspectors were not allowed to touch children, and inspections were done with children fully clothed. In 1915, the New York Board of Education introduced a new requirement that all children entering school must undergo a physical examination without clothing. This requirement met some resistance, with critics declaring it immoral to strip children for medical purposes and asserting that school physical examinations were an intrusion and a "violation of personal liberty, and hence contrary to the principles of a free government" (Duffy, 1974).

The prevalence of tuberculosis in the United States had a significant impact on school health during the early part of the century. Particularly notable was the development and spread of "open-air classrooms"—wide open to the outside air, even in the middle of winter—in all major cities, under the supervision of both medical and education personnel. In 1915, the National Tuberculosis Association enlisted school children in the Christmas Seal drive. A child who bought or sold 10 cents worth of seals was enrolled as a "Modern Health Crusader" and received a certificate with four "health rules." Crusaders also kept a personal record of how well they carried out 11 daily "health chores."[1] In the first year of the program, 100,000 children became "crusaders," and the drive was endorsed by the National Education Association and the National Congress of Parents and Teachers (Means, 1975).

Throughout the late nineteenth century and early twentieth century, the temperance movement also had an influence on school health programs, stressing that children should learn about the effects of alcohol, tobacco, and narcotics on the human system. As a result of this effort, a

---

[1]The list of these health chores gives a revealing look at what were considered to be significant health issues for children in that era. These daily chores were as follows:

1. Wash hands before each meal; clean fingernails.
2. Brush teeth after breakfast and the evening meal.
3. Carry handkerchief and use it to protect others when coughing or sneezing.
4. Avoid accidents; look both ways when crossing the street.
5. Drink four glasses of water, but no tea, coffee, or any harmful drink.
6. Eat three wholesome meals; drink milk.
7. Eat some cereal or bread, green (watery) vegetable and fruit, but no candy or "sweets" unless at the end of the meal.
8. Go to the toilet at regular times.
9. Sit and stand straight.
10. Spend 11 hours in bed, with windows open.
11. Have a complete bath and rub yourself dry.

majority of states passed legislation mandating such instruction, which was often incorporated into the physiology and hygiene curricula. Physical training—commonly called "gymnastics"—also began to be introduced into schools during this period. The early leaders in the physical education movement had medical degrees, and there was much discussion about the new profession of physical education being a blend of the medical and educational fields. Physical training was often associated with instruction in temperance and hygiene; other topics of focus in the early years of physical education included anthropometrical measurement, gymnastic systems, athletics, folk dancing, and military drill—although military activities fell out of favor around the turn of the century (Lee and Bennett, 1985).

The range of school-linked health services was broad in the early twentieth century, and school-based medical and dental clinics sprang up to provide services, especially to indigent students. These services were sometimes overpromised and touted as a panacea for eliminating school failure and delinquency, providing equal educational opportunity, and reaching parents to make them more responsible citizens. Although free school clinics were frequently denounced by the medical establishment as socialized medicine, dentists tended to support free school dental clinics. Many dentists considered children to be "troublesome patients; moreover, parents demanded lower fees for children's care, and they often refused to pay the dentist's bill for that care" (Tyack, 1992).

The extent of the medical services provided was so broad that sometimes even minor surgery was performed in schools. For example, in New York City in 1906, when the parents of large numbers of children who needed their tonsils and adenoids removed could not afford carfare to the nearest dispensary, several volunteer physicians performed this surgery on 83 children at Public School 75. Unfortunately, a rumor subsequently spread that "school doctors were slitting the throats of school children as a prelude to a general massacre of the Jews," and several riots resulted. These riots were found to be instigated by the "snip doctors," private physicians who performed the same surgery for a fee and resented the schools doing the work for free (Duffy, 1974).

In the period between the 1890s and World War I, the impetus for many health and social services in education came from outside the schools. In the 1890s, schools in Boston and Philadelphia were early pioneers in establishing cooperative programs with philanthropic organizations to provide school lunches to fight malnutrition and hunger and their consequent effect on learning. In many cities, women's clubs provided school meals, transportation, and special classes for sickly or handicapped children, as well as education and recreation programs during the summer and out-of-school hours. Settlement-house workers developed model programs for social work and for vocational counseling, generally staffed by volunteers or supported by charitable contributions. Visiting teachers, the forerunner of school social workers, worked with families—especially immigrant families—to help them adjust and to find needed resources and worked with educators to help them deal with the greater diversity of students coming into the classroom. Vocational guidance counselors, the forerunners of school guidance counselors, attempted to link students with jobs and to connect the school with the overall economy (Tyack, 1992).

School Health from World War I to the 1960s

World War I marked a turning point in the history of school health programs. Prior to this period, programs had a narrow focus emphasizing inspection, hygiene, negative messages, and didactic instruction about anatomy and physiology. However, the advent of the war made the problems of poverty more visible: malnutrition, poor physical condition, and the abysmal state of the health and welfare of many of the country's children. New health promotion philosophies and movements began to spring up to replace the outmoded methods; these new approaches were based on using motivational psychology and an understanding of behavior. During the years immediately following World War I, the image of modern school health programs began to emerge.

The Influence of Reports and Publications

Following World War I, the Child Health Organization was one of the most active groups devoted to the health of children, and the organization conducted "a nationwide campaign to raise the health standard of the American School Child." This distinguished group began as an outgrowth of the Committee on War Time Problems of Childhood, and its members were leaders in the fields of medicine, education, public health, psychology, and other arts and sciences. The organization's primary focus was on the development of improved health practices, and its approach was enlightened and progressive. Recognizing the motivating effect of stimulating students' interest, the organization promoted a positive approach to health and influencing behavior. It printed and distributed teaching materials for students, provided speakers, and published a large volume of material on school health. In 1922, in collaboration with the U.S. Department of the Interior and the Bureau of Education, the organization published and widely distributed *The Rules of the Health Game*[2] (Means, 1975).

In 1918, the Commission on the Reorganization of Secondary Education of the National Education Association (NEA) published the pivotal report *The Cardinal Principles of Secondary Education.* This report established a new framework for contemporary secondary education in the United States and listed seven main objectives of education: health, command of fundamental processes, worthy home membership, vocation, citizenship, use of leisure, and ethical character (Commission on the Reorganization of Secondary Education, 1981). The NEA had also joined with the American Medical Association (AMA) in 1911 to sponsor what would be for more than a half century one of the most influential groups in the development of school health: the Joint Committee on Health Problems of the National Education Association and the American Medical Association. Prior to 1920, this group published the report *Minimum Health Requirements for Rural Schools.* The Joint Committee strongly promoted the emerging concept of coordinated effort for health in schools. In a 1927 paper, *Health Supervision and Medical Inspection of Schools*, the group declared (Means, 1975):

> As yet, states have been slow in providing for coordination between the medical service or supervision, the physical education, and health education programs. Such a step is necessary for the proper functioning of any program of health supervision.

It is ironic that almost 70 years later, coordination of these programs is still considered lacking.

Early in the 1920s, the NEA–AMA Joint Committee on Health Problems in Education reported the results of a nationwide survey of the status of health education in 341 city schools. The findings are particularly interesting in light of the current U.S. Public Health Service's *Healthy People 2000*, which calls for this goal: "Increase to at least 75 percent the

---

[2]Despite the progressive tone to the publication, the "rules" still seem antiquated by modern standards. The "rules" are as follows:

1. Take a full bath more than once a week.
2. Brush the teeth at least once every day.
3. Sleep long hours with windows open.
4. Drink as much milk as possible, but no coffee or tea.
5. Eat some vegetables or fruit every day.
6. Drink at least four glasses of water a day.
7. Play part of every day out of doors.
8. Have a bowel movement every morning.

proportion of the nation's elementary and secondary schools that provide planned and sequential kindergarten through grade 12 quality school health education" (U.S. Department of Health and Human Services, 1991). In the 1920s, more than 73 percent of the surveyed schools taught health directly under the name of "health" or "hygiene," while 108 cities reported correlating content in their health curriculum to such other subjects as language, civics, reading, physical education, general science, and art. Daily inspection for health habits was reported by 69 percent of the 341 cities, and nearly 30 percent of elementary schools reported having organized student clubs for the promotion of health (Means, 1975).

In 1928, the *Sixth Yearbook* of the Department of Superintendents of the National Education Association outlined the following content guidelines for health education (Means, 1975):

- Mental hygiene must be emphasized and protected.
- The establishment of health habits depends upon the pupil's understanding something of the function of his own body.
- A discussion of the causes of disease merits a place in the secondary school program.
- A thorough study of nutrition should be placed in the upper grades.
- Posture should be emphasized.
- The hygiene of the home should be taught.
- Sex hygiene cannot be overlooked.

School health became the focus of a variety of agencies and professional organizations between the 1930s and 1960s, and many important documents emphasizing a range of health issues were published during this period. Nationally and at state levels, maternal and child health agencies sponsored numerous conferences to improve school health services by linking them to other community health efforts. Particularly significant health education reports include *Suggested School Health Policies*, published by the National Committee on School Health Policies of the National Conference for Cooperation in Health Education, and *Health Appraisal of School Children*, published by the NEA–AMA Joint Committee on Health Problems in Education. Other agencies and organizations publishing important reports on school health during this period included the U.S. Public Health Service, the U.S. Office of Education, the American Association of School Administrators, and various affiliates of the National Education Association (Means, 1975).

School health services research was also under way during this period and resulted in the publication of reports on such topics as staffing patterns for school health services, effective strategies for referral and follow-up of students with positive screening results, and the beneficial impact of nursing services on school attendance.

The Nature of School Health Programs from World War I to the 1960s

Between 1918 and 1921, almost every state enacted laws related to health education and physical education for school children (Kort, 1984). During the following decades, the health education curriculum became stabilized and more fully developed. Topics such as nutrition, personal health habits, diseases, exercise, alcohol and tobacco, family health, and sex education became common. The importance of the cooperation of schools with other community agencies and of parental involvement became increasingly acknowledged. The significance of the health of the teaching force became recognized, both so that the teachers would be able to cope with the demands of the job and so that they could better serve as role models of health and vigor for the students (Means, 1975).

Safety problems and conditions that surfaced during World War I stimulated the scientific study of safety and the introduction of safety into the school environment and curriculum. Fire drills began to be prescribed, and safety instruction included such topics as fire prevention, traffic safety, and bicycle safety. Increasingly, safety education became integrated into classroom health education (with the exception of driver training, which developed later and is often organized and staffed separately).

When many of the World War I draftees failed their physical examinations, there was a move to require physical education "without military features" in schools in an attempt to improve the physical condition of children and young people (Lee and Bennett, 1985). Similarly, when many World War II draftees were found to suffer from nutritional deficiencies, the federal government in 1946 passed the National School Lunch Act to provide funds and surplus agricultural commodities to assist schools in serving nutritious hot lunches to school children. It was not until 1966, however, that a pilot school breakfast program was established, and the program was not made permanent until 1975.

School-based medical inspections and screening continued into the 1930s, but typically there was a lack of follow-up to correct defects. In an attempt to remedy the situation, in 1936, in New York City Board of Education set aside a day as Health Day, during which teachers checked children's height, weight, vision, hearing, and teeth. Teachers then had the responsibility for trying to get any defects corrected (Duffy, 1974). Unfortunately, the teachers' work duplicated the efforts of the Health Department. In response, New York City devised the Astoria Plan, an experimental program designed to coordinate all school health services and eliminate duplication; this plan is discussed in the next section.

During this period, the NEA–AMA collaboration defined the role of schools in providing health services. Health services should focus on the prevention of health problems through conducting screening activities, establishing a healthful environment, providing for immediate care in the instance of problems, and referring children to professionals and facilities that could handle more complex health problems. Many school systems had physicians coordinating the health service programs. It was assumed that most students had family doctors for primary care services, and the appropriate role of schools was to inform parents of problems and advise them when it was necessary to take their children to the doctor. Although collaboration between the medical and educational sectors occurred throughout this period, clearly boundaries were also being established to limit the range of health services that should be available in schools (Lynch, 1977; Walker et al., 1990).

This philosophy of discouraging the delivery of primary health services in the schools was the basis for the traditional configuration of school health services between the 1920s and the 1970s (Walker et al., 1990). Although health education was considered an important and legitimate function of the school, when it came to providing services the school acted primarily as a link between students and the community's health services resources. Typically, a school nurse and/or aide, sometimes under the supervision of a part-time physician, was responsible for first aid, immunization, screening, referral, recordkeeping, and follow-up. Over the years, these school-based health services became institutionalized into the educational bureaucracy and were often no longer under the purview of the medical community. As a result, school health policy and the responsibilities of school health personnel became increasingly prescribed by those with an education background rather than health training (Lynch, 1977).

These decades saw a continual decline in the diagnostic and treatment aspect of school health services. A 1930 White House Conference on Child Health and Protection called for the elimination of treatment in schools and for school physicians and nurse supervisors to increase contact with physicians in private practice. School dentistry during this period changed from restorative treatment to dental health education and inspection. The 1948 National School Health Bill, which was designed to provide federal aid to school health, was defeated partly because of the opposition of the medical profession whose members feared that funds would be provided for services to students who would otherwise have paid private practitioners (Solloway et al., 1995). It was not until the 1960s that concern for the health and welfare of children and young people led to a reconsideration of the possibility of delivering diagnostic and treatment services at the school site. A classic report appearing in the 1970s signified the return to more substantial health services in schools (Leeds et al., 1980).

Research and Experimentation

The period around World War I saw the beginning of many research studies and demonstration projects in school health (Means, 1975). One of the earliest was the Locust Point Demonstration, which was launched in 1914 in Locust Point, a highly underprivileged section of Baltimore, under the direction of a school physician, school nurse, and school principal. The program's team approach was successful in improving the health of children and teachers, and the project attracted visitors from near and far to learn about the new methods and approaches. Another early demonstration conducted in 1917 in Framingham, Massachusetts, was primarily concerned with tuberculosis prevention and resulted in increased school appropriations for health education and physical education; the project was financed by the Metropolitan Life Insurance Company and carried out by the National Tuberculosis Association.

A number of school health demonstration projects and studies were carried out during the 1920s, 1930s, and 1940s. These included such examples as the School Health Study of the American Child Health Association (begun in 1926); the Ohio Research Study (1929–1932); the Cattaragus County Studies (begun in 1931); the School-Community Health Project, funded by the W.K. Kellogg Foundation (begun in 1942); and the California School-Community Health Project (launched in 1944).

One of the most intensive research efforts was the Astoria Plan, carried out in the Astoria Health District of New York City from 1936 to 1940, which was supported by the American Child Health Association, Metropolitan Life Insurance Company, Milbank Memorial Fund, and the U.S. Children's Bureau. Directed by the public health leader Dorothy B. Nyswander, the study had five objectives: (1) to determine whether prevailing methods used to discover children needing medical or dental care were satisfactory and, if not, to find what methods could be substituted; (2) to make inquiries into the nature of the cumulative health records of the children examined; (3) to find out just how the teacher, nurse, and physician were working together; (4) to find out the ways in which the staff made use of its time; (5) and to find out how physicians and nurses, immured in old practices, could be educated to new ways of work and thought (Means, 1975).

Under the Astoria Plan, services became more streamlined and efficient. Routine but cursory annual physical examinations were replaced by detailed examinations when the child first entered school and thereafter only when the conferring teacher and nurse deemed it necessary. The nurse and teacher would periodically discuss the health condition of each student, and physicians were freed to give attention to those children who most needed help. Parents were included in the nurse–teacher conference, thus ensuring follow-up treatment, and emphasis was placed on having at least one parent present during any physical examination. In one of the program's major accomplishments, education and prevention began to be recognized as being just as important as diagnosing defects and disease. A possible downside was the burden placed on teachers to recognize student health problems and report them to the school nurse and parents.

By 1941, the Astoria Plan was institutionalized throughout New York City, and *Solving School Health Problems*, which described the details and outcomes of research on the plan, was released in 1942 (Means, 1975).

National Conferences and Collaboration

Since World War I, several White House Conferences have been convened that relate directly to school health issues. These include the Conference on Child Welfare (1919); the White House Conference on Child Health and Protection (1930); the White House Conference on Children in a Democracy (1940); the Mid-Century White House Conference on Children and Youth (1950); the Golden Anniversary Conference on Children and Youth (1960); the White House Conference on Food, Nutrition, and Health (1969); and the White House Conference on Children and Youth (Children's Conference, December 1970, and Youth Conference, February 1971). Each of these landmark conferences resulted in specific recommendations and suggested programs related to school health services, health instruction, and a healthy school environment (Means, 1975).

Throughout this period, numerous other important national conferences devoted to school health have occurred (Means, 1975). In 1947, for example, the American Medical Association, through its Bureau of Health Education, inaugurated a continuing series of conferences that brought together leaders from medicine, allied health professions, and education to focus on school health work. The first national conference on undergraduate and graduate professional preparation in school health education was held in 1948, which has been followed by a variety of other conferences on the preparation of educators. This attention culminated in the development by the Association for the Advancement of Health Education (AAHE) of the current National Council for the Accreditation of Teacher Education guidelines on the preparation of health education specialists, and in the development of guidelines on the health education preparation of elementary teachers by AAHE and the American School Health Association. In 1950, standards for school health services were reviewed and revised by the American Public Health Association, the American Nurses Association, and the American School Health Association.

School Health from the 1960s to the Present

With the advent of the Great Society programs in the 1960s, the education and health scene experienced another major change. The Great Society and War on Poverty programs marked a new level of federal involvement in the schools and made new health and social services funds available. Relevant legislation passed in the 1960s and 1970s included Head Start, Medicaid, the Elementary and Secondary Education Act, the Community Health Center Program, the Education for All Handicapped Children Act, and the Child Nutrition Act that established the School Breakfast Program and the Nutrition Education and Training Program, and permanently authorized reimbursements for school lunches served to needy students.

Title I of the Elementary and Secondary Education Act tripled the number of school nurses, and a new nursing role—the school nurse practitioner—began to emerge in the late 1960s. At that time, issues of diagnosis and treatment in nontraditional health facilities surfaced, and the prevailing belief was that such activities were not permissible in schools by any primary care provider, including physicians. However, a state-by-state survey released in 1972 and sponsored by the Robert Wood Johnson Foundation failed to uncover any legislation that would prohibit the delivery of these services in schools. As a result, the clinical functions of school nurses were expanded to include primary care services with the nurses working in close collaboration with physicians. The introduction of school nurse practitioners into schools resulted in reaching students in need of primary care, an increase in problem resolution rates, and greater accuracy in excluding students from school for illness and injury (Hilmar and McAtee, 1973; Kohn, 1979; Silver et al., 1976).

The most significant school health education initiative of the 1960s was the School Health Education Study. This study defined health as a dynamic, multidimensional entity and outlined 10 conceptual areas of focus that over the years have often been translated into 10 instructional content areas. These conceptual areas include such themes as human growth and development, personal health practices, accidents and disease, food and nutrition, mood-altering substances, and the role of the family in fulfilling health needs. The primary publication from this initiative, *School Health Education Study: A Summary Report*, provided the basis for most of the current legislation on school health education (Sliepcevich, 1964). Numerous additional publications resulted from nearly 10 years of this activity, including curriculum designs and teacher–student resource guides that address the 10 instructional content areas of health education across all grade levels.

The new social morbidities of children and young people began to increase in visibility beginning in the 1950s and 1960s. Mental, social, and emotional health became issues, and schools began to attempt to deal with delinquency, narcotic addiction, and the inability of students to adjust to the regular school environment. The 1960 White House Conference on Children and Youth had youths participating for the first time; the conference was profoundly concerned with drug abuse, increases in the incidence of venereal diseases, illegitimate births, and inadequate opportunities for youth employment (University of Colorado, Office of School Health, 1991).

Although the Great Society programs of the 1960s and 1970s brought an influx of funding for school health, many of these programs focused largely on disadvantaged and special populations. As these programs grew, the perceived importance of school health for mainstream students may have begun to decline. In addition, with the publication of *A Nation at Risk* (Goldberg and James, 1983) and the emergence of the "back to the basics" movement during the early 1980s, the role of health and physical education in the curriculum also came under question. Should these courses be considered part of the core curriculum or did they intrude on and distract from "academics"?

Since the mid- to late-1980s, however, there has been a resurgence of concern for the health and welfare of children and families, with renewed focus on the potential for schools to address health and social problems. Examples of recent significant activities in school health include the following:

- the School-Based Adolescent Health Care Program, begun in 1986 by the Robert Wood Johnson Foundation, which catalyzed the rapid proliferation of school-based clinics;
- the establishment in 1987 of the National Commission on Children, a bipartisan group created by public law "to serve as a forum on behalf of the children of the Nation;" the commission published its seminal report, *Beyond Rhetoric*, in 1991 (National Commission on Children, 1991);
- the creation of the Division of Adolescent and School Health (DASH) of the Centers for Disease Control and Prevention (CDC) in 1988, and the associated increase in funding of school health initiatives and demonstration projects;
- the launching of the U.S. Public Health Service's *Healthy People 2000* initiative, which includes a set of nearly 300 national health promotion and disease prevention objectives to be achieved by the year 2000.

One-third of these objectives can be influenced significantly or achieved in or through the schools (McGinnis and DeGraw, 1991);

 • the National Education Goals, a bipartisan effort begun at a national governors' summit in 1989; among their directives, the goals call for (National Education Goals Panel, 1993, 1994) students to start school with the healthy minds, bodies, and mental alertness necessary for learning; the development of safe and disciplined school environments that are free of drugs and alcohol, including the development of comprehensive K–12 drug and alcohol prevention education programs in every school district; access for all students to physical education and health education to ensure that students are healthy and fit; and increased parental partnerships with schools in order to promote the social, emotional, and academic growth of children;

 • the organization in the early 1990s of a federal Interagency Committee on School Health and a National Coordinating Committee on School Health;

 • significant reports during the late 1980s and early 1990s on the health status of children and young people from organizations such as the American Medical Association, the National Association of State Boards of Education, the National School Boards Association, the Office of Technology Assessment of the U.S. Congress, the Carnegie Corporation, and the Council of Chief State School Officers (Lavin et al., 1992); numerous reports from the Maternal and Child Health Bureau, especially in relation to students with special health care needs, have also provided valuable assistance to school health planners (much of this material can be accessed through local and state health department maternal and child health offices);

 • the issuance by the American Medical Association in 1992 of Guidelines for Adolescent Preventive Services (GAPS), which calls for all adolescents aged 11 to 21 to have an annual preventive services visit to a physician who will address both the biomedical and the psychosocial aspects of health, with emphasis on health guidance and screening for risky behaviors such as sexual activity, substance abuse, eating disorders, learning difficulties, abuse, and emotional problems (American Medical Association, 1992);

 • since the beginning of 1994, a number of national conferences and reports have focused on the importance of improving access to comprehensive health and social services for children and families as a means of improving the health, welfare, and educational achievement of children;[3]

---

[3]One important event was "Principles to Link By," a conference in early 1994 attended by over 50 national organizations, including such wide-ranging groups as the American

recent legislation contains new provisions encouraging access to comprehensive services through school-based and school-linked approaches;[4]

• the formation of the National Nursing Coalition for School Health, with representatives from the American School Health Association, the American Nurses Association, the National State School Nurse Consultants Association, the American Public Health Association, and the National Association of School Nurses; in 1994 the coalition convened a national conference to examine future issues and priorities in school nursing (National Nursing Coalition for School Health, 1995);

• the establishment of the Healthy Schools, Healthy Communities initiative by the U.S. Public Health Service's Maternal and Child Health Bureau and the Bureau of Primary Health Care, to support and strengthen school-based health centers;

• the organization of the National Assembly on School-Based Health Care in 1995 (*Adolescent Medicine*, 1995); this group is establishing standards for school-based health centers and developing strategies for expanding and financing school-based health services; and

• the development of national standards in many fields related to school health, including health education (Joint Committee on National Health Education Standards, 1995), physical education (National Association for Sport and Physical Education, 1995), school nursing (Proctor et al., 1993), and school foodservice and nutrition practices (American School Food Service Association, 1995).

What Have We Learned from the History of Health Programs in the Schools?

Today, some observers question whether school health programs and school-accessed comprehensive services for families go well beyond the intended function of the schools. A review of history shows, however, that for more than a century, schools been called on to play an important role in addressing health and social needs due to their strategic ability to reach children and families. The potential for schools to provide more

---

Academy of Pediatrics, Council of Governor's Policy Advisors, American Medical Association, National School Boards Association, National Parent Teachers Association, National Education Association, and the American Association of School Administrators (American Academy of Pediatrics, 1994a).

[4] This legislation includes the Human Services Reauthorization Act (which reauthorized Head Start), the Goals 2000: Educate America Act, the Improving America's Schools Act (which reauthorized the Elementary and Secondary Education Act), the School-to-Work Opportunities Act, the Violent Crime Control and Law Enforcement Act of 1994, and the Family Preservation Act.

than mere academic preparation continues to be rediscovered, and today's renewed efforts in school health could be regarded as not new in concept but simply updated to reflect the needs of the times. There is a parallel, for example, between today's HIV (human immunodeficiency virus) and AIDS (acquired immunodeficiency syndrome) instruction and yesteryear's curriculum in physiology and hygiene, today's school-based clinics and yesteryear's medical inspections, and today's family services programs and yesteryear's of visiting teachers home visits to immigrants in urban tenements.

History also shows that controversy is not new to school health programs. Today's issues of local control of education and resistance to well-intended mandates imposed from above were also prominent a century ago. For example, at the turn of the twentieth century when the New York State Legislature proposed a bill to provide for sanitation, ventilation, and fire protection in schoolhouses in cities with populations of more than 5,000, the bill was easily defeated with charges that "it smacked of interference and paternalism in local affairs" (Duffy, 1974). These charges are echoed today as some individuals and communities resist directives about school health programs imposed from above, especially directives pertaining to such controversial aspects of programs as sex education or mental health counseling.

Other conflicts mirroring contemporary issues have surfaced periodically over the years. The New York free lunch program of the early twentieth century was criticized for the "hysterical sentimentality" over needy children, and later budgetary cuts led to farming out the lunch program to concessionaires whose sole motivation was making a profit. When free dental care for New York children was advocated in the early 1900s, the *New York Times* argued that this tendency toward "free everything" would only lead to socialism. Some considered the mandatory inspections of children at the turn of the century immoral and a violation of personal liberty. The debate about the proper role of the schools in providing primary care, begun in the 1920s during the period of the NEA–AMA collaboration, continues into this era of managed care.

The problems that confronted school health programs a hundred or more years ago—disease, physical defects, poor sanitation, inadequate nutrition, poverty, parental illiteracy, exploitation of children—were as critical in their time as current problems are today. However, yesterday's problems lent themselves more readily to well-defined permanent solutions—immunizations, eyeglasses, better personal health habits and nutrition, improved sanitary conditions, child labor laws. In contrast, many of today's new social morbidities are amorphous, chronic rather than acute, mental as much as physical. Individual behavior and societal norms have replaced disease pathogens and sanitation as major contributors to health problems, and solutions are not clear-cut. The schools of yesteryear were not expected to solve the health and social problems of the day by themselves; the medical, public health, social work, legislative, and phil-anthropic sectors all pitched in. Given the scope and complexity of the health problems of today's children and young people, it is again likely that schools will not be able to provide solutions without the cooperation and support of families, community institutions, the health care enter-prise, and the political system.

THE COMPREHENSIVE SCHOOL HEALTH PROGRAM

School health programming has evolved into today's concept of a comprehensive school health program. As the Institute of Medicine (IOM) committee began its study, it became clear that there were many descrip-tions about what a comprehensive school health program is and what outcomes it is expected to produce. In its interim statement, the commit-tee considered these issues, and the following sections extends that dis-cussion.

Goals and Desired Outcomes

The committee believes that the overarching goals of a comprehen-sive school health program are to enable all students to achieve and main-tain an optimal state of health and well-being, reach their full academic potential, and develop into healthy productive adults who take personal responsibility for their own health.

In its interim statement (IOM, 1995), the committee described the following set of optimal outcomes for CSHPs—a vision of what these programs might be able to achieve. These optimal outcomes are catego-rized into three general areas: (1) student outcomes, (2) programmatic and organizational outcomes, and (3) community outcomes.

Student Outcomes

Students will assume personal responsibility for avoiding behaviors that compromise physical, social, and emotional well-being and for en-gaging in health-promoting behaviors. Students' health needs—preven-tive, emergency, acute, and chronic—will be addressed to allow students to reach the highest possible level of educational achievement and per-sonal health. Particular attention will be given to the health component of Individualized Education Plans of students with special health care needs who require special education and related services.

Programmatic and Organizational Outcomes

The relationship between health status and educational achievement will be evident in the policies and programs of the school. The school's health emphasis will be integrated across all activities. Linkages among program components, disciplines, and participating agencies will be clearly defined and regularly evaluated. Individual and group health problems will be identified and managed with appropriate prevention, assessment, intervention or referral, and follow-up measures. Services will be organized to provide appropriate and timely responses to emergency, acute, and chronic health problems. The school's education and health programs will be continually reexamined and reformed as necessary to enhance student health, performance, and achievement.

Community Outcomes

The community will be actively involved in determining the design of a school health program and in supporting and reinforcing the goals of the program. This design will include assurance that schools are safe, with an environment conducive to learning and health promotion, and that policies and procedures are in place to enhance the use of schools as a community resource for health. All health-related programs delivered by the school and by community members through the schools will enhance the health status of the students and result in an improvement of the health and quality of life of the community.

The Need for a Definition

Early in its study, the committee encountered a variety of terminologies to describe school health programs and realized that there was not a single universally adopted model or definition for the term *comprehensive school health program*. According to recent common usage, a CSHP refers to an overall school health program, of which school health education and school health services are each components. However, some use the term "comprehensive school health education" to refer to an overall program and consider school health services to be a component of comprehensive school health education. (For example, the commissioned paper by Mary Ann Pentz in Appendix A.) Others use the term "school health services" to describe an overall program and consider health education to be a component of school health services. (For example, see the list of Maine integrated services in Appendix G-1 and Solloway et al., 1995.)

For the sake of consistency, the committee determined that it was necessary to establish its own working definition of the term *comprehen-*

sive school health program to serve as the basis for further work. In developing that definition, the committee examined previous models and definitions of school health programs that have evolved into today's concept of a CSHP. The provisional definition and relevant background information on previous models were presented in the committee's interim statement, and the following section reviews and expands on that discussion.

Previous Definitions and Models of School Health Programs

The Three-Component Model

The three-component model is considered the traditional model of school health programs. Originating in the early 1900s and evolving through the 1980s, this model, as shown in Table 2-1, defines a school health program as consisting of the following three basic components:

1. **health instruction**, accomplished through a comprehensive health education curriculum that focuses on increasing student understanding of health principles and modifying health-related behaviors;
2. **health services**, focused on prevention and early identification and remediation of student health problems; and
3. **a healthful environment**, concerned with the physical and psychosocial setting and such issues as safety, nutrition, foodservice, and a positive learning atmosphere.

The Eight-Component Model

In the 1980s, the three-component model was expanded to include additional components (Allensworth and Kolbe, 1987; Kolbe, 1986). According to this model, a comprehensive school health program contains the following eight essential components:

1. **Health education** consists of a planned, sequential, K–12 curriculum that addresses the physical, mental, emotional, and social dimensions of health.
2. **Physical education** is a planned, sequential, K–12 curriculum promoting physical fitness and activities that all students could enjoy and pursue throughout their lives.
3. **Health services** focuses on prevention and early intervention, including the provision of emergency care, primary care, access and referral to community health services, and management of chronic health conditions. Services are provided to students as individuals and in groups.
4. **Nutrition services** provides access to a variety of nutritious and

TABLE 2-1 Three-Component Model of the School Health Program

ORGANIZATION

Health Services	Health Instruction	Healthful Environment
Appraisal Aspects	*Planned Instruction*	*Physical Environment*
Health examination, dental examination; teacher health assessment, vision testing, hearing testing, height and weight measurement, cleanliness inspection, guidance and supervision, teacher health	Practices, attitudes, knowledge	Site, plant plan, heating, ventilation, lighting, water, lunchroom facilities, sewage disposal
	Correlated Instruction	
	Arts, social studies, sciences	*Mentally Healthy Environment*
Preventive Aspects	*Integrated Learning*	Pupil status, pupil–teacher relationships, provision for individual differences, curriculum adaptation, atmosphere of mutual respect
Communicable disease control, safety, emergency care, first aid	Personal experiences, pupil–teacher relationships, classroom experiences, school experiences	
Remedial Aspects	*Incidental Instruction*	*Practices*
Follow-up services, correction of remediable defects, practitioner services, school functions	Personal experiences, classroom experiences, school activity, community events	Schedules, time allotments, activity and rest, fire protection safety, inspection, housekeeping

NOTE: For purposes of planning and administration, three distinct phases of the program are recognized, but in actual function, the three phases constitute a cohesive integrated contribution to the total school program.

SOURCE: Adapted from Stone, 1990. Reprinted with permission. American School Health Association, Kent, Ohio.

appealing meals, an environment that promotes healthful food choices, and support for nutrition instruction in the classroom and cafeteria.

5. **Health promotion for staff** provides health assessments, education, and fitness activities for faculty and staff, and encourages their greater commitment to promoting students' health by becoming positive role models.

6. **Counseling, psychological, and social services** include school-based interventions and referrals to community providers.

7. **Healthy school environment** addresses both the physical and the psychosocial climate of the school.

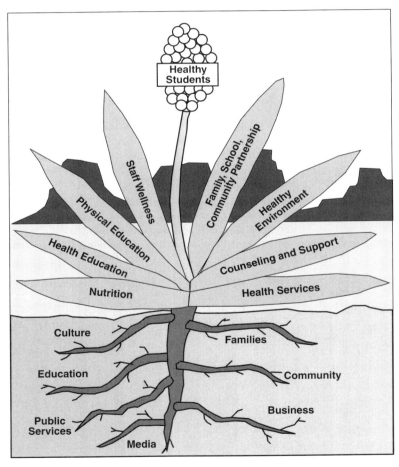

8. **Parent and community involvement** engages a wide range of resources and support to enhance the health and well-being of students.

The CDC's Division of Adolescent and School Health has promoted the eight-component model, which has received widespread attention and adoption by many states in recent years. Some states have even developed their own logo to depict the model; New Mexico, for example, represents the eight components as leaves of a yucca plant, the state flower, as shown in Figure 2-1.

FIGURE 2-1 Eight-component model. SOURCE: New Mexico Healthier Schools: A Model of Comprehensive School Health, State of New Mexico.

Related Models and Definitions

In recent years, additional models, definitions, and descriptions of school health programs have emerged that build upon previous models. Several examples are discussed below.

- Nader (1990) has proposed that the school is one locus of a broad range of health and educational activities that are carried out by a diverse group of health and educational personnel based both in the community and in the school. This model emphasizes that the school, community, and family or friends are the three important systems supporting children's health status and educational achievement. Further, the media—including educational, electronic, and print media—play a prominent role in influencing health-related behaviors. This model is shown in Figure 2-2. According to this model, the first steps in developing a CSHP

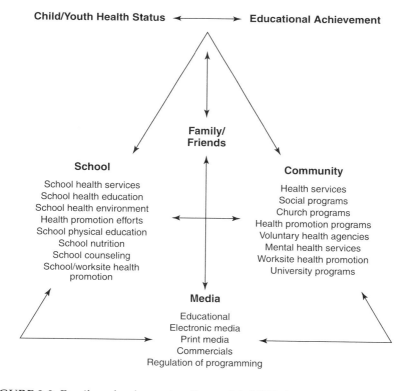

FIGURE 2-2 Family–school–community model. SOURCE: Nader, 1990. Reprinted with permission. American School Health Association, Kent, Ohio.

are to establish community linkages and carry out a community needs and resources assessment. These steps will then lead to the implementation and expansion of school health services, school health education, and a healthful school environment.

• The ACCESS model—Administration, Community, Curricula, Environment, School, Services—regards the school as an institution that is a microcosm of society where students spend much of their developmental years (Stone, 1990). This model calls for five "keystones" or interrelated areas, with interactive pathways between the areas, as shown in Figure 2-3.

According to this model, the administration and community keystones are overarching and should be developed first to provide an administrative structure and base of support for the other areas. The environmental keystone should be developed next, for it sets a tone for students and school personnel. Once these three areas have been developed, the remaining areas of curricula and services can be added with optimal effect, for then there will be consistency between what is learned in the classroom and what takes place outside the classroom. Another distinguishing feature of this model is that the word "promotion" has been added to its title to give "school health promotion program," to reflect more accurately the nature of the program and of the public health movement in this country.

• The Illinois Department of Health has recently developed a model of a CSHP as part of its long-range plan for school health (Edwards, 1992). This model consists of six critical elements: (1) management, (2) health promotion and education, (3) school health services, (4) healthy and safe environment, (5) integration of school and community programs, and (6) specialized services for students with special needs. This model is shown in Figure 2-4.

The distinguishing characteristics of this model include the importance of the management role in coordinating and integrating the other critical elements, and the emphasis on students with special health care needs.

• Allensworth (1993) has described a CSHP by what it does, rather than by listing what it contains. According to this model, a comprehensive school health program focuses on priority behaviors that interfere with learning and long-term well-being; fosters the development of a supportive foundation of family, friends, and community; coordinates multiple programs within the school and community; uses interdiscipli-

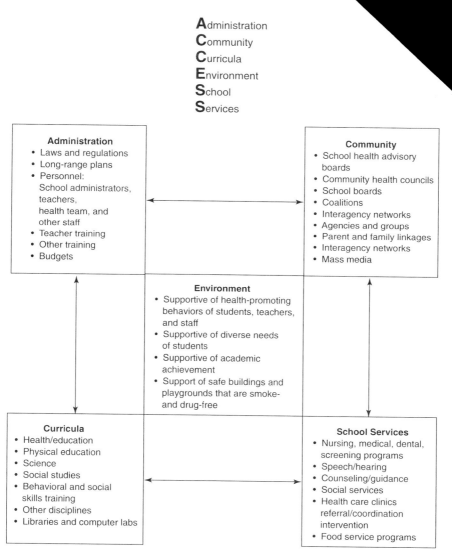

Administration
Community
Curricula
Environment
School
Services

Administration
- Laws and regulations
- Long-range plans
- Personnel:
  School administrators,
  teachers,
  health team, and
  other staff
- Teacher training
- Other training
- Budgets

Community
- School health advisory boards
- Community health councils
- School boards
- Coalitions
- Interagency networks
- Agencies and groups
- Parent and family linkages
- Interagency networks
- Mass media

Environment
- Supportive of health-promoting behaviors of students, teachers, and staff
- Supportive of diverse needs of students
- Supportive of academic achievement
- Support of safe buildings and playgrounds that are smoke- and drug-free

Curricula
- Health/education
- Physical education
- Science
- Social studies
- Behavioral and social skills training
- Other disciplines
- Libraries and computer labs

School Services
- Nursing, medical, dental, screening programs
- Speech/hearing
- Counseling/guidance
- Social services
- Health care clinics referral/coordination intervention
- Food service programs

FIGURE 2-3 ACCESS model. SOURCE: Stone, 1990. Reprinted with permission. American School Health Association, Kent, Ohio.

nary and interagency teams to coordinate the program; uses multiple intervention strategies to attain programmatic goals; promotes active student involvement; solicits active family involvement; provides staff development; and accomplishes health promotional goals via a program planning process.

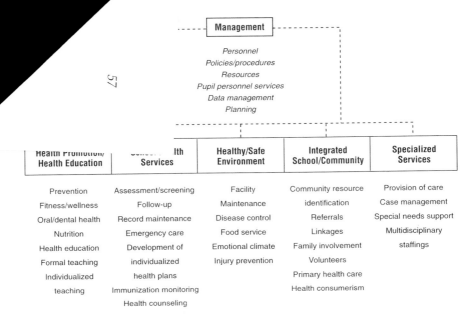

FIGURE 2-4 Illinois Department of Health model. SOURCE: Wallace et al., 1992. Reprinted with permission from Third Party Publishing, Oakland, California.

• International models of school health programs often include the school as an element of a country's primary health care system (Edwards, 1992). Although each country's approach to primary health care may vary, school programs throughout the world typically include components of preventive, promotive, curative, and rehabilitative services. Another prominent feature in many countries is the strong collaboration between the school nurse and the physician, with both health professionals often available to the school, on either a full- or a part-time basis.

In 1992, the European Network of Health Promoting Schools was initiated "to foster and sustain innovation, disseminate models of good practice, and make opportunities for health promotion in schools more equitably available throughout Europe" (Hirsch, 1995). The network of school health educators is a joint project of the World Health Organization, the Council of Europe, and the Commission of the European Communities and is active in 34 countries. Each participating school develops programs that include health education, a health-promoting environment, and linkages with families and community resources. Collaboration at all levels is emphasized, and best practices are shared and disseminated through cross-border workshops and major international meetings.

The prominent role of the school in many international health efforts is facilitated by two conditions that exist in many countries but not in the United States: health care is an entitlement, and the educational system is nationalized.

Full-Service Schools

A recent model in the evolution of school health programs is the full-service school (Dryfoos, 1994). A full-service school is the center for collocating—locating together in one place—a wide range of health, mental health, social, and/or family services into a one-stop, seamless institution. The exact nature and configuration of services and resources offered will vary from place to place, but services should thoroughly address the unique needs of each particular school and community—hence the title "full-service schools."

According to this model, a full-service school provides a quality education for students that includes individualized instruction, team teaching, cooperative learning, a healthy school climate, alternatives to tracking, parental involvement, and effective discipline. The school and/or community agencies provide comprehensive health education, health promotion, social skills training, and preparation for the world of work.

A distinguishing feature of this model is the broad spectrum of services to be provided at the school site by community agencies. Some examples of these various services include health services such as health and dental screening and services, nutrition counseling, and weight management; mental health services such as individual counseling, crisis intervention, and substance abuse treatment and follow-up; and family welfare and social services such as family planning, childcare, parent literacy, employment training, legal services, recreational and cultural activities, basic services for housing, food, and clothing.

Definition of the Joint Committee on Health Education Terminology

In 1990, the Association for the Advancement of Health Education convened a committee of delegates from the Coalition of National Health Organizations[5] and the American Academy of Pediatrics. The charge to

---

[5]Members of the coalition are the American Public Health Association, School Health Education and Services Section and the Public Health Education and Health Promotion Section; American College Health Association; American School Health Association; Association for the Advancement of Health Education; American Alliance for Health, Physical Education, Recreation and Dance; Association of State and Territorial Directors of Public Health Education; Society for Public Health Education, Inc.; and Society of State Directors of Health, Physical Education and Recreation.

this Joint Committee on Health Education Terminology was to review and update earlier terminology and to provide definitions for new terms currently used in the health education field. The Joint Committee defined a CSHP as follows (Joint Committee on Health Education Terminology, 1991):

> A comprehensive school health program is an organized set of policies, procedures, and activities designed to protect and promote the health and well-being of students and staff which has traditionally included health services, healthful school environment, and health education. It should also include, but not be limited to, guidance and counseling, physical education, food service, social work, psychological services, and employee health promotion.

The Committee's Provisional Definition

After review of previous models and definitions, the committee proposed the following provisional definition of a CSHP, which was presented in its interim statement (IOM, 1995):

> A **comprehensive** school health program is an **integrated** set of **planned, sequential, school-affiliated strategies, activities, and services** designed to promote the optimal physical, emotional, social, and educational **development** of students. The program **involves** and is **supportive of families** and is **determined** by the **local community** based on community **needs, resources, standards, and requirements**. It is **coordinated** by a **multidisciplinary team** and **accountable** to the community for program **quality** and **effectiveness**.

Each term printed in bold was further described and discussed in the interim statement. A brief summary of that discussion follows:

Comprehensive means inclusive, covering completely and broadly, and refers to a broad range of components. It should be emphasized, however, that programs and services actually delivered *at* the school site may not provide complete coverage by themselves but are intended to work with and complement the efforts of families, primary sources of health care, and other health and social service resources in the community to produce a continuous and complete system to promote and protect students' health.

Integrated means formed, coordinated, or blended into a functioning or unified whole. It is assumed that when the various elements of CSHPs are integrated, they mutually reinforce and support each other, producing a whole that is greater than the sum of its separate parts in meeting the health needs of students and fostering student health literacy.

Planned implies a deliberate design, a detailed formulation of a program of action. Planning involves developing an orderly arrangement of program strategies, activities, and services, after careful consideration of needs and resources, in order to meet the needs of students and their families. The planning process should involve a broad range of stakeholders and should begin with local needs and resources assessment. Planning should also include ongoing evaluation and means for continuous program improvement.

Sequential implies a deliberate ordering or succession of program elements, so that each successive event builds upon previous student experience and is compatible with a student's developmental status.

School-affiliated refers to activities that take place at the school site (school based), that take place off-site but are associated with the school (school linked), or that have any other connection with the schools.

Strategies, activities, and services refer to approaches, methods, actions, and interventions for the purpose of accomplishing program goals and objectives. **Strategies** are the overall approach or network of related methods and processes, carefully designed to achieve desired goals. **Activities and services** are those specific and concrete actions carried out as part of a strategy.

Development refers to the process of growth, advancement, and maturation. Optimal **development** implies setting children on a course of growth and maturation that will lead to a healthy adulthood.

Involve means to engage as a participant, to include. **Supportive of families** implies helping, assisting, or advocating, to keep families as a key foundation, with family defined in its broadest context as a unit consisting of one or more children plus parent(s), guardian, or other care provider(s). Involving the family implies that the family has knowledge about the CSHP and participates in community deliberations to determine needs and to design program strategies, activities, and services. When properly designed and sensitive to community concerns, CSHPs provide family support by reinforcing community values and providing access to health and social services, both for students and possibly for other family members.

Determine means to come to a decision by investigation, reasoning, or calculation, to settle or decide by choosing among alternatives or possibilities.

The **local community** refers to the wide range of stakeholders—parents, students, educators, health and social service personnel, insurers, business and political leaders, and so forth—at the particular site where the program will be implemented.

Needs refer to the lack of something desirable or useful and to conditions requiring relief or remediation. **Resources** refer to the strengths and available sources of relief or recovery upon which the community can draw in meeting identified needs. **Standards and requirements** involve both professional and legal criteria and community ethics, mores, and values.

Coordinated means brought into combined action to cause separate elements to function in a smooth concerted manner. Coordination implies a formal relationship and blurring of boundaries between coordinating partners, although partners can still retain their identity and affiliation to their profession.

Multidisciplinary team involves individuals with different backgrounds, skills, and knowledge working together. Even in a small or isolated school, it should be possible to find two or more individuals with different disciplinary backgrounds to coordinate the program and link it to the community.

Accountable means that those involved in the program are responsible and answerable to the community and that they must provide information on program implementation, outcomes, and financial matters to allow for informed decisionmaking.

Quality refers to the degree of competence and excellence of the program; **effectiveness** has to do with producing the desired result: improved health and educational outcomes. Quality and effectiveness are interrelated in CSHPs—the existence of one implies the presence of the other.

The Definition Revisited

With the benefit of knowledge and insight gained during the course of its study, the committee reexamined its original provisional definition of a CSHP and determined that it was still valid and useful. The definition is flexible, not overly prescriptive, and emphasizes what the committee believes are the crucial features of a CSHP—family and community involvement, multiple interventions, integration of program elements, and collaboration across disciplines. The various definitions and models of CSHPs are not separate and distinct, and considerable commonality exists among them. The committee believes that there is no single "best" definition or model for a CSHP but that programs must be tailored to meet each community's needs, resources, perspectives, and standards. It is important to move beyond definitions and models to examine essential program elements and approaches for program design and implementation. The remainder of this chapter provides a brief overview of key program elements found in virtually all program models.

Key Elements of a Comprehensive School Health Program

Community Participation and Focus

The essential foundation for any successful CSHP is built from the involvement of a wide range of community stakeholders—parents, students, educators, health and social service personnel, insurers, and business and political leaders. This involvement can be effectively organized and channeled through the formation of some type of "community school health coordinating council." The first step under the leadership of the council should be to assess the priority health-related needs and problems of children and young people in that community. Are they related to poor dietary habits and physical fitness, stress, violence, substance abuse, risky sexual behavior, deteriorating family conditions, lack of access to medical care, or other factors? Next, an assessment should be made of resources available to deal with these needs. Chances are that many resources already exist and merely need to be reconfigured, rejuvenated, or made more accessible. To provide focus, it is important to identify at the onset a few key indicators that will be monitored to track program impact—perhaps improved attendance or academic achievement, increased physical fitness scores, decreased teen pregnancy or drug abuse, fewer hospital emergency room visits, or an increase in the number of families with a medical "home."

Once the foundation of community support and the program focus have been established, the actual program will certainly consist of a collection of program elements or components, which ideally should work in an integrated fashion to address identified community needs. As mentioned previously, all program models share many common components. The committee does not believe it fruitful to attempt to rank components in order of importance or to prioritize which should be implemented first. Each community may have different priorities, and furthermore, the resources and infrastructure for many of these components are already in place. All that may be needed is a reinvigoration and refocusing of current efforts—and the development of linkages and mutual support among the component parts.

The most prominent program components found in virtually every recent model of school health program are described below. The following discussion is intended simply to provide a brief overview, not an exhaustive analysis. Each of these components has its own wide literature[6] that should be consulted for an in-depth understanding of that component.

---

[6]*Guidelines for Comprehensive School Health Programs* from the American School Health Association (1994) gives a concise summary of each of the components of the eight-

School Environment

Physical Environment. School buildings and grounds should be clean, safe, and secure. Regulations from the Occupational Safety and Health Administration and others must be followed in ensuring a safe and healthful environment. Building design should ensure adequate ventilation, lighting, noise abatement, and heating and cooling, with provisions for complying with federal Americans with Disabilities Act mandates. Environmental hazards—such as asbestos, lead, and radon—must be given attention, and school sources of pollution—science laboratories, art classes, shop and vocational classes—should be governed by appropriate policies and receive constant vigilance. Safety and sanitation measures are established, understood, and followed. Emergency disaster plans are in place and emergency drills are held periodically. Policies are in place to ensure safe transportation practices that address such transportation modes as cars, buses, bicycles, skateboards, and walking. Staff and students are made aware of safety, first aid, and infection control equipment and procedures. Buildings, equipment, and grounds are kept clean, in good repair, and free of hazards that foster infection and handicaps.

As a result of the 103d Congress considering 66 bills that referenced the "school environment" and 51 that were directed at the goal of "safe schools," the Office of Technology Assessment of the U.S. Congress was asked to prepare the report *Risks to Students in Schools* (Office of Technol-

---

component model. Excerpts from this document are found in Appendix B. The following documents are also suggested as an introduction to the various components and as a source of references to the primary literature and research in these fields:

• The *Guidelines* documents from the CDC: At the time of writing of this report, guidelines for tobacco prevention programs had been released (CDC, 1994). Guidelines for school health programs to promote healthy eating and guidelines for school and community health programs to promote physical activity among youth were scheduled to be released in 1997, and guidelines for school health education were under development.

• *Principles and Practices of Student Health,* edited by Wallace et al. (1992), is a three-volume compendium of papers on all aspects of student health programs.

• *School Health: Policy and Practice* was issued by the Committee on School Health, American Academy of Pediatrics (1993).

• *The School Health Challenge* is a document from ETR Associates (Cortese and Middleton, 1994).

• In addition, CDC's DASH is supporting the development of a series of papers, under the direction of the Education Development Center, that examine in depth each of the individual components of the eight-component model and how the components fit together to make an integrated program. Drafts are expected to be available for discussion in late 1997, and a monograph containing all papers is expected to be released in the fall of 1997.

ogy Assessment, 1995). This document describes regulations and risks pertaining to environmental hazards, such as asbestos and lead; exposure to infectious agents, such as influenza virus and disease-causing bacteria; unintentional injuries, such as sports and playground accidents; and intentional injuries, such as homicide and fighting.

Policy and Administrative Environment. Rules and regulations are established to promote the physical, psychological, and social health of students. Health and safety promotion is prominent. A smoke-, drug-, weapon-, and violence-free environment is enforced, with clear and reasonable penalties. Extracurricular sports and physical fitness activities are promoted for all students, and healthful foods are sold in the school lunch, school breakfast, and a la carte options in the school cafeteria, as well as through vending machines, school events, or fund-raising drives. Schedules are designed not merely to improve efficiency but also to reduce stress; for example, class release times may be staggered to minimize crowding in halls and avoid unnecessary sources of conflict, and lunch periods may be scheduled to provide adequate time to enjoy healthful meals. When appropriate, students have input in establishing policies and discipline procedures, and discipline is administered in a fair and evenhanded manner. A consistent process is in place for reporting, analyzing, and preventing injuries and health problems.

Psychosocial Environment. Students and staff function in a supportive atmosphere that encourages open communication, respects individual differences, and promotes each student's reaching full academic and social potential. The diverse needs of individual students are addressed, and families are kept informed and involved. There is a collaborative rather than adversarial spirit among students and staff, and a sense that everyone is pulling together toward the same goals. A cooperative, not overly competitive, atmosphere exists in academic instruction. Expectations are high, but students are not left to flounder or fall through the cracks. Academic assistance is easily available and actively promoted for those students needing additional help. Faculty and staff take the initiative to look for and help resolve student problems that may affect learning, morale, and well-being. Policies related to provision of services for at-risk students, such as free and reduced-price meals, are made in ways that do not stigmatize recipients. A crisis response system is established to support students in the event of violence, suicide, disaster, or other incident.

The psychosocial environment has been shown to have a significant impact on student achievement and functioning. It has been speculated that in some situations, a healthful psychosocial environment may be as important—or even more important—than classroom health education in keeping students away from drugs, alcohol, violence, risky sexual behavior, and the rest of today's new social morbidities (Carnegie Council on Adolescent Development, 1995). Studies have also shown that families of students can be reached and can benefit from an improved school psychosocial environment (Comer, 1988).

Many authorities believe that for all children and young people to have a chance to succeed, significant changes are required in the environment in which students are educated and in the way schools are structured. In quality schools, the staff has high expectations for all students, student receive support and nurturing, and students are involved in significant and worthwhile activities. Schools are responsive to a wide range of students' needs and interests, and meaningful involvement of families is sought and supported. Change in the school structure and climate is seen as the ultimate intervention to insure the long-term "health" of students. Examples of endeavors promoting these principles include the following:

- *The School Development Program*, founded by James Comer of the Yale University Child Study Center, focuses on school-based management and parental involvement to improve the education of disadvantaged students (Comer, 1984, 1988). Each participating school is governed by an elected School Advisory Council that includes the principal, teachers, teacher aides, and parents. A mental health team, comprising the school psychologist and other support personnel, provides direct services to children and advises school staff and parents. A parent is employed to work in each classroom on a part-time basis, and parents are encouraged to volunteer as teacher aides and librarians, publish newsletters, and organize social activities. A social skills curriculum has been developed that integrates the teaching of basic skills with teaching of "mainstream" arts and social skills. According to Comer, the strength of this project is its focus on the entire school rather than on any one particular aspect, and its attention to institutional change rather than to individual change.

- *Success for All*, initiated by Robert Slavin and colleagues at the Johns Hopkins University, restructures the entire school to do "everything" necessary to ensure that all students will be performing at grade level by the end of third grade (Slavin et al., 1992). Interventions include a half-day preschool and full-day kindergarten, a family support team, an effective reading program with reading tutors, individual academic plans based on frequent assessments, a full-time program facilitator and coordinator, training and support for teachers, and a school advisory committee that meets weekly. The family support team works full-time in each school and consists of social workers, attendance workers, and a parent liaison worker. The team provides parenting education and support assistance for day-to-day problems such as nutrition, getting glasses, attendance, and problem behaviors. Family support teams are also responsible for developing linkages with community resources.

• *Turning Points*, led by the Carnegie Council on Adolescent Development, focuses on early adolescence, a critical and pivotal developmental period (Carnegie Council on Adolescent Development, 1989). The project is based on the premise that a serious mismatch exists between the organization and curriculum of most middle grade schools and the intellectual and emotional needs of young adolescents, which results in increased alienation, substance abuse, absenteeism, and school dropouts. The project is restructuring a set of middle schools with the following characteristics. There will be "Schools-Within-a-School" that has students and teachers grouped together in teams, with every student known well by at least one adult. There will be a core academic program that emphasizes critical thinking, citizenship values, a healthy life-style, and responsible and ethical behavior. Cooperative learning will be used, and tracking will be eliminated. The staff will be expert in teaching young adolescents, and the staff will be empowered to make decisions and create the environment necessary for students to succeed. Emphasis will be placed on health and fitness as a means to improve academic performance, and every school will have a health coordinator, access to health care and counseling, and a health-promoting environment. Finally, families and the community will be involved with the operation of the school.

Health Promotion for Staff. Staff health promotion frequently receives low priority among school health issues, and research on its impact is scarce. A few studies, however, have shown that staff health promotion programs are feasible and produce improvement in morale, absenteeism, perceptions of well-being, attitudes toward personal health, and even quality of classroom instruction. (Belcastro and Gold, 1984; Falck and Kilcoyne, 1984; Jamison, 1993; Maysey, 1988)   Another benefit of staff health promotion may be a decrease in group health insurance costs.

Healthy People 2000 calls for employee health promotion for all worksites (U.S. Department of Health and Human Services, 1991). Employers are encouraged to provide physical activity and fitness programs, nutrition education and weight management programs, blood pressure and cholesterol education and control activities, stress management, policies limiting smoking, and aggressive prevention and intervention programs for drug and alcohol abuse. The Health Insurance Association of America has outlined reasons why health promotion for school employees is a particularly strategic investment (Allensworth et al., 1994). For example, health promotion would have a significant impact on overall health care costs; reduce absenteeism and hiring of substitute teachers, improving instruction for students; improve employee morale by demonstrating a commitment to their well-being; create a "multiplier effect" as staff become positive role models for students and reinforce consistent CSHP health-enhancing messages; take advantage of existing school-based facilities and resources; and encourage the school to develop "open-door" policies and become the focus for community-wide health promotion activities.

Education

The two educational components of CSHPs are physical education and health education. In addition, health topics may be integrated into other curricular areas. The following is a brief overview of these educational components; Chapter 3 provides a more in-depth discussion.

Physical Education. Physical education involves a planned, sequential, developmentally appropriate, K–12 curriculum that provides cognitive and affective content and physical activity. Content areas include motor skills; physical fitness; rhythm and dance; games; team, dual, and individual sports; tumbling and gymnastics; and aquatics. Most states mandate the minimum time per week spent in physical education and the number of years that students must be enrolled.

While debate continues over whether the essential purpose of physical education is to teach motor skills or promote fitness, the concept of health-related fitness is emerging to bridge the gap between skills and fitness[7] (Simons-Morton, 1992). The focus in physical education is shifting away from competitive sports and athletic performance to cultivating an interest and sense of self-efficacy in physical activities that students can enjoy and pursue throughout adulthood.

Physical activity in youth is associated with higher levels of health and physical fitness, greater resistance toward cigarette and alcohol use, and possibly enhanced academic achievement and cognitive functioning. Physical activity levels tend to decline steadily during adolescence, especially among girls, although *how* physical activity tracks into an adult life-style is not well understood. It is established, however, that merely engaging in physical activity during youth will not protect against risks brought on by a sedentary life-style as an adult; physical activity must be

---

[7] The cultivation of finely tuned motor skills does not always translate into overall fitness and desirable health practices—note the physical condition and behaviors of certain highly skilled professional sports figures.

sustained throughout adulthood. A sedentary life-style in adults is associated with higher risk for coronary heart disease, hypertension, non-insulin-dependent diabetes mellitus, and certain cancers; evidence also suggests that physical activity may reduce risks for osteoporosis and obesity and relieve symptoms associated with anxiety and depression (CDC, 1997).

Health Education. Health education consists of a planned, sequential, developmentally appropriate K–12 curriculum that deals with the physical, mental, emotional, and social dimensions of health, provided by qualified teachers prepared to teach the subject. The goal of health education is to empower students with the necessary knowledge and skills to maintain and improve their health, adopt healthful behaviors, avoid health-threatening behaviors, and become health literate consumers and decisionmakers. The CDC's School Health Policies and Programs Study (SHPPS)[8] examined the most commonly required topics in health education across the country; these findings are shown in Table 3-10 (see Chapter 3). SHPPS found that a large majority of schools require instruction in such areas as the prevention of alcohol and other drug use, HIV and other sexually transmitted diseases, and tobacco use; dietary behaviors and nutrition; human growth and development; and human sexuality.

Issues in health education are complicated, and national consensus is slow to emerge on the position of health education in the overall curriculum. Questions continue to be raised about what topics should be taught in health education, who should teach them and when, how conflicts over controversial topics can be resolved, and what outcomes can reasonably be expected and measured. These questions are considered in Chapters 3 and 6.

Other Curricular Areas. Other subject matter areas—home economics, science, mathematics, language arts, social studies, visual and performing arts, vocational education—can use health-related topics to reinforce the school health message and also capture student interest in these other subjects. Health topics seem relevant to students, whereas other academic

---

[8]The School Health Policies and Programs Study was carried out in 1994 to examine policies and programs across multiple components of school health programs at the state, district, school, and classroom levels. The October 1995 issue of the *Journal of School Health* is devoted to a summary report of SHPPS findings and includes separate analyses of school health education (Collins et al., 1995); school physical education (Pate et al., 1995); school health services (Small et al., 1995); school health services (Small et al., 1995); school foodservice (Pateman et al., 1995); and school health policies prohibiting tobacco use, alcohol and other drug use, and violence (Ross et al., 1995).

subjects may seem abstract and remote.[9] Science is a logical area to connect with health because most health practices and health problems have a scientific basis. The National Science Education Standards call for students to understand science in its personal and social perspectives, including science in health. These standards contain extensive references to health, including basic body functions, cardiovascular fitness, nutrition, sexuality, the scientific basis for disease, problems with substance abuse, accident prevention and safety, risks and personal decisionmaking (National Research Council, 1996).

Science is not the only subject that can be enhanced and made more relevant using health topics. In mathematics, elementary students can collect and use the information on nutrition labels to devise a well-rounded diet for themselves, and secondary students can examine the mathematical models for the spread of contagious disease. Language arts classes can analyze the persuasive effects of the media on health behaviors or write letters to politicians and the media about student health concerns. Visual and performing arts classes, including dance, drama, music, and visual arts, can encourage students to enhance mental health through expression of personal feelings; awareness of health issues can be promoted through student expression and interpretation in these various art media. Social studies classes can explore how nutrition and disease shaped history, discuss the advantages and disadvantages of prohibition and current implications for controlling other substances, or debate the ethics of withholding health care and other benefits to those suffering from conditions caused by deliberately engaging in risky behavior.

It should be emphasized that the inclusion of health topics in other curricular areas should *enhance*, but not replace, the health education curriculum.

Services

Presented below is a brief summary of the types of services typically found in school health programs. These services represent a complex area, and issues of concern include determining the appropriate range and configuration of school-based services, interaction between the school and other community providers, qualifications and training of service deliv-

---

[9]In a related situation, the American Association for the Advancement of Science was recently concerned with increasing the scientific knowledge of low-literate adults. In surveys, these adults expressed a lack of interest in science but indicated that health was highly relevant to daily life. Consequently, materials were developed that taught scientific concepts through health topics, and these materials are currently in use in adult education centers throughout the country.

ery personnel, scientific validity of mandated services, financing, evaluation, and controversial aspects of certain services. Chapter 4 focuses on services, and these issues are discussed in greater depth there.

Health Services. Health services are designed to evaluate, protect, and promote student health. SHPPS has described school health services as a "coordinated system that ensures a continuum of care from school to home to community health care provider and back" (Small et al., 1995). The goals and program elements of school health services vary at the state, community, school district, and individual school levels, but some common elements exist across the country. A recent national school health survey, *A Closer Look*, reported on the most frequently provided health services in schools (Davis et al., 1995). The results are shown in Table 4-1 (see Chapter 4). Two health services are provided almost universally by school districts—first aid and administration of medications. Other commonly provided services include screenings—height, weight, vision, and hearing—and services mandated by law for children with disabilities and special needs.

School health services are provided by nurses, physicians, dentists, and other allied health personnel in settings ranging from a health aide's office in the school to a full-blown school-based clinic providing a wide range of primary care services. Depending on the community, certain basic health services may be considered the responsibility of the school system, such as the provision of school nurses or health aides. However, more extensive ventures—school-based clinics, for example—are often initiated and managed in cooperation with the school by groups outside education, such as a health department, community clinic, or hospital.

Counseling, Psychological, and Social Services. These services promote the mental, emotional, and social health of students and deal with problems that interfere with teaching and learning. Services include individual or group assessment, interventions, and referrals. School staff and families of students may also receive these services, and services for special education students are an important focus.

These services bridge the gap between the school's academic program and the mental and emotional health of students and their families. Professionals in these fields work closely with each other and with school health personnel, teachers and administrators, families, and community agencies. They frequently serve as brokers in linking community health and social service resources to the school site.

In this era of emphasis on academic standards and limited financial resources, counseling, psychological, and social services are sometimes seen as outside the mainstream and are threatened by cutbacks. However, these services address today's new social morbidities that prevent students from achieving at their highest potential, and the extent of the problems may not be recognized. It is estimated that 12 to 20 percent of our nation's children and adolescents suffer from one or more diagnosable mental disorders, and many others are at risk due to violent neighborhoods, parental abuse or neglect, and risky and dangerous behavior (IOM, 1994). In fact, it has been suggested that fully 40 percent of all students are in "very bad educational shape" and "at risk of failing to fulfill their physical and mental promise" (Hodgkinson, 1993). It is also important to realize that all students—not simply low-income or low-achieving students—are vulnerable to mental and emotional problems. A recent national survey of high-achieving high school students indicated that more than 50 percent report violence at their school, 29 percent have considered committing suicide, 81 percent report that it is easy to get alcohol and 77 percent say alcohol is very common at parties, 25 percent have engaged in sexual intercourse, and 11 percent have tried marijuana. More than 30 percent of these high-achieving students say their home life is less than "happy and close most of the time" (Who's Who Among American High School Students, 1994). Given this context, it has been proposed that counseling, psychological, and social services receive increased emphasis in school reform and restructuring, as an essential "enabling" component to address factors that interfere with students' learning and performance (Adelman, in press).

Nutrition and Foodservice. The school foodservice not only provides nutritious and appealing meals but also helps students develop lifelong healthful eating habits. Evidence shows that dietary behaviors tend to stay constant over time, and poor eating habits established in childhood tend to persist through adulthood (CDC, 1996). A poor diet contributes to the development of four of the nation's ten leading causes of death: coronary heart disease, stroke, diabetes, and certain types of cancer. Other detrimental conditions associated with diet are hypertension, obesity, osteoporosis, and poor oral health. Also, the number of overweight children and adults has increased significantly in the last decade, and eating disorders and unsafe weight loss methods have become more prevalent as well.

Nutrition education is critical at all levels, even in early childhood and elementary schools, in order that students develop healthful dietary habits and understand the influence of nutrition on health. Nutrition education should be part of classroom health education, and nutrition should be introduced into other subjects such as science, physical education, and home economics. In providing a variety of nutritious and appealing meals, the school foodservice serves as a laboratory to reinforce the lessons learned in the classroom.

Research has shown that children's cognitive, behavioral, and physical performance are impaired by poor nutrition (Center on Hunger, Poverty, and Nutrition Policy, 1993; CDC, 1996). School meals that meet U.S. Department of Agriculture (USDA) dietary guidelines play a significant role in providing good nutrition. The School Nutrition Dietary Assessment Study (Burghart and Devaney, 1995) found that students who ate the school lunch had higher intakes of key nutrients than students who made other choices. A study of low-income elementary students found that participation in the school breakfast program led to increased standardized test scores and decreased absenteeism and tardiness (Meyers et al., 1989).

The concept of foodservice is not limited to the reimbursable school meal program for which the USDA establishes nutrition standards. High-quality local standards are needed for *all* food available on the school campus—including food sold through vending machines and special events—and for the environment in which these foods are made available to students. Although the immediate goal of the school foodservice may be the provision of student meals, the ultimate goals are providing education and establishing lifelong healthful dietary habits.

Comprehensive Family Services. Access may be provided through the school to a wide range of health and social services for students and their families, especially in disadvantaged communities. Examples of services include health and dental care, adult literacy programs, employment training, family counseling, child care, legal services, recreation and culture, and provision of basic needs in housing, food, and clothing. Providing access to services through the school does not necessarily require an increase in overall budgets for these services. Typically, many of these services already exist but in a fragmented manner, and families often find the system difficult to access and navigate. Collocating and coordinating comprehensive services through a familiar neighborhood institution such as the school has been found to improve access, increase efficiency, and facilitate follow-up (Wagner et al., 1994). Comprehensive school-affiliated family services are increasingly considered to be an important means for reaching families and for improving academic, health, and social outcomes for students[10] (American Academy of Pediatrics, 1994a, 1994b;

---

[10]As examples, the Goals 2000 legislation calls for states to involve parents and other community representatives in developing the state's educational improvement plan, which should include such strategies as increasing the access of all students to health and social services in convenient sites designed to provide "one-stop shopping" for parents and students. The Improving America's Schools Act, which reauthorizes the Elementary and Secondary Education Act (ESEA), allows local districts to set aside 5 percent of ESEA funds for the coordination of services.

Bruininks et al., 1994; U.S. Department of Education and U.S. Department of Health and Human Services, 1993; U.S. Department of Education, 1995). Although seeming ambitious, comprehensive school-affiliated family services are not a new idea; many schools were providing access to a similar range of services in poor urban and rural areas a century ago (Tyack, 1992).

Integration of Comprehensive School Health Programs with Community Health Efforts

Early in its study, the IOM committee sensed that school programs working in isolation are likely to have limited effect without community support and reinforcement. To examine this premise further, a paper on integrating school and community health efforts was commissioned; the paper is found in its entirety in Appendix A. (Note that in this paper the author uses the terminology "comprehensive school health education" to refer to what the committee has called a "comprehensive school health program.") The paper reviews the results of selected studies on school-based programs, community programs, and programs integrating the efforts of schools and communities. Examples of community participation and mechanisms for interfacing the school and community are also discussed. Results suggest that combined school–community programs yield higher levels of participation, implementation, and dissemination; greater effects on the more serious levels of health risk (e.g., on daily smoking compared to monthly smoking); and effects on parents as well as youth, perhaps longer effects than are currently obtainable from most school programs alone. The author notes that in the programs analyzed, the assumption of the need for integrating school and community efforts has usually been based on practical considerations and common wisdom rather than on theory or empirical evidence. The author also points out knowledge gaps and the limitations of existing studies, and suggests directions for future research.

Integration of the Elements of a Comprehensive School Health Program

Integration—the blending of program components into a unified whole—is an elusive concept. A single standard process for achieving and recognizing "integration of components" does not exist, because each situation is unique. Integration might be considered a topic that is "hard to define, but you recognize it when you see it." Consider the following simple example pertaining to nutrition that illustrates the practical meaning of the term integration:

Lessons on nutrition in the health education classroom are supported by a school foodservice that serves healthful, well-balanced meals and labels the nutritional content of cafeteria selections to increase nutrition awareness. Classroom lessons are also strengthened by school policies requiring that foods available through vending machines, special events, and fund-raising drives meet a high standard of nutrition. School nurses and counselors promote awareness about weight management and eating disorders, and provide assistance for students and staff with problems in this area. Students with special conditions, such as diabetes, have dietary provisions prescribed by a physician and arranged by the school nurse and foodservice or by a community dietitian if the school lacks the required expertise. Physical education instructors help students understand the relationship between caloric intake and energy expenditure and between nutrition quality and physical stamina and performance. Nutrition-related topics also enhance instruction in other subject matter areas, such as science, mathematics, and social studies. Community-wide campaigns promote nutrition awareness so that healthy eating habits acquired in school will be reinforced outside school; restaurant and fast-food outlets promote healthful choices, and grocery stores publicize healthful selections and provide recipes and tips for healthful family meal planning.

The conventional wisdom is that when the various elements of a CSHP are integrated, they will mutually reinforce and support each other and produce a whole that is greater than the sum of its separate parts. The concept and desired outcomes of integration are simple to recite, but integration is a difficult and sophisticated process to implement and measure—"the reality lags far behind the vision" (Education Development Center, 1995). While exemplary individual program components exist in many schools and various states and communities are making progress in establishing CSHPs, truly comprehensive and integrated programs do not yet appear to be widespread.[11] Although individual program components have been studied separately and many are reasonably well understood, the committee could find no record of systematic research on the integration of multicomponent programs. There is a dearth of *scientific* analysis of what exactly constitutes integration of components, whether integration actually enhances the effects of separate components, and what the most effective strategies are for achieving integration and measuring its impact. This lack of evidence is not surprising, given the scarcity and complexity of programs and limited program resources. Research

---

[11]The committee did not attempt to carry out a national search for comprehensive school health programs. However, informal feedback from the Infrastructure States—demonstration sites for comprehensive school health programs sponsored by DASH/CDC—indicates that progress is being made, but CSHPs are not yet a widespread institutionalized phenomenon.

on the process and effectiveness of individual components—a particular health education curriculum, health services intervention, or modification of school environment—is difficult enough; even more so is the study of any synergism among them.

Since individual programs are idiosyncratic and not easily replicable, research and evaluation that attempt to detect the effects of integration per se or to detect the specific contribution of individual or various combinations of factors to the overall program are not likely to be fruitful. The pragmatic approach to integration of program components at the local level is to make certain that each individual component is designed to address identified needs and implemented according to effective practices, and that systematic and regular communication occurs among all stakeholders. Then, if indicators are moving in the right direction at the desired rate, this should be sufficient evidence for a community to declare that its program is effective. Additional issues and dilemmas involved in evaluating comprehensive integrated programs are discussed further in Chapter 6.

SUMMARY

Schools have a long history of providing health education, services, and outreach to families. A vision of what schools might be able to do to promote health, education, and family well-being has led to the concept of a CSHP. Although exemplary individual program components exist in many schools, truly comprehensive and integrated programs are not yet widespread. Various models for CSHPs exist, but most of the basic elements or components tend to be similar. There is no "best" model or standard algorithm for establishing a program—it must be specifically tailored to fit each particular community. Active community involvement is key, and the integration of school programs with other community efforts appears to produce more positive results than school or community programs operating in isolation.

REFERENCES

Adelman, H.S. In press. *Restructuring Education Support Services: Toward the Concept of the Enabling Component.* Kent, Ohio: American School Health Association.
Adolescent Medicine. 1995. 20(10):1–4.
Allensworth, D.D. 1993. Expansion of comprehensive school health: What works. Paper presented at the Institute of Medicine Workshop, Integrating Comprehensive School Health Programs in Grades K–12, Washington, D.C., May.
Allensworth, D.D., and Kolbe, L.J. 1987. The comprehensive school health program: Exploring an expanded concept. *Journal of School Health* 57(10):409–411.

Allensworth, D.D., Wolford Symons, C., and Olds, R.S. 1994. *Healthy Students 2000: An Agenda for Continuous Improvement in America's Schools.* Kent, Ohio: American School Health Association.

American Academy of Pediatrics, Committee on School Health. 1993. *School Health: Policy and Practice.* Elk Grove Village, Ill.: American Academy of Pediatrics.

American Academy of Pediatrics. 1994a. *Principles to Link By: Integrating Education, Health, and Human Services for Children, Youth, and Families.* Report of the Consensus Conference. Washington, D.C.

American Academy of Pediatrics. 1994b. Statement by the Task Force on Integrated School Health Services. *Pediatrics* 94(3):400–402.

American Medical Association. 1992. *Guidelines for Adolescent Preventive Services.* Chicago: American Medical Association, Department of Adolescent Medicine.

American School Food Service Association. 1995. *Keys to Excellence: Standards of Practice for School Food Service and Nutrition.* Alexandria, Va.: American School Food Service Association.

American School Health Association. 1994. Guidelines for Comprehensive School Health Programs. Kent, Ohio: American School Health Association.

Belcastro, A., and Gold, R. 1984. Teacher stress and burnout: Implications for school health personnel. *Journal of School Health* 53(7)404–407.

Bruininks, R.H., Frenzel, M., and Kelly, A. 1994. Integrating services: The case for better links to schools. *Journal of School Health* 64(6):242–248.

Burghart, J., and Devaney, B., eds. 1995. The school nutrition dietary assessment study. *American Journal of Clinical Nutrition* 61:1(Suppl.).

Carnegie Council on Adolescent Development. 1989. *Turning Points: Preparing American Youth for the 21st Century.* Washington, D.C.: Carnegie Corporation.

Carnegie Council on Adolescent Development. 1995. Personal communication with Turning Points Evaluator.

Center on Hunger, Poverty, and Nutrition Policy. 1993. Statement on the Link between Nutrition and Cognitive Development in Children. Medford, Mass.: Tufts University School of Nutrition.

Centers for Disease Control and Prevention. 1994. Guidelines for school health programs to prevent tobacco use and addiction. *Morbidity and Mortality Weekly Report* 43(RR–2):1–18.

Centers for Disease Control and Prevention. 1997. Guidelines for school and community health programs to promote physical activity among youth. *Morbidity and Mortality Weekly Report.*

Centers for Disease Control and Prevention. 1996. Guidelines for school health programs to promote healthy eating. *Morbidity and Mortality Weekly Report* 45(RR-9).

Collins, J.L., Small, M.L., Kann, L., Pateman, B.C., Gold, R.S., and Kolbe, L.J. 1995. School health education. *Journal of School Health* 65(8):302–311.

Comer, J.P. 1984. Improving American Education: Roles for Parents. Hearing Before the Select Committee on Children, Youth, and Families. Washington, D.C.: U.S. Government Printing Office.

Comer, J.P. 1988. Educating poor minority children. *Scientific American* 259(5):42–48.

Commission on the Reorganization of Secondary Education. 1981. *Cardinal Principles of Secondary Education.* Bulletin #35. Washington, D.C.: Bureau of Education.

Cortese, P., and Middleton, K., eds. 1994. *The Comprehensive School Health Challenge.* Santa Cruz, Calif.: Education, Training, and Research Associates.

Davis, M., Fryer, G.E., White, S. and Igoe, J.B. 1995. A Closer Look: A Report of Select Findings from the National School Health Survey 1993–1994. Denver, Colo.: Office of School Health, University of Colorado Health Sciences Center.

Dryfoos, J.G. 1994. *Full-Service Schools: A Revolution in Health and Social Services for Children, Youth, and Families*. San Francisco, Calif.: Jossey-Bass.

Duffy, J. 1974. *A History of Public Health in New York City, 1866–1966*. New York: Russell Sage Foundation.

Education Development Center. 1995. The Status of School Health: Annex 1 to the Working Paper of the World Health Organization Expert Committee on Comprehensive School Health Education and Promotion. Newton, Mass.: Education Development Center.

Edwards, L.H. 1992. Organizational models for school health. In *Principles and Practices of Student Health, Volume Two: School Health*, H.M. Wallace, K. Patrick, G.S. Parcel, and J.B. Igoe, eds. Oakland, Calif.: Third Party Publishing.

Falck, V., and Kilcoyne, M. 1984. A health promotion program for school personnel. *Journal of School Health* 54(6):239–242.

Goldberg, M., and James, H. 1983. A nation at risk: the report of the National Commission on Excellence in Education. *Phi Delta Kappan* 65(1):14-18.

Hilmar, N.S., and McAtee, P. 1973. The school nurse practitioner and her practice: A study of nurses in elementary schools. *Journal of School Health* 43(7):431–441.

Hirsch, D. 1995. Health-Promoting Schools: From Ideas to Action. Frontiers in Education: Schools as Health Promoting Environments. Review of conference held in Geneva, Switzerland, February, 1995, jointly sponsored by the Johann Jacobs Foundation and the Carnegie Corporation.

Hodgkinson, H.L. 1993. American education: The good, the bad, and the task. *Phi Delta Kappan* 74:619–623.

Institute of Medicine. 1994. *Reducing Risks for Mental Disorders*. Washington, D.C.: National Academy Press.

Institute of Medicine. 1995. *Defining a Comprehensive School Health Program: An Interim Statement*. Washington, D.C.: National Academy Press.

Jamison, J. 1993. Health education in schools: A survey of policy and implementation. *Health Education Journal* 52(2):59–62.

Joint Committee on Health Education Terminology. 1991. Report of the 1990 Joint Committee on Health Education Terminology. *Journal of Health Education* 22(2):99–108.

Joint Committee on National Health Education Standards. 1995. *National Health Education Standards: Achieving Health Literacy*. Atlanta, Ga.: American Cancer Society.

Kohn, M.A. 1979. School Health Services and Nurse Practitioners: A Survey of State Laws. Washington, D.C.: Center for Law and Social Policy.

Kolbe, L.J. 1986. Increasing the impact of school health promotion programs: Emerging research perspectives. *Journal of Health Education* 17(5):47–52.

Kort, M. 1984. The delivery of primary health care in American public schools, 1890–1980. *Journal of School Health* 54(11):453–457.

Lavin, A.T., Shapiro, G.R., and Weill, K.S. eds. 1992. *Creating an Agenda for School-Based Health Promotion: A Review of Selected Reports*. Boston: Harvard School of Public Health.

Lee, M., and Bennett, B. 1985. Centennial articles. *Journal of Physical Education, Recreation and Dance Centennial Issue* 56(4):19–27.

Leeds, S., Heneson-Walling, R., and Shwab, J. eds. 1980. EPSDT: *A Guide for Educational Programs*. Washington, D.C.: U.S. Government Printing Office.

Lynch, A. 1977. Evaluating school health programs. In *Health Services: The Local Perspective*, A. Levin, ed. New York: Academy of Political Science; *Proceedings of the Academy of Political Science* 32(3):89–105.

Maysey, D.L. 1988. School worksite wellness programs: A strategy for achieving the 1990 goals for a healthier America. *Health Education Quarterly* 15(1):53–62.

McGinnis, J.M., and DeGraw, C. 1991. Healthy Schools 2000: Creating partnerships for the decade. *Journal of School Health* 61(7):292–297.

Means, R.K. 1975. *Historical Perspectives on School Health*. Thorofare, N.J.: Charles B. Slack.

Meyers, A.F., Sampson, A.D., Weitzman, M., Rogers, B.L., and Kayne, H. 1989. School breakfast program and school performance. *American Journal of Diseases and Children* 143: 1234.

Nader, P.N. 1990. The concept of comprehensiveness in the design and implementation of school health programs. *Journal of School Health* 60(4):133–138.

National Association for Sport and Physical Education. 1995. *Moving into the Future: National Standards for Physical Education: A Guide to Content and Assessment*. St. Louis, Mo.: Mosby.

National Commission on Children. 1991. *Beyond Rhetoric: A New American Agenda for Children and Families*. Washington, D.C.: U.S. Government Printing Office.

National Education Goals Panel. 1993. *The National Education Goals Report: Building a Nation of Learners*, Volume One: *The National Report*. Washington, D.C.: U.S. Government Printing Office.

National Education Goals Panel. 1994. *The National Education Goals Report: Building a Nation of Learners*. Washington, D.C.: U.S. Government Printing Office.

National Nursing Coalition for School Health. 1995. School health nursing services: Exploring national issues and priorities. *Journal of School Health* 65(9):370–389.

National Research Council. 1996. *National Science Education Standards*. Washington, D.C.: National Academy Press.

Office of Technology Assessment, Congress of the United States. 1995. *Risks to Students in School*. OTA–ENV–633. Washington, D.C.: U.S. Government Printing Office, September.

Pate, R.R., Small, M.L., Ross, J.G., Young, J.C., Flint, K.H., and Warren, C.W. 1995. School physical education. *Journal of School Health* 65(8):312–318.

Pateman, B.C., McKinney, P., Kann, L., Small, M.L., Warren, C.W., and Collins, J.L. 1995. School food service. *Journal of School Health* 65(8):327–332.

Pigg, R.M. 1992. The school health program: Historical perspectives and future prospects. In *Principles and Practices of Student Health, Volume Two: School Health,* H.M. Wallace, K. Patrick, G.S. Parcel, and J.B. Igoe, eds. Oakland, Calif.: Third Party Publishing.

Proctor, S.T., Lordi, S.L., and Zarger, D.S. 1993. *School Nursing Practice Roles and Standards*. Scarborough, Maine: National Association for School Nurses.

Ross, J.G., Einhaus, K.E., Hohenemser, L.K., Greene, B.Z., Kann, L., and Gold R.S. 1995. School health policies prohibiting tobacco use, alcohol and other drug use, and violence. *Journal of School Health* 65(8): 333–338.

Silver, H.K., Igoe, J.B., and McAtee, P. 1976. The school nurse practitioner: Providing improved health care to children. *Pediatrics* 58(4):580–584.

Simons-Morton, B.G. 1992. Health-related physical education. In *Principles and Practices of Student Health, Volume Two: School Health,* H.M. Wallace, K. Patrick, G.S. Parcel, and J.B. Igoe, eds. Oakland, Calif.: Third Party Publishing.

Slavin, R.E., Madden, N.A., Karweit, N.L., Dolan, L.J., and Wasik, B.A. 1992. *Success for All: A Relentless Approach to Prevention and Early Intervention in Elementary Schools*. Arlington, Va.: Educational Research Service.

Sliepcevich, E. 1964. School Health Education Study: A Summary Report. Washington, D.C.: School Health Education Study.

Small, M.L., Majer, L.S., Allensworth, D.D., Farquhar, B.K., Kann, L., and Pateman, B.C. 1995. School health services. *Journal of School Health* 65(8):319–326.

Solloway, M.R., Pine, Y., and Anderson, E. 1995. Health supervision and school health services for children. In *Child Health Supervision*, M.R. Solloway and P.P Budetti, eds. Arlington, Va.: National Center for Education in Maternal and Child Health.

Stone, E.J. 1990. ACCESS: Keystones for school health promotion. *Journal of School Health* (60)7:298–300.

Tyack, D. 1992. Health and social services in public schools: Historical perspectives. *The Future of Children: School Linked Services*, R.E. Behrman, ed. Los Altos, Calif.: Center for the Future of Children, David and Lucille Packard Foundation 2(1):19-31.

U.S. Department of Education. 1995. *School-Linked Comprehensive Services for Children and Families: What We Know and What We Need to Know.* Washington, D.C.: U.S. Department of Education, SAI 9503025.

U.S. Department of Education and U.S. Department of Health and Human Services. 1993. *Together We Can: A Guide for Crafting a Profamily System of Education and Human Services.* Washington, D.C.: U.S. Government Printing Office.

U.S. Department of Health and Human Services, Public Health Service. 1991. *Healthy People 2000: National Health Promotion and Disease Prevention Objectives.* DHHS Publication No. (PHS) 91-50213, Washington, D.C.: U.S. Government Printing Office.

University of Colorado Health Sciences Center, Office of School Health. 1991. The Community Health Nurse in the Schools. Denver, Colo.: University of Colorado Health Sciences Center.

Wagner, M., Golan, S., Shaver, D., Newman, L., Wechsler, M., Kelley, F. 1994. *A Healthy Start for California's Children and Families: Early Findings from a Statewide Evaluation of School-Linked Services.* Menlo Park, Calif.: SRI International.

Walker, D.K., Butler, J.A., and Bender, A. 1990. Children's health care and the schools. In *Children in a Changing Health System: Assessments and Proposals for Reform*, M.J. Schlesinger and L. Eisenberg, eds. Baltimore: Johns Hopkins University Press.

Wallace, H.M., Patrick, K., Parcel, G.S., and Igoe, J.B., eds. 1992. *Principles and Practices of Student Health, Volume Two: School Health.* Oakland, Calif.: Third Party Publishing.

Who's Who Among American High School Students. 1994. Twenty-Fifth Annual Survey of High Achievers. Views on Education, Social and Sexual Issues, Drugs. Lake Forest, Ill.: Educational Communications. Health, State of New Mexico.

3

Education

As discussed in Chapter 2, the educational realm of comprehensive school health programs (CSHPs) includes two curricular components with a health focus: physical education and health education. These should be perceived as distinct courses or programs within the school curriculum. Although physical education and health education may have differences in their conceptual basis and approach, they share the common goal of enabling students to take personal control of factors that affect their health. Both fields are currently undergoing change, with new developments informed by research. This chapter will review the state of physical education and health education, and examine how these two curricular areas can contribute to a comprehensive school health program.

THE ROLE OF PHYSICAL EDUCATION IN COMPREHENSIVE SCHOOL HEALTH PROGRAMS

Introduction

The physical education instructional program is an integral part of a comprehensive school health program, because it teaches the knowledge and skills that lead to a physically active life-style and reinforces positive health behaviors (McGinnis et al., 1991). Research has confirmed a direct relationship between a physically active life-style and the long-term health status of individuals. A sedentary life-style as an adult leads to premature mortality and morbidity. The sedentary are more likely to experience coronary heart disease (Berlin and Colditz, 1990; Powell et al., 1987), hypertension (Paffenbarger et al., 1986; Blair et al., 1988), certain cancers (Kohl et al., 1988; Lee et al., 1992), osteoporosis (Cummings et al., 1985), and obesity (King and Tribble, 1991). The ultimate consequence of increased numbers of sedentary adults is an increase in the number of premature deaths. A study released in 1986 estimated that approximately 257,000 deaths in the nation could be attributed to a sedentary life-style, making this a risk factor equal to or greater than that attributed to obesity, elevated cholesterol, or hypertension (Hahn et al., 1986). Epidemiologic studies estimate that all-cause mortality rates are at least two to three times greater for sedentary persons than for those who are active (Centers for Disease Control and Prevention, 1997).

Light to moderate physical activity for adults can have significant health benefits and reduce the chronic diseases associated with a sedentary life-style (Leon, 1989; Leon et al., 1987; Sallis et al., 1986). Since regular exercise increases functional capacity and reduces many risk factors for chronic disease (McGinnis, 1992; Pate et al., 1995; Powell et al., 1989), it is prudent to provide children with the information and skills necessary to maintain a physically active life-style. Physical education programs in schools should prepare children for a lifetime of physical activity (Sallis and McKenzie, 1991).

Recognition of the link between physical education and public health is not a recent phenomenon. Lemuel Shattuck's pioneering 1850 Report to the Sanitary Commission of Massachusetts, described in Chapter 2, included physical training as part of the plan for improving public health (Means, 1975; Pate et al., 1995). Physical education has long been justified on the basis of broad physical, social, and moral developmental goals, although to date the major focus has often been on team and competitive sports. Even large-scale fitness testing programs in the recent past assessed sport-related skills rather than health-related fitness (Ross and Gilbert, 1985; Ross and Pate, 1987; Sallis and McKenzie, 1991). In a review of physical education's role in public health, Sallis and McKenzie noted:

> In a society in which adult sedentary behavior contributes substantially to the epidemic of cardiovascular and other chronic diseases, there is a rationale for shifting the orientation of physical education to a health focus. . . . Health-related physical education programs should focus on maximizing the participation of all children, whether they are athletically gifted, clumsy, disinterested, or obese. Physical education in schools is the only preparation most children will have in how to develop an active life-style. . . .

Quality Physical Education

The physical education instructional program makes a unique contribution to the health and education of students by promoting the development of a physically educated person who has skills necessary to perform a variety of physical activities, is physically fit, participates regularly in physical activity, knows the implications of and benefits from involvement in physical activities, and values physical activity and its contributions to a healthful life-style (National Association for Sport and Physical Education, 1992).

The goals of the physical education program are the attainment of appropriate levels of physical fitness and the development and refinement of motor skills that support a physically active life-style and safe, efficient movement. Skillful movement is a fundamental part of everyday life. It is a prerequisite for health-related physical activities and supports safety and self-confidence in work-related performance and recreational pursuits.

The recently released National Standards for Physical Education identify the psychomotor, cognitive, and affective aspects of physical education that all students should know and be able to do as a result of a quality physical education program (National Association for Sport and Physical Education, 1995). According to these standards, the physically educated person does the following:

1. Demonstrates competency in many movement forms and proficiency in a few movement forms.
2. Applies movement concepts and principles to the learning and development of motor skills.
3. Exhibits a physically active life-style.
4. Achieves and maintains a health-enhancing level of physical fitness.
5. Demonstrates responsible personal and social behavior in physical activity settings.
6. Demonstrates understanding and respect for differences among people in physical activity settings.
7. Understands that physical activity provides opportunities for enjoyment, challenge, self-expression, and social interaction.

The relationship between quality school physical education and health status was also recognized by the developers of *Healthy People 2000*, the national decade-long public—private initiative to improve the health of the nation (U.S. Department of Health and Human Services, 1991). Two of the *Healthy People 2000* national health objectives focused on physical activity in schools:

1.8 Increase to at least 50 percent the proportion of children and adolescents in Grades 1 through 12 who participate daily in school physical education,

1.9 Increase to at least 50 percent the proportion of school physical education class time that students spend being physically active, preferably engaged in lifetime physical activities.

Quality physical education programs should be taught by qualified physical educators and include a planned, sequential curriculum that incorporates the seven national standards for physical education into a program of developmentally appropriate movement experiences for all students.

Health-Related Physical Fitness

Health-related physical fitness refers to performance levels in one or more of these fitness components: muscular strength and endurance, cardiovascular endurance, flexibility, and body composition. Health-related physical fitness is the aspect of a quality physical education program most readily identified as physical education's contribution to public health. However, the use of fitness scores to measure the impact of the physical education experience on public health is shortsighted. Physical fitness scores are a time-bound measure. They are important in describing current health status but not future health status. The importance of motor skill development must also be emphasized. A child who does not develop a level of confidence and competence as a skillful mover will probably choose not to pursue a lifetime of physical activity and may incur unnecessary injuries through poor, inefficient movement patterns.

Research

Participation in moderate to vigorous physical activity provides considerable health benefits for children and youth (Blair et al., 1989; Cale and Harris, 1993; McKenzie et al., 1992; Simons-Morton et al., 1988), as well as for adults. Relationships have been established between children's physical activity and obesity (Berkowitz et al., 1985; Saris et al., 1980; Sasaki et al., 1987), high-density lipoprotein (HDL) cholesterol (Durant et al., 1983), blood pressure (Hofman et al., 1987; Panico et al., 1987), and cardiovascular fitness (Duncan et al., 1983; Dwyer et al., 1983; Maynard et al., 1987; Siegel and Manfrede, 1984). Exercise training produces improved physical fitness in students (Mahon and Vaccaro, 1989; Pate and Ward, 1990; Pate et al., 1995). More than 100 large population-based studies on the relation of physical activity or fitness to health have been published in the peer-reviewed literature, most during the past 20 years; examples are summarized in Table 3-1. Youth physical activity has also been linked to improved mental health, cognitive functioning, and academic performance; and involvement in physical activity and sports has been associated with a decrease in smoking, alcohol consumption, and drug use and abuse (CDC, 1997; Shephard et al., 1984).

It is well accepted that physical activity has significant health benefits, but the levels of activity required in childhood to achieve those benefits are not fully understood (Sallis and McKenzie, 1991). Furthermore, there is currently little research to directly link students' current or future physical fitness levels to the physical activity that occurs in physical education classes. Although the relationship between school physical education and active adult life-styles is not fully understood, many believe that increasing a person's ability to move competently and confidently may increase their willingness to become more physically active.

Current Practice

A nationwide assessment of physical education programs at the state, district, and school levels was recently completed by the Centers for Disease Control and Prevention (CDC) as part of the School Health Policies and Programs Study (SHPPS)[1] (Pate et al., 1995). This assessment shows that current instructional practices in physical education do not meet the standards identified by the national health objectives *Healthy People 2000* nor the National Standards for Physical Education. According to SHPPS data, most states (94 percent) and school districts (95 percent) require physical education. Yet 80 percent of states and 83 percent of all districts allow students to be excused from physical education classes for reasons such as parents' requests (65 percent of middle schools, 42 percent of secondary schools), physical disability (58 percent of middle schools, 59 percent of secondary schools), and participation in other activities such as band, chorus, or cheerleading (30 percent of middle schools, 23 percent of secondary schools). Even if no exemptions were approved, the number of students participating in daily physical education remains less than optimal. In middle school, less than one-half of the students (47 percent) are required to attend physical education each year (Table 3-2). Of those who

---

[1]The School Health Policies and Programs Study was carried out in 1994 to examine policies and programs across multiple components of school health programs at the state, district, school, and classroom levels across the country. The October 1995 issue of *The Journal of School Health* is devoted to a summary report of SHPPS findings and includes separate analyses of school health education; school physical education; school health services; school foodservice; and school health policies prohibiting tobacco use, alcohol and other drug use, and violence.

TABLE 3-1A Illustrative Studies Regarding Physical Activity and Physical Education

Study

Cohen, C.H. 1995. The effect of a three-year physical fitness program on the body composition and lifestyle behaviors of middle school students. *RQES Supplement*, March.

Ignico, A.A. 1994. A longitudinal study of the fitness levels of children enrolled in daily versus twice weekly physical education. *RQES Supplement*, March.

Sallis, J.F., Simons-Morton, B.G., Stone, E.J., Corbin, C.B., Epstein, L.H., Faucette, N., Ianotti, J.D., Killen, R.C., Klesges, Petray, C.K., Rowland, T.W., and Taylor, W. 1992. Determinants of physical activity and interventions in youth. *Med. Sci. Sports Exerc.* 24:S248–S257.

Taylor, W., and Baranowski, T. 1991. Physical activity, cardiovascular fitness, and adiposity in children. *RQES* 62:157–163.

Pate, R.R., Dowda, M., and Ross, J.G. 1990. Associations between physical activity and physical fitness in American children. *AJDC* 144:1123–1129.

Dennison, B.A., Straus, E.D., Mellits, E.D., and Charney, E. 1987. Childhood physical fitness tests: Predictor of adult physical activity? *Pediatrics* 82:324–330.

Gruber, J.J. 1986. Physical activity and self-esteem development in children, A meta-analysis. Pp. 30–48 in *Effects of Physical Activity on Children* (The American Academy of Physical Education Papers, No. 19), G.A. Stull an H.M. Eckert, eds. Champaign, Ill.: Human Kinetics.

Iverson, D.C., Fielding, J.E., Crow, R.S., and Christenson, G.M. 1985. The promotion of physical activity in the United States population: The status of program in medical, worksite, community, and school settings. *Public Health Reports* 100:212–224.

Caspersen, C.J., Powell, K.E., and Christenson, G.M. 1985. Physical activity, exercise, and physical fitness: Definitions and distinctions for health-related research. *Public Health Reports* 100:126–131.

Corbin, C.B., and Pangrazi, R.P. 1991. Are American children and youth fit? *RQES* 63(2):96–106.

Principal Findings

The study supports the position that life-style behaviors are established very early in life; therefore intervention programs must be implemented early on in elementary school in order to have a significant effect.

The findings suggest that school physical education program can make a significant contribution to children's fitness levels, particularly in the area of cardiovascular endurance.

This study reports that directed interventions increased physical activity in 4th-grade children. Interventions included teacher training, family support, incentives and focus on enjoyment.

Obese children are less active than non-obese children. Results indicate that physical activity is positively related to cardiovascular fitness in more obese children.

Physical activity and fitness are positively associated but directionally is not clear.

Childhood fitness results did not predict levels of adult physical activity consistently.

Positive fitness and regular physical activity participation are associated with positive self-concepts in children.

The Statement on Exercise by the American Heart Association references this study under the area of implementation of exercise programs—schools as a study that demonstrates that organized school programs not only are feasible but can also be successful.

This article provides working definitions of and distinctions among physical activity, exercise, and physical fitness.

This article reviews several large-scale studies from perspective of accepted standards that have evolved since 1985. Most children meet some fitness criteria; many do not meet recommended standards in all fitness components (muscular strength and endurance, cardiovascular endurance, flexibility and body composition). Authors conclude that children have more health-related fitness than earlier studies indicated.

continued on next page

TABLE 3-1A Continued

Study

Sallis, J.F., ed. 1994. *Special Issue Pediatric Exercise Science* 6(4), November.

Kuntzleman, C.T., and Reiff, G.G. 1992. The decline in American children's fitness levels. *RQES* 63(2):107–111.

Oded, B. 1990. Disease specific benefits of training in the child with a chronic disease: What is the evidence? *Pediatric Exercise Science* 2:384–394.

Updyke, W.F., and Willet, M.S., eds. 1989. *Physical Fitness Trends in American Youth.* Washington, DC: Chrysler-AAU Physical Fitness Program.

Ross, J.G., and Pate, R.R. 1987. The National Children and Youth Fitness Study II. A summary of findings. *JOPERD* 58:51–56.

are required to take physical education each year, less than one-half (45 percent) are required to take physical education daily (Table 3-3). At the high school level, few schools require four years of physical education (Table 3–2). One-quarter of schools (26 percent) require three years; 25 percent require two years; 37 percent require one year; and 9 percent require less than one year. Only 67 percent of the classes at the secondary level are five days per week (Table 3-2) (Pate et al., 1995).

Not only do most schools provide students with less daily exposure to physical education than the national health objectives have set as appropriate, but the instructional activities most commonly included in physical education classes are not the recommended lifetime physical activities or activities ensuring moderate aerobic exercise for all participants; but rather they are competitive sport activities (Table 3-4). Basketball, volleyball, baseball, and football were the top four activities presented in class (Pate et al., 1995). Another way to assess the quality of physical education classes is to identify the time that students are actively

---

Principal Findings

This issue devoted to review of literature relating to physical activity and adolescence and consensus statement on guidelines for adolescent activity. Includes two recommendations: (1) all adolescents should be physically active daily or nearly every day as part of play, games, sports and transportation, recreation, physical education, or planned exercise in context of family, school and community activities; (2) adolescents should engage in three or more sessions per week of activities that last 20 minutes or more at a time and that require moderate to vigorous levels of exertion.

As fitness levels increase, positive changes in risk factors (HDL, triglycerides, body composition, blood pressure) also occur.

There appear to be some benefits of physical activity and improved physical fitness for children with certain specific chronic diseases, but insufficient data and uncontrolled studies limit conclusive results.

Results of this study indicate decline in some fitness measures for school-age youth.

Children receive more of their physical education time from a specialist, are more likely to attend schools that conduct fitness tests, are less likely to take physical education outdoors, and spend less time at recess. School factors tend to be unrelated to body composition. Other factors related to student fitness include the child's activity level, as rated by the teacher, television watching time, receipt of physical activity through community organizations, and parental exercise habits.

---

engaged in moderate to heavy physical activity. Parcel et al. (1987) and Faucette et al. (1990) observed and coded activity levels during physical education sessions in elementary classes. The average child was vigorously active for only two minutes (Parcel et al., 1987). Children were usually engaged in game play that required only a few to be active while the majority awaited their turn (Faucette et al., 1990). Recently, however, the Child and Adolescent Trial for Cardiovascular Health (CATCH) has shown that it is possible to increase significantly the intensity of physical activity in physical education classes; in CATCH intervention schools, students spent 40 percent of class time in moderate to vigorous physical activity (Luepker et al., 1996).

Scheduling and environmental factors may make physical education less appealing for students. For example, students may not look forward to physical education class early in the day, especially in hot humid weather, if there is no opportunity to shower and change their clothes. The status of physical education in the curriculum may also be ques-

TABLE 3-1B   Studies Supporting the Contribution of Physical Activity to Academic Achievement

Study

Kirkendall, D.R. 1986. Effects of physical activity on intellectual development and academic performance. Pp. 49–63, in: Effects of Physical Activity on Children (The American Academy of Physical Education Papers, No. 19), G.A. Stull and H.M. Eckert eds. Champaign, Illinois: Human Kinetics.

Shepard, R.J., Volel, M., Lavallee, H., LaBarre, R., Jequier, J.C., and Rajic, M. 1984. Required physical activity and academic grades: A controlled study. Pp. 58–63 in J. Ilmarinen and I. Vaelimaeki eds., Children and sport: Paediatric work physiology. Berlin, Germany: Springer-Verlag.

Moore, J.B., Guy, L.M., and Reeve, T.G. 1984. Effects of the capon perceptual-motor program on motor ability, self-concept, and academic readiness. Perceptual and Motor Skills 58:71–74.

Thomas, J.R., Chissom, B.S., Steward, C., and Shelly, F. 1975. Effects of perceptual motor training on preschool children: A multivariate approach. *RQES* 46:505–513.

Lipton, E.D. 1970. A perceptual-motor development program's effect on visual perception and reading readiness of first grade children. *RQES* 41:402–405.

Kuntzleman, C.T., and Reiff, G. 1992. American Children's Fitness Levels. *RQES* 63:107–111.

Rowland, T.W. 1990. *Exercise and Children's Health*. Champaign, IL: Human Kinetics: Chapter 8.

American Academy of Pediatrics. 1987. Physical Fitness and the Schools. Pediatrics 80(3).

McKenzie, T.L., Faucette, F.N., Sallis, J.F., Roby, J.J. and Kilody, B. 1993. Effects of curriculum and inservice program on the quantity and quality of elementary physical education classes. *RQES* 64:178–187.

tioned because physical education is not mentioned in the National Education Goals as one of the core subjects in which students should demonstrate competence (although one of the expanded objectives of Goal 3 states that "all students will have access to physical education and health education to ensure they are healthy and fit") (National Education Goals Panel, 1994). Thus, in this era of increased emphasis on academic rigor and standards, students, parents, and other educators may perceive that

Principal Findings

This article reviews literature relating to cognitive development and physical activity. Indicates that while not conclusive, consistent and positive correlations are found between physical activity and academic achievement.

The Trois Riveres study in Canada demonstrated significant gains in academic performance during a six-year elementary program as a result of increased time for physical education and concomitant 13% decrease in time for academic instruction.

The results of this study supported increase in self-concept and reading readiness based on participation in perceptual-motor program.

A perceptual motor training program appeared to facilitate limited, positive short term gains in academic ability.

Physical education programs that focused on directionality of movement increased reading readiness in selected full class groups.

Fitness levels of children are not increasing. Many children do not have fitness levels high enough to sustain good health.

Suggests positive benefits of physical activity to various psychological factors which may influence success in academic settings (these include depression, anxiety, self-esteem). There is no evidence to suggest that physical activity reduces academic achievement.

This is a position statement advocating daily physical education and physical activity in the schools.

Targeted health-related objectives and teacher training increased student activity and lesson quality for 4th grade students when compared to control classes. Classes taught by specialist physical educators further improved lesson quality.

physical education is less important than other "academic" subjects. The committee does not wish to engage in a debate over such artificial issues as whether physical education is an "academic" subject or its relative importance compared to other subjects. The point is that physical education and physical activity are very important to students' current and future health, and a choice should not have to be made between physical education and other "academic" subjects. Room should be made in the

TABLE 3-1C   Articles Defining the Role of Physical Education in
Public Health

Article
Sallis, J.F., and McKenzie, T.L. 1991. Physical education's role in public health. *RQES* 62:124–137, June.
McGinnis, J.M., Kanner, L., and DeGraw, C. 1991. Physical education's role in achieving national health objectives. *RQESs* 62:138–142, June.
Nelson, M.A. 1991. The role of physical education children's activity in the public health. *RQESs* 62:148–150, June.
Haywood, K.M. 1991. The role of physical education in the development of active lifestyles. *RQES* 62:1515–1516, June.
Pate, R.R., Corbin, C.B., Simons-Morton, B.G., and Ross, J.G. 1987. Physical education and its role in school health promotion. *Journal of School Health* 57(10).
Simons-Morton, B.G., O'Hara, D.G., Simons-Morton, D.G., and Parcel, G.S. 1987. Children and fitness: A public health perspective. *RQES* 58:295–303.

NOTE: CDC = Centers for Disease Control and Prevention.
             EDC = Education Development Center.
             RQES = Research Quarterly on Exercise and Sport.

schedule for physical education and physical activity, and additional
opportunities for physical activity outside the regular school schedule
should be provided and encouraged.

Personnel Providing Physical Education

The SHPPS study (Pate et al., 1995) found that one-half of all physical
education classroom teachers at the middle and secondary levels majored
in physical education. Approximately another 25 percent majored in
health and physical education, which means that one-fourth of the classroom teachers of physical education do not have the specialized training
necessary to be quality physical educators. This gap in training is verified
by the fact that 25 percent of physical education teachers were not certi-

---

Purpose/Scope/Content

This article identifies physical education as an important vehicle to support increased physical activity to support positive health. Physical education should have objective of increasing life-long physical activity. Authors advocate strong public health focus for school physical education and shift from sport focus.

This article addresses the physical activity and fitness goals of HP2000 and the role of physical education programs in attaining the objectives.

The article urges additional research about amount and intensity of exercise needed to support health of children and cooperation of medical and physical education community to increase health-related benefits of physical education classes.

This reviews the developmental perspective in relation to a health-related physical education program. Suggests alternative perspective to Sallis and McKenzie for increasing health-related activity in the comprehensive physical education program.

In this article, the authors promote the concept of health-oriented physical education, discuss professional standards, examine the current status of physical education programs, and discuss trends affecting physical education. Recommendations to make physical education more effective are provided.

Documents level of physical activity in selected physical education classes as less than moderately vigorous and urges that structured physical activity and physical education programs be enjoyable and moderately vigorous.

SOURCE: Adapted from information provided by the National Association for Sport and Physical Education, Reston, Virginia.

fied by the state agency in either physical education or health and physical education. SHPPS did not examine the certification status of elementary physical education teachers, but it is likely no better than that of middle and secondary teachers. The physical education profession has taken the position that elementary physical education should be taught by teachers certified in physical education (National Association for Sport and Physical Education, 1994). A rationale for this position is that inappropriate or improperly taught physical education for young children could possibly cause harm and lead to permanent injury. The actual qualifications of those who teach elementary physical education no doubt vary considerably from state to state, for each state has its own laws and certification standards.

SHPPS reported that during the past two years, six in ten classroom

TABLE 3-2 Requirements for Physical Education Classes—by Number of Years for Middle and Secondary Schools

	Districts Requiring Physical Education (%)	
Number of Years	Middle School (92%)	Secondary School (93%)
Less than 1 year	5	9
1 year	20	37
2 years	24	25
3 years	47	26
Other not determined	5	4

SOURCE: Pate et al., 1995.

physical education teachers attended staff development programs. The most common topic was "teaching sports or activities" (Table 3-5). When asked which topics they would like as staff development programs, the teachers identified developing individualized fitness programs (45 percent), increasing student's physical activity in physical education class (41 percent), increasing students' physical activity outside physical education class (35 percent), and involving families in physical activity (32 percent). Only 27 percent identified teaching sports or activities as a desired staff development program. The desire for less training on teaching sports and more training on teaching fitness and promoting physical activity within and without the classroom may indicate a recognition by the teaching staff of changing priorities and a desire to use physical education as a public health strategy (Pate et al., 1995).

Most (95 percent) junior and senior high schools employed a variety of strategies to promote physical activity at school. Approximately three-fourths of the schools provided intramural and interscholastic sports and 30 percent implemented fitness activities such as Jump Rope for Heart (Pate et al., 1995). Many (77 percent) physical education classroom teachers conducted fitness testing that included tests of abdominal strength (98 percent), upper body strength (97 percent), flexibility (85 percent), and body composition or lean body mass (49 percent).

Findings Regarding Physical Education

Physical education's unique contribution to students—and to

TABLE 3-3   Percentage of All Required Physical Education Courses, by Days per Week and Minutes per Class Period[a]

Number of Days per Week	Less Than 30 Minutes	30–45 Minutes	46–60 Minutes	61–90 Minutes	More Than 90 Minutes
1 or 2	0.0	49.5	30.4	18.2	1.9
2 days one week and 3 days the next week	0.0	54.7	34.3	8.1	3.0
3 or 4	0.0	53.0	40.4	5.6	1.0
5	0.6	30.2	66.4	2.5	0.3

[a]School Health Policies and Programs Study, 1994.

SOURCE: Pate et al., 1995.

TABLE 3-4   Percentage of all Physical Education Courses in Which More Than One Class Period Was Devoted to Each Activity—by Activity[a]

Activity	All Courses (%)
Basketball	86.8
Volleyball	82.3
Baseball/softball	81.5
Flag/touch football	68.5
Soccer	65.2
Jogging	46.5
Weightlifting or training	37.3
Tennis	30.3
Aerobic dance	29.6
Walking quickly	14.7
Swimming	13.6
Handball	13.2
Racquetball	4.9
Hiking/backpacking	3.0
Bicycling	1.3

[a]School Health Policies and Programs Study, 1994.

SOURCE: Pate et al., 1995.

TABLE 3-5 Percentage of Lead Physical Education Teachers and Physical Education Classroom Teachers Who Received Training During the Past Two Years or Wanted In-Service Training—by Topic[a]

Topic	Lead Physical Education Teachers (%)		Physical Education Classroom Teachers (%)	
	Who Received Training	Who Wanted Training	Who Received Training	Who Wanted Training
Developing individualized fitness programs	26.7	41.1	21.5	44.5
Fitness testing—administration and use	21.1	26.9	16.9	20.9
Increasing students' physical activity in physical education class	25.0	37.6	27.6	41.1
Increasing students' physical outside physical education class	15.4	33.4	12.6	34.7
Involving families in physical activity	9.7	35.3	5.9	32.1
Staff wellness	29.3	23.9	25.6	21.1
Teaching sports or activities	46.3	21.2	41.6	26.6

[a]School Health Policies and Programs Study, 1994.

SOURCE: Pate et al., 1995.

CSHPs—is to impart the knowledge, skills, and values necessary to be physically competent in many situations over the course of a lifetime. The skills and attitudes acquired in a quality physical education program reinforce the messages promoted in other parts of a CSHP—the importance of physical fitness, self-discipline, good nutrition, respect for self and others, avoiding health-threatening behavior, and adopting health-promoting behavior.

The committee believes that the recommendations found in the National Standards for Physical Education (National Association for Sport and Physical Education, 1995) **provide a sound framework to ensure that these goals are attained. In addition, the committee supports the following recommendations for physical education developed through the SHPPS analysis** (Pate et al., 1995):

1. Provide more emphasis on lifetime physical activities.
2. Increase inservice training opportunities for physical education staff.
3. Promote collaboration between physical education staff and staff from other CSHP program components.
4. Increase the number of schools that require daily physical education.
5. Increase the number of schools requiring physical education in each grade.

Finally, the committee believes that physical activity must not be limited to a formal class in the curriculum; physical activity must be a family and community priority and extend beyond the school walls and the school day. Thus, **the committee welcomes the following recommendations from the CDC Guidelines for School and Community Health Programs to Promote Physical Activity Among Youth (CDC, 1997), which emphasize the following ideas:**

1. **Policy:** Implement policies to promote enjoyable, lifelong physical activity through physical activity instruction and physical and social environments that encourage physically active life-styles. [The guidelines include such wide-ranging policies as providing physical activity instruction and programs that meet the needs and interests of all students, regardless of gender, culture, physical competence, physical disability, cognitive disability, and chronic health conditions; employing properly prepared physical education teachers, coaches, and physical activity program directors, and preparing volunteer coaches to have appropriate qualifications for sports and recreation programs; establishing discipline policies that do not include the use of physical activity as a

form of punishment; and promoting effective relationships between school and community recreation and sports programs.]

2. **Curriculum:** Implement coordinated physical activity curricula through pre-K to grade 12 school physical education programs and health education programs that are consistent with national education standards.

3. **Physical Education Instruction:** Implement school physical education programs that emphasize enjoyable participation in physical activity and promote the acquisition of the knowledge, attitudes, behavioral skills, and participation competencies needed for adoption of physically active life-styles.

4. **Health Education Instruction:** Implement school health education programs that provide students with knowledge, attitudes, and behavioral skills needed for adoption of physically active life-styles.

5. **School-Based Programs and Facilities:** Provide extracurricular physical activity programs that meet the needs and interests of all students, and assure access to spaces and facilities that promote safe, enjoyable physical activity. [The guidelines state that these extracurricular activities should include noncompetitive activities that meet the needs and interests of the largest possible percentage of students and that community resources should be used to deliver school-based physical activity programs, school facilities should be made available for community-based physical activity programs, and students should actively be connected to community-based physical activity programs.]

6. **Community-Based Programs and Facilities:** Provide developmentally appropriate recreation and youth sport programs that are attractive to all youth, and assure easy public access to spaces and facilities that promote safe, enjoyable physical activity.

7. **Parental Involvement:** Parents and other guardians should be involved in physical activity instruction and physical activity programs, and should ensure that their children regularly participate in physical activities in which they experience enjoyment and success. [The guidelines stress that parents should serve as role models for physical activity and plan family activities that include physical activity.]

8. **School and Community Health Services:** Physicians, school nurses, and others who provide health services to children and youth should assess physical activity habits and promote physical activity participation in their patients.

9. **Training:** Provide education, recreation, and health care professionals and volunteer coaches with training programs that emphasize the development of the knowledge and skills they need to effectively promote enjoyable, lifelong physical activity among youth.

10. **Evaluation:** Evaluate school physical education programs, health education programs, and school and community physical activity programs and facilities at regular intervals.

THE ROLE OF HEALTH EDUCATION IN COMPREHENSIVE SCHOOL HEALTH PROGRAMS

Introduction

No knowledge is more crucial than knowledge about health. Without it, no other life goal can be successfully achieved. (Boyer, 1983)

This concept is the driving force for the development and implementation of sound school health education programs throughout the United States. School health education is an integral component of a comprehensive school health program and is defined as "the development, delivery, and evaluation of a planned instructional program and other activities for students preschool through grade 12, for parents and for school staff, and is designed to positively influence the health knowledge, attitudes, and skills of individuals" (Joint Committee on Health Education Terminology, 1991). In 1990, the Centers for Disease Control and Prevention prepared an interim operational definition of health education that identified its instructional elements as the following (Collins et al., 1995):

1. A documented, planned, and sequential program of health education for students in grades K through 12.

2. A curriculum that addresses and integrates education about a range of categorical health problems and issues.

3. Activities to help young people develop the skills they will need to avoid behaviors that result in unintentional and intentional injuries; alcohol and other drug use; tobacco use; sexual behaviors that result in human immunodeficiency virus (HIV) infection, other sexually transmitted diseases (STDs), and unintended pregnancies; imprudent dietary patterns; and inadequate physical activity.

4. Instruction provided for a prescribed amount of time at each grade level.

5. Management and coordination in each school by an education professional trained to implement the program.

6. Instruction from teachers who have been trained to teach the subject.

7. Involvement of parents, health professionals, and other concerned community members.

8. Periodic evaluation, updating, and improvement.

The value of health education in promoting the health of young people and contributing to the overall public health mission is articulated in *Healthy People 2000*, which identified nine national health education objectives to be attained by the year 2000 (U.S. Department of Health and Human Services, 1991). Eight of the nine objectives refer to specific topics to be covered in the health education curriculum. The remaining objective

(8.4) is an overarching objective that calls for increasing to at least 75 percent the proportion of the nation's elementary and secondary schools that provide planned and sequential health instruction from kindergarten through grade 12. The other eight objectives are as follows:

> 2.19   Increase to at least 75 percent the proportion of the nation's schools that provide nutrition education from preschool through grade 12, preferably as part of quality school health education.
>
> 3.10   Establish tobacco-free environments and include tobacco use prevention in the curricula of all elementary, middle, and secondary schools, preferably as part of quality school health education.
>
> 4.13   Provide to children in all school districts and private schools primary and secondary school education programs on alcohol and other drugs, preferably as part of quality school health education.
>
> 5.8   Increase to at least 85 percent the proportion of people aged 10 through 18 who have discussed human sexuality, including values surrounding sexuality, with their parents and/or have received information through another parentally endorsed source, such as youth, school, or religious programs.
>
> 7.16   Increase to at least 50 percent the proportion of elementary and secondary schools that teach nonviolent conflict resolution skills, preferably as a part of quality school health education.
>
> 9.18   Provide academic instruction on injury prevention and control, preferably as part of quality school health education, in at least 50 percent of public school systems (grades K through 12).
>
> 18.10   Increase to at least 95 percent the proportion of schools that have age-appropriate HIV education curricula for students in grades 4 through 12, preferably as part of quality school health education.
>
> 19.12   Include instruction in sexually transmitted disease transmission prevention in the curricula of all middle and secondary schools, preferably as part of quality school health education.

Instructional Focus

Although formal health education programs were often present in schools prior to the 1960s, it was not until the School Health Education Study (SHES), conducted from 1964 to 1972, that the concept of a "comprehensive" health education instructional program was defined and put into action (Sliepcevich, 1964). The SHES initiative developed 10 conceptual areas that represented the broad spectrum of learning necessary to develop and preserve individual, family, and community health. The 10 conceptual areas were adopted readily by both health educators and general educators, and the SHES outcomes became the basis of nearly all health education curricula and legislation in the United States during the

1970s and 1980s. Often, the 10 conceptual areas were translated into 10 content areas when discussed in legislation and curriculum frameworks at the state and local education agency levels. These 10 areas became known as the "traditional" 10 content areas of health education. Although there is some variation from state to state, the major content areas usually include (Joint Committee on Health Education Terminology, 1991) community health, consumer health, environmental health, family life, mental and emotional health, injury prevention and safety, nutrition, personal health, prevention and control of disease, and substance use and abuse.

Recently, CDC has identified six factors that are the major contributors to morbidity and mortality among school-aged children and adolescents (Kann et al., 1995). The CDC recommends that these be the priority areas for health education instruction: sexual behaviors that result in HIV infection, other STDs, and unintended pregnancy; alcohol and other drug use; behaviors that result in unintentional and intentional injuries; tobacco use; dietary patterns that result in disease; and sedentary life-style.

Desired Practice in Health Education

National Standards for Health Education

As is the case with physical education, the status of health education in the curriculum is sometimes questioned by school policy makers because health was not originally mentioned in the National Education Goals as one of the core subjects in which students should demonstrate competence. However, with each updated report of the National Education Goals Panel, language has been added emphasizing the importance of health education and other essential components of a CSHP (National Education Goals Panel, 1994). In particular, two of the objectives under Goal 3, Student Achievement and Citizenship, are (1) all students will be involved in activities that promote and demonstrate good citizenship, good health, community service, and personal responsibility; and (2) all students will have access to physical education and health education to ensure that they are healthy and fit. In addition, the National Education Goals call for students to start school with the healthy minds, bodies, and mental alertness necessary for learning; safe, disciplined, and healthful environments that are free of alcohol, drugs, crime, and violence; the development of a comprehensive K–12 drug and alcohol prevention education program in every school district; a drug and alcohol curriculum, which should be taught as an integral part of sequential, comprehensive health education; and increased parental partnerships with schools in order to promote the social, emotional, and academic growth of children.

In the spring of 1995, the Joint Committee on National Health Education Standards released the *National Health Education Standards*, which are designed to help students achieve the National Education Goals and the national health goals set forth in *Healthy People 2000: National Health Promotion and Disease Prevention Objectives*. The overarching goal of the *National Health Education Standards* is the development of health literacy. Health literacy is "the capacity of individuals to obtain, interpret, and understand basic health information and services and the competence to use such information and services in ways which enhance health" (Joint Committee on National Health Education Standards, 1995). Four characteristics were identified as being essential to health literacy. The health-literate person is (1) a critical thinker; (2) a responsible, productive citizen; (3) a self-directed learner; and (4) an effective communicator.

The document presents seven standards and a series of performance indicators that are recommended to be assessed at grades 4, 8, and 11. Once curricula have been redesigned to attain the performance indicators for each standards, it is anticipated that students will be able to do the following (Joint Committee on National Health Education Standards, 1995):

1. Comprehend concepts related to health promotion and disease prevention.

2. Demonstrate the ability to access valid health information and health promoting products and services.

3. Demonstrate the ability to practice health-enhancing behaviors and reduce health risks.

4. Analyze the influence of culture, media, technology, and other factors on health.

5. Demonstrate the ability to use interpersonal communication skills to enhance health.

6. Demonstrate the ability to use goal setting and decision-making skills to enhance health.

7. Demonstrate the ability to advocate for personal, family, and community health.

Since the National Health Education Standards have recently been released at the time of writing this report, only a few curricula have been redesigned or developed based on the standards. Such redesign is one of the intended outcomes of the standards development and the concurrent health education assessment initiative. Probably the outcome that has been most often assessed in the past is the ability of a curriculum to increase knowledge about concepts related to health promotion and disease prevention. However, the new health education standards focus on the development of skills to enhance healthy choices, not just the acquisition of knowledge. Of increasing importance is the ability of a health education curriculum to achieve the standard to "demonstrate the ability to practice health-enhancing behaviors and reduce health risks." Although behavior change as an outcome for health education can be found in textbooks written at midcentury as one of the three desirable outcomes in health education (changes in knowledge, attitudes, and behavior), not until 1979 when the Surgeon General's report *Healthy People* (U.S. Department of Health and Human Services, 1979) revealed that 50 percent of premature death and illness was caused by life-style choices, did a focus on behavior become prepotent. Health educators and public health officials began to shift their emphasis to behavioral outcomes, once it was established that knowledge alone does not change behavior.[2]

Effective Curricula

Desired practice in health education requires that effective curricula be selected and implemented by well-prepared teachers. There have been a number of studies demonstrating the effectiveness of health education curricula that target a single specific behavior (Glynn, 1989; Stone et al., 1989), as well as studies of programs that use a comprehensive health education curriculum to prevent or reduce certain debilitating behaviors such as tobacco, alcohol, and drug use; imprudent dietary behaviors; physical inactivity; and inappropriate sexual behaviors (Botvin and Eng, 1982; Connell et al., 1985; Ross et al., 1989; Williams et al., 1983). Table 3-6 identifies some illustrative studies of the outcomes of various health education curricula. Two large-scale evaluations have found that (1) students' knowledge of health behaviors increases after instruction; (2) students' behaviors, especially those related to substance abuse, become more health enhancing; (3) "booster sessions" are required up to two or three years after the initial program to maintain the desired effect; (4) greater changes in behavior occur after 50 hours of instruction; and (5) teachers who received training implement the curriculum with more fidelity and achieve more positive effects than teachers who do not receive training (Connell et al., 1985; Ross et al., 1991).

Two systems are currently in place for curriculum developers to disseminate exemplary evaluated curricula. One method is to apply to the U.S. Department of Education National Diffusion Network. If the developer can demonstrate strong evaluation data that establish the impact of the curriculum, it may be "accepted" into the National Diffusion Network and dissemination funding can be obtained. Another means is to submit detailed evaluation results to the Division of Adolescent and School

---

[2]Chapter 6 further examines the issue of behavior change as a feasible and realistic outcome of health education.

TABLE 3-6   Illustrative Prevention Programs in Health Education

Name	Targeted Population Group or Sample Size When Project Began	Grade Levels
Growing Healthy	N = 30,000	4–7
Know Your Body	N = 2,283; 1,105	K–6
Teenage Health Teaching Modules	Unknown	7–12
Go for Health	Unknown	3–4
Cardiovascular Heart Healthy Eating and Exercise	Unknown	4–5
Hearty Heart	Unknown	3

Risk Factors Addressed	Outcomes for Total Intervention	References
Unhealthy behaviors	Increased health knowledge, attitudes, and behaviors; reduction in smoking; improved reading scores; positive changes in health practices among parents	Connell et al., 1985; Owen et al., 1985
Substance abuse, nutrition, safety, physical activity, dental health, environmental health	Lower cigarette smoking onset, reduced saturated fat consumption, increased carbohydrate consumption; reduction in total cholesterol and blood pressure	Bush et al., 1989a, 1989b; Walter, 1989; Walter and Wynder, 1989; Walter et al., 1989; Resnicow et al., 1989; Taggart et al., 1990; Resnicow et al., 1991; Resnicow et al., 1992; Resnicow et al., 1993a, b
Substance abuse, nutrition, safety	Increases in health knowledge; health attitudes were unchanged among THTM schools but deteriorated among control schools; increased abstinence from cigarette and smokeless tobacco use, illegal drugs and alcoholic drinks in past 30 days	Nelson et al., 1991; Ross et al., 1991; Errecart et al., 1991; Gold et al., 1991
Cardiovascular risk factors	Moderate to vigorous physical activity increased, self-reported salt use declined, selections of fresh fruits and vegetables increased significantly	Parcel et al., 1989; Simons-Morton et al., 1991
Decrease consumption of saturated fats, cholesterol, sodium, and sugar; increase consumption of complex carbohydrates; increase physical activity	38% increase in heart healthy foods found in student lunches, observed changes in physical activity minimal	Coates et al., 1981
Lack of nutrition knowledge, poor eating habits by students and parents	Reduction in total fat, Reduction in total fat, monosaturated fat; increased intake of complex carbohydrates; parents had more healthy foods on shelves.	Crockett et al., 1989; Perry et al., 1989

TABLE 3-6 Continued

Name	Targeted Population Group or Sample Size When Project Began	Grade Levels
Pawtucket Heart Health Progam	N = 105	7–12
Stanford Adolescent Heart Health Program	N = 1,447	9–10
Nutrition in a Changing World	N = 880	3–5
Nutrition for Life	N = 1,863	7–8
Postponing Sexual Involvement	Unknown	8
Peer Power and ADAM	Unknown	6–8
Reducing the Risk	N = 586	10
San Francisco AIDS Prevention Education Curricula	N = 639	6–12

NOTE: Programs described in this table represent only a sample of school health programs that have been evaluated. No attempt has been made by the IOM Committee on Comprehensive School Health Programs in Grades K-12 to determine the quality and validity of the methods of evaluation or the findings of these programs. The findings presented are based

Risk Factors Addressed	Outcomes for Total Intervention	References
Cardiovascular disease	Reduced blood cholesterol.	Gans et al., 1990
Cardiovascular disease, smoking, physical activity, nutrition, stress	Increased knowledge, increased physical activity, better resting heart rates, enhanced body mass index and triceps skin fold thickness, increased nutritional choices	Killen et al., 1988; 1989
Nutrition	Increased nutrition knowledge, improvement in eating behaviors	Shannon and Chen, 1988
Nutrition	Improvements in nutrition knowledge behavior and attitude scores	Devine et al., 1992
Premature sexual activity and pregnancy, STDs		Howard and McCabe, 1990
Premature sexual activity, school dropout	Rates of sexual abstinence doubled, improved school attendance, reading and math ability more likely to remain at or above grade level than for controls	Ounce of Prevention Fund, 1990
Sexual behavior	Delays in sexual involvement, increase in knowledge, increase in discussion of abstinence with parents	Kirby et al., 1991
Sexual knowledge	Increased knowledge about AIDS transmission, increased acceptance of persons who have AIDS	DiClemente et al., 1989

on other publications or reports. Inclusion of these program descriptions and evaluations in this report does not imply endorsement by the committee or the U.S. Public Health Service, Department of Health and Human Services, who provided the publication from which this information was compiled.

SOURCE: Adapted from U.S. DHHS, 1993.

Health (DASH) at CDC for inclusion in the "Programs That Work" project. Through these mechanisms, state and local school agencies can identify health education curricula they may wish to adopt and/or adapt for their needs.

Assessment

Special attention tends to be given to those school subjects that are tested in major local, state, and national assessments. Teachers and schools are pressured to increase student performance in reading, mathematics, or whatever other subject needs improving, and considerable class time and teacher preparation is often devoted to the effort. Unfortunately, health education is not typically tested in major assessment programs, and the lack of this driving force may contribute to indifference about health education on the part of school administrators, teachers, parents, and students.

The situation may be changing, however, as a result of collaborative efforts between the Council of Chief State School Officers (CCSSO) and participating states (Council of Chief State School Officers, 1994). The CCSSO began the State Collaborative on Assessment and Student Standards (SCASS) project in 1991 to identify and develop assessment measures in the area of science. In 1992, SCASS was extended to the field of health education, and many states have joined the effort. The project is using the new National Health Education Standards and emerging state frameworks to develop materials, resources, and strategies for meaningful assessment of what students should know and be able to do as a result of state-of-the-art health education. The project will develop assessment strategies for both classroom and large-scale assessment. The vision of many health educators is that performance assessment of student health knowledge and skills will become an expectation in state and national testing programs, just as assessment in reading or mathematics is expected, resulting in increased implementation of health education at the local level as an integral part of the total instructional program.

Well-Prepared Health Education Teachers

The Association for the Advancement of Health Education (AAHE), in collaboration with the National Council for Accreditation of Teacher Education (NCATE), has developed standards for preservice preparation of health education teachers (American Alliance for Health, Physical Education, Recreation, and Dance, 1995). Unfortunately, less than one-half of middle and secondary health education teachers are state certified (Collins et al., 1995), and few elementary teachers have had any preservice preparation in health education teaching methodology. Even certified teachers may not have had the benefit of a preservice program that meets the AAHE-NCATE standards. Further, health education is undergoing important changes as curricula, pedagogy, and assessment are becoming aligned with the National Health Education Standards and as new research on effective approaches is published. Consequently, professional development programs (also called staff development or inservice programs) are crucial to enable current teachers to implement state-of-the-art health education. Teachers of health education must be given opportunities and should be expected to participate in ongoing, discipline-specific inservice programs in order to stay abreast of new developments in their field.

The literature on professional development confirms that even among enthusiastic teachers, successful implementation and maintenance of new curricula and teaching practices do not always follow successful initial training (Gingiss, 1992). Transfer of training—the critical link between learning in the staff development program and application in the work setting—depends on whether teachers are able and motivated to apply the skills and strategies learned in the program. Follow-up is critical to assist teachers as they confront the reality of working with colleagues who did not attend the staff development program. The more complex the required outcomes, the greater are the need for and benefits of follow-up programs (Gingiss et al., 1991). Follow-up should provide opportunities for teacher collaboration since peer coaching is an effective strategy for maintaining and improving effective practice (Bennett, 1987; Sparks, 1986). Computer network discussion groups can also provide support, especially for isolated health education teachers, and can serve as a forum for exchanging new ideas and approaches.

Although the above could be considered general issues in professional staff development regardless of the field, these issues are particularly important for health education teachers as they attempt to implement new curricula and assessment strategies. Like teachers in other disciplines, health education teachers are expected to impart knowledge; however, probably more so than in other disciplines, health education teachers are also expected to influence present and future behavior, in and out of school—a competence not easily acquired and put into practice.

Time

Studies have shown that a considerable number of hours of health education are required for behavior change to occur. In 1991, the National School Boards Association reported on research pertaining to the time necessary for effective health education. One study showed that 1.8 hours of health instruction per week over the school year produces measurable increases in student knowledge and improved attitudes about health, as well as some behavior change. Another study demonstrated that health knowledge begins to increase after 15 hours, particularly in grades 4 to 7; 45 to 50 hours were needed to begin to affect attitudes and practices, with maximal learning and attitude or behavior changes occurring after about 60 hours of instruction in a given year (National School Boards Association, 1991). The issue of required "dosage" to produce behavioral change is further examined in Chapter 6, which notes that while there may be uncertainties with regard to the specific number of hours of "clock time" needed, a brief exposure to individual health topics is not likely to be effective. More intensive exposure and follow-up "booster sessions" in subsequent years are often necessary to produce sustained effects.

Unfortunately, the time spent in health education falls far short of what is necessary. Typically, at the elementary level, health topics are woven into the general curriculum as time and teacher interest dictate; at each of the middle and secondary levels, often only a single semester of health education is required.

Current Practice in Health Education

As described earlier, in 1994 the CDC commissioned a nationwide survey, the SHPPS, that examined school health at the state, district, and school levels. This section reviews and analyzes some of the SHPPS findings about health education curricula and teachers (Collins et al., 1995) and offers some comparisons with the *Healthy People 2000* goals (U.S. Department of Health and Human Services, 1991).

Curriculum

SHPPS found that 90 percent of states and school districts required or mandated health education programs at some level. At the elementary level, only 10 percent of states require a separate course; at the middle or junior high level the number rises to 28 percent; and at the secondary level, 55 percent require a separate class for health education (Table 3-7). Among school districts, 19 percent require a separate health education course at the elementary level; 44 percent require a separate course at the middle school level; and 66 percent require a separate course at the secondary level. Typically at the secondary level, health education classes last only a semester (44 percent of all schools). However, approximately 20 percent of the schools require a year's course work at the secondary

TABLE 3-7 Percentage of All States and Districts Specifying How Health Education Must Be Offered—by Type of Delivery and Grade Level[a]

Type of Delivery	States Specifying at Each Level (%)			Districts Specifying at Each Level (%)		
	Elementary School	Middle–Junior High School	Senior High School	Elementary School	Middle–Junior High School	Senior High School
As a separate course devoted almost entirely to health topics	9.8	27.5	54.9	18.7	43.9	65.9
As a course split equally between health education and physical education	2.0	15.7	17.6	9.1	23.3	10.7
As lessons taught as part of the school curriculum	35.3	11.8	7.8	44.5	13.8	12.4
Not specified	66.7	47.1	17.6	15.6	19.5	1.4

[a]School Health Policies and Programs Study, 1994.

SOURCE: Collins et al., 1995.

level. An additional course beyond the semester is required by 13 percent of schools. Unfortunately, three-fourths of schools allow students to be exempted from all or part of required health education courses. Although 90 percent of schools require health education at some level, there is no state that requires health education at *every* grade level. The goal in *Healthy People 2000* states that 75 percent of the nation's elementary and secondary schools should provide planned, sequential health instruction in grades K–12. This goal remains elusive.

The three specific content areas that are required most often by the state educational agency are HIV-AIDS prevention education (79 percent), prevention of drug and alcohol abuse (75 percent), and tobacco use

TABLE 3-8 Percentage of States and Districts Requiring That Each Health Education Topic Be Taught and Percentage of All Schools Including Each Topic in a Required Course—by Topic[a]

Topic	States Requiring Topic (%)	Districts Requiring Topic (%)	Schools Including Topic (%)
Alcohol and other drug use prevention	75.0	86.0	90.4
Community health	54.8	73.5	58.9
Conflict resolution, violence prevention	38.5	61.0	48.0
Consumer health	55.8	70.6	56.6
Cardiopulmonary resuscitation	37.5	61.9	48.0
Death and dying	25.0	54.1	52.5
Dental and oral health	51.2	78.2	56.7
Dietary behaviors and nutrition	68.9	80.1	84.3
Disease prevention and control	68.9	81.3	84.5
Emotional and mental health	64.4	76.8	73.8
Environmental health	59.1	70.5	59.9
First aid	55.8	73.9	58.8
Growth and development	62.2	79.5	80.2
HIV prevention	78.7	83.0	85.6
Human sexuality	48.9	76.0	80.0
Injury prevention and safety	62.2	74.5	66.2
Personal health	63.0	81.2	79.0
Physical activity and fitness	65.2	81.9	77.6
Pregnancy prevention	43.9	72.1	69.3
Sexually transmitted disease prevention	65.1	80.9	84.1
Suicide prevention	37.8	66.7	58.1
Tobacco use prevention	71.7	83.2	85.6

[a]School Health Policies and Programs Study, 1994.

SOURCE: Collins et al., 1995.

prevention (72 percent). These are also the topics most often required at the district and school levels (Table 3-8). A variety of content areas are required through state legislation and/or school district codes. As a general rule, districts require more topics than do the state, although this requirement is not always fulfilled at the school level (Table 3-8). Two-thirds of the districts required that instruction be offered on 19 of the 22 topics listed on the SHPPS questionnaire (Table 3-8). At the school level, 86 percent required the topic of HIV prevention, close to the *Healthy People 2000* goal of 95 percent. Additionally, 84 percent of schools required instruction in STD prevention. Among school districts, 90 percent required alcohol and other drug prevention education, which approaches the *Healthy People 2000* goal of 100 percent; 86 percent of schools required tobacco use prevention, compared to the *Healthy People 2000* goal of 100 percent, and 80 percent of schools required course work on human sexuality, close to the *Healthy People 2000* goal of 85 percent. Injury prevention education was required by 60 percent of the schools, which actually exceeded the *Healthy People 2000* goal of 50 percent. Although these topics were required by the school's curricular document, teachers at the classroom level did not always comply and teach that which was required (Table 3-9).

The SHPPS study interviewed classroom health teachers at the middle or junior high and senior high school level to assess the actual practice of health education at the classroom level. Approximately one-half of the teachers (46.9 percent) taught a course that focused exclusively on health education. The remaining (53.1 percent) infused health education content into a course that focused primarily on another subject. Both types of health education teachers were asked to identify the topics that were addressed in their classes that focused on the priority health issues—unintentional and intentional injury, tobacco use, alcohol and other drug use, sexual behaviors, HIV infection and AIDS, dietary behaviors, and physical activity (Table 3-9). Those teachers who infused health education into other subjects covered numerous topics, but the teachers who taught a separate and distinct course provided much more health content to their students.

The SHPPS survey of the required course work at the state, district, and school levels reveals that at least on paper, schools have come very close to achieving some of the course work identified as essential by *Healthy People 2000* in certain areas (Table 3-8). A better assessment of actual progress, however, would be to review the amount of instruction on each topic by "infusion" teachers, since this approach was used by more than 50 percent of the schools. Table 3-9 lists the percentage of infused and classroom health teachers who spent more than one class period on particular health topics. One limitation to the data is that the

TABLE 3-9 Percentage of All Health Education Classroom Teachers and Infused Classroom Teachers Who Taught and Spent More Than One Class Period on Health Education Topics—by Topic[a]

	Health Education Classroom Teachers (%)		Infused Classroom Teachers (%)	
	Teaching Topic	Spending More Than One Class Period on Topic	Teaching Topic	Spending More Than One Class Period on Topic
Alcohol and other drug use prevention	79.3	77.5	62.8	50.9
Community health	37.4	32.0	28.0	17.5
Conflict resolution/ violence prevention	37.4	31.7	34.7	24.4
Consumer health	33.6	27.5	30.9	20.4
Cardiopulmonary resuscitation	36.8	31.8	14.8	7.3
Death and dying	28.6	19.1	29.3	17.9
Dental and oral health	49.0	31.4	33.1	14.8
Dietary behaviors and nutrition	66.8	64.2	54.0	46.0
Emotional and mental health	67.8	65.6	41.5	28.6
Environmental health	35.3	29.4	43.8	34.8
First aid	43.9	41.5	23.6	15.8
Growth and development	57.2	52.9	61.6	55.1
HIV prevention	83.6	44.7	71.5	24.1
Human sexuality	52.1	46.0	51.4	43.8
Injury prevention and safety	36.1	31.7	30.8	20.6
Personal health	47.7	44.1	41.9	33.6
Physical activity and fitness	44.4	41.4	31.6	21.9
Pregnancy prevention	38.9	30.9	33.8	19.6
Sexually transmitted disease prevention	54.2	47.6	41.5	26.9
Suicide prevention	38.0	28.9	16.1	6.8
Tobacco use prevention	58.9	52.9	44.8	28.4

[a]School Health Policies and Programs Study, 1994.

SOURCE: Collins et al., 1995.

SHPPS study did not assess the actual time that each topic received, only the number of classroom periods in which the topic was discussed.

Other goals outlined in *Healthy People 2000* were not close to being achieved, by either infused or regular health education teachers. In infused classrooms, 63 percent taught the topic of HIV prevention, which falls short of the *Healthy People 2000* goal of 95 percent, 63 percent taught alcohol and other drug prevention, far short of the *Healthy People 2000* goal of 100 percent. In infused classrooms, only 45 percent taught tobacco use prevention, compared to the *Healthy People 2000* goal of 100 percent, 51 percent taught human sexuality compared to the *Healthy People 2000* goal of 85 percent, and 31 percent taught injury prevention compared to the *Healthy People 2000* goal of 50 percent. While 84 percent of schools reported including dietary behaviors and nutrition among health education topics, only 46 percent of infused classroom teachers reported spending more than one class period on the topic, in contrast to the *Healthy People 2000* goal that 75 percent of schools provide nutrition education from preschool through grade 12. In general, examination of the number of infusion teachers who spent more than one class period on important topics—which is critical for behavior change—shows that the gap between goals and infusion practice is considerable; even though they fell short of the *Healthy People 2000* goals, teachers assigned to a dedicated health education course provided significantly more instructional time on these priority areas than did the infused health teachers (Table 3-9).

Qualifications of Health Teachers

In many states, specific certification to teach health education is available, but separate certification is more common at the secondary (grades 6–12) level than at the elementary level. According to the SHPPS study (Collins et al., 1995), 67 percent of states required certification for secondary health teachers and only three states required certification for elementary health education teachers. Nationwide, only 5 percent of all health teachers and 1 percent of teachers who infuse health content into another subject majored in health education as part of their college preservice teacher training. An additional 28 percent of classroom teachers had a joint major in health and physical education, and another 14 percent had a minor in health education. Teachers who infused health education in their classroom most often majored in biology or another science field.

The infusion approach is an area of concern, particularly since it is the predominant mode of health instruction. While connecting health to other curricular areas can increase relevance for students, infusion courses are taught primarily by teachers not trained in health, and health messages may be buried among other topics. Further, these teachers are likely to teach only what they know about health education, and this knowledge may be superficial or even incorrect.

Although health education teachers may have had limited preservice preparation in the field, 48 percent of classroom health teachers had accumulated enough credits to be certified, although only 9 percent of the infused health teachers were certified in health or a combination of health and physical education. Despite the inadequacies in preparation, there is not an overwhelming demand for staff development (Table 3-10). Given that most teachers of health education did not major in this field during their college preservice experience, it might be concluded that the lack of interest results from a naivete of the potential and complexities of health education or possibly from the fact that current health teachers would rather teach other courses and can see no value in improving their skills in this area. Hamburg (1994) notes lack of teacher training as a significant obstacle to the implementation of quality health education programs. The results of the SHPPS study underscore this observation and reinforce the need for more inservice programming in the short run and the hiring of appropriately prepared professionals in health education in the long run.

Research on Effectiveness of Health Education

Health education approaches are based on various models of behavior change, some of which have proved more effective than others, and our understanding of this theoretical base is still evolving. Social learning theory, which addresses the behavior of social groups and the dynamic interaction of the individual within the larger social context, is emerging as a dominant theoretical framework for health education. An extensive discussion of social learning theory and other models of health behavior change is found in Appendix C.

Lessons Learned

Health education is a relatively young discipline, and its practice is only beginning to have a rich tradition upon which to build (Gold, 1994). Prior to 1970, there were no rigorous studies that examined the effectiveness of school health curricula (Cortese, 1993). Since 1970, there have been hundreds of effectiveness studies, many under well-controlled conditions.

Gold (1994) has reviewed the science base for health education and identified some of the major studies that document effectiveness; Table 3-11 provides a listing of some of these major studies. In writing a commissioned textbook article on school health education, Gold (1994) proposed the following lessons learned, gleaned from a review of the scientific literature on health education:

• Significant improvements in outcomes are achieved with attention to multiple-risk behaviors, rather than focusing on separate categorical behaviors.
• Although most health education programs and interventions are

based on several behavior theory constructs, it is not yet possible to identify which are most important.

• School health instruction based on skills training, peer involvement, social learning theory, and community involvement has the greatest impact.

• Environmental variables influence the prevalence and consequences of behavior choices.

• Social support affects all phases of behavior change.

• Significant benefits can come from the active and appropriate engagement of parents and families in prevention programs.

• It is important to focus on comprehensive efforts in schools, including teaching reform, cooperative learning strategies, policy issues, and interpersonal relationships.

• Appropriate attention must be paid to literacy and to social, cultural, gender, and ethnic diversity in program planning.

• Teacher training is required for effective educational programs.

• The characteristics of the individual influence the success of potential interventions.

• Relapse prevention efforts are necessary to sustain behavior changes.

The U.S. Department of Education's Comprehensive School Health Education Program commissioned three papers to identify the research base for school health education; the papers were published by the department and later by the *Journal of School Health* (Allensworth, 1994; DeGraw, 1994; English, 1994). An analysis of the common themes of these papers suggests that a new paradigm of school health education is emerging, which moves away from an exclusive focus on the traditional ten content areas that have been in place since the SHES initiative of the 1960s (Jackson, 1994). According to the analysis, school health education is moving as follows:

• from school-based to school-wide and community-wide programs (Allensworth, DeGraw),

• from an instructional focus on the traditional 10 content areas to a focus on needs-driven and health-enhancing behaviors and skills that influence life-style changes (Allensworth, DeGraw, English),

• from a focus on providing health information to a focus on changing health-related behavior in priority areas of vulnerability (Allensworth, DeGraw),

• from a health content instruction model in the classroom to a health

TABLE 3-10 Percentage of Lead Health Education Teachers, Health Education Classroom Teachers, and Infused Classroom Teachers Who Received Training During the Past Two Years or Wanted Training—by Topic[a]

Topic	Lead Health Education Teachers (%)		Health Education Classroom Teachers (%)		Infused Classroom Teachers (%)	
	Who Received Training	Who Wanted Training	Who Received Training	Who Wanted Training	Who Received Training	Who Wanted Training
Alcohol and other drug use prevention	33.4	23.2	29.6	23.0	17.0	25.0
Community health	6.8	5.7	4.1	6.7	3.1	7.3
Conflict resolution, violence prevention	18.0	25.1	13.3	21.3	14.5	24.6
Consumer health	4.4	7.2	2.9	6.6	0.9	6.4
Cardiopulmonary resuscitation	43.8	18.6	36.7	19.1	27.8	21.0
Death and dying	7.2	11.9	2.8	12.2	4.4	13.6
Dental and oral health	0.7	3.3	1.6	3.0	0.6	2.9

Dietary behaviors and nutrition	17.3	14.1	13.7	13.2	7.5
Disease prevention and control	12.8	7.0	10.3	7.0	10.4
Emotional and and mental health	15.9	22.1	10.2	21.3	24.8
Environmental health	7.1	9.9	4.9	12.3	13.7
First aid	30.5	12.5	24.5	14.2	16.5
Growth and development	7.3	5.7	5.5	6.2	9.9
HIV prevention	44.2	22.9	38.6	30.5	24.9
Human sexuality	19.3	14.4	17.0	15.6	16.6
Injury prevention and safety	12.1	5.6	9.2	5.0	7.9
Personal health	7.8	5.0	5.2	3.2	7.1
Physical activity and fitness	16.4	6.7	11.5	7.9	9.1
Pregnancy prevention	13.5	12.6	8.4	10.4	11.0
Sexually transmitted disease prevention	26.7	18.5	21.3	19.2	16.2
Suicide prevention	13.0	24.5	7.9	25.7	23.0
Tobacco use prevention	15.7	6.7	11.3	6.7	8.2

[a]School Health Policies and Programs, 1994.

SOURCE: Collins et al., 1995.

TABLE 3-11 Selected Summary of Pertinent Research Literature

Selected Lessons Learned	Citations
Significant improvements in outcomes are achieved with attention to multiple-risk behaviors	Dwyer et al., 1991; Johnson, 1992; Kottke et al., 1985; Lorion and Ross, 1992; Puska et al., 1981; Shane and Kaplan, 1988; Wynne, 1989
The reasons people make changes in health-related behaviors are varied and individualized	Davis et al., 1987; Iverson et al., 1989; Wynne, 1989
Although most health education programs and interventions are based on several behavior theory constructs, it is not yet possible to identify which are most important	Elders et al., 1993, Hansen and Graham, 1991; Lefebvre et al., 1987; McCaul and Glasgow, 1985; Pentz et al., 1989; Puska et al., 1988; Resnicow and Botvin, 1993; Resnicow et al., 1993c; Sussman et al., 1993
School health instruction based on skills training, peer involvement, social learning theory, and community involvement has the greatest impact	Botvin and Eng, 1982; Flay, 1985; Glider et al., 1992; Hansen et al., 1988; Johnson et al., 1986; Johnson, 1992; Murray et al., 1987; Schinke et al., 1985; Thomas et al., 1992
Self-monitoring may enhance behavior change efforts	Bertera and Cuthie, 1984; King et al., 1988; Koegel et al., 1986
Environmental variables influence the prevalence and consequences of behavior choices	Decker et al., 1988; Hoadley et al., 1984; Marburger and Friedel, 1987; Mayer et al., 1986; Pentz et al., 1989; Seekins et al., 1988; Simons-Morton et al., 1991; Taggart et al., 1990; Wagner and Winnett, 1988
Relapse prevention efforts are necessary to sustain behavior changes; however, little is known about factors influencing relapse for specific behaviors	Vaillant, 1988
Social support affects all phases of behavior change	Lewis et al., 1990; Broadhead et al., 1989; Morisky et al., 1985
The characteristics of the individual influence the success of potential interventions	Holloway et al., 1988; Jarvik and Schneider, 1984; Klesges et al., 1988
Significant benefits can come from the active and appropriate engagement of parents and families in prevention programs	Bruce and Emshoff, 1992; DeMarsh and Kumpfer, 1986; Freedman, 1988; Johnson, 1992; Kumpfer, 1987; Perry et al., 1989; Resnicow et al., 1993c; Ruch-Ross, 1992; Springer et al., 1992

TABLE 3-11   Continued

Selected Lessons Learned	Citations
After-school programs have substantial potential to contribute to the health of youth	Ross et al., 1991
It is important to focus on comprehensive efforts in schools, including teaching reform, cooperative learning strategies, policy issues, and interpersonal relationships	Collins, 1991; Hawkins et al., 1986; Johnson, 1992; Knight, 1991; Lewis et al., 1990; Nader, 1990; Pentz et al., 1989; Simons-Morton et al., 1991
Appropriate attention must be paid to literacy, and to social cultural, gender, and ethnic diversity in program planning	*Advertising Age*, 1990; Conner and Conner, 1992; Hall and Reyes, 1992; Ireland, 1990; Isikoff, 1989; Jones et al., 1992; Marin and Marin, 1991; Oyemade and Brandon-Monye, 1990; Rana et al., 1992; Shane and Kaplan, 1988; Smith, 1992; Terry et al., 1992
Teacher training is required for effective educational programs	Gingiss, 1992; Koenig, 1992; McKenzie et al., 1993; Perry et al., 1990; Rohrbach et al., 1993; Ross et al., 1991; Taggart et al., 1990; Tortu and Botvin, 1989
Early detection and prevention of risk are necessary	Starfield, 1989
The potential exists for creative school–community linkages	Kelder et al., 1993; Murray et al., 1987; Pentz et al., 1989; Perry et al., 1992; Shane and Kaplan, 1988

SOURCE: Adapted from Gold, 1994.

promotion model that involves a variety of strategies by an interdisciplinary team (Allensworth, DeGraw, English),

• from a school health program that ignores media and its influence to a health promotion program that designs strategies to negate directly the negative messages of media and that develops media campaigns to promote positive health-enhancing messages (Allensworth),

• from a school health classroom approach to an interdisciplinary—interagency team approach within the community (Allensworth, DeGraw, English),

• from an approach based on curriculum and program decisions derived from professional and personal preferences to curricula and program decisions based on sound education theory, research-mediated standards for student outcomes, effective health education programs, and behavioral change theories and knowledge (Allensworth, DeGraw, English), and

• from a focus on teaching skills in isolation through categorical areas to a focus on teaching generic skills identified as promoting adoption of health-enhancing behaviors. Generic personal and social skills that should be taught include refusal skills, problem-solving, decisionmaking, media analysis, assertiveness skills, communication, coping strategies for stress, and behavioral contracting (Allensworth, Degraw, English).

Cost-Effectiveness

Rigorous experimental studies have not been undertaken to establish the cost-effectiveness of school health education. However, Rothman and coworkers (1993) have developed mathematical models to predict what benefit-cost ratio might possibly be achieved from exemplary state-of-the-art health education programs dealing with smoking, other substance abuse, and sexual behavior leading to unplanned pregnancy and STDs, including HIV or AIDS. For their analysis, the authors examined studies of selected exemplary programs that had been reported in the literature to produce positive behavior change among adolescents. Criteria for program selection in this analysis included the following: outcomes were measured longitudinally (12 or more months of behavioral data); the program was classroom based and offered during school hours; results had been reported since 1982; and a control or comparison group was used. Program costs included such variables as instructor salary and benefits, teaching and training time, and curriculum materials. Program effectiveness included both the initial effectiveness rates and the decay effects found in the actual studies. Direct and indirect benefits involved estimates of avoided morbidity and mortality. Highlights of their calculations are described below.

Substance Abuse: Substance abuse in the Rothman et al. (1993) study refers primarily to alcohol abuse. Benefits were defined as averted costs associated with adolescent avoidance of substance abuse. Direct benefits were those associated with avoidance of hospitalizations for which the primary or secondary diagnoses were related to substance abuse, and indirect benefits included the avoidance of such events as motor vehicle injuries and crime-related loss of productivity and social expenditures. The benefit-to-cost ratio was 5.69 for substance abuse education.

Smoking: Benefits involved averted costs associated with the life-long treatment of smoking-related diseases. The benefits of tobacco avoidance education far exceeded that for other areas, even with high program costs, with a benefit-to-cost ratio of 18.86.

Sexual Behavior: The benefits included averted medical costs due to avoiding STDs and postponing pregnancy, as well as averted indirect costs associated with public support, food stamps, and Medicaid. The resulting benefit-to-cost ratio was 5.10.

Overall Program: The overall benefit-to-cost ratio of exemplary school health education is estimated to be 13.84, indicating that the value of the benefits accrued (i.e., costs avoided) is almost 14 times the cost of the program. The authors conclude the following:

> The potential benefits of an exemplary integrated school health educa-
> tion program, relative to the costs on implementing it, are very high,
> even under conservative assumptions, such as lower program effects,
> higher teacher salaries, and a big decay of program effects. These results
> compare favorably with other benefits cost studies of social and health
> programs, such as the measles, mumps and rubella vaccination program
> which shows a benefit cost ratio of 14.0; a pertussis vaccination program
> with a ratio of 11.1; a work site blood pressure control program with a
> ratio of 1.89 to 2.72; and a work site health promotion program with a
> ratio of 3.4.

Public Perceptions of Health Education

In the past decade, two major studies have described how parents, students, and teachers perceive health education. The first study was conducted in 1988 by Louis Harris and Associates, Inc. and sponsored by the Metropolitan Life Foundation. The results appear in *Health: You've Got to be Taught* (Harris, 1988). In this poll, 82 percent of the students indicated that they had experienced health education as a separate subject in school, 32 percent thought that their health classes were "more interesting than other classes;" and another 45 percent felt they were at the same interest level as other classes. Ninety-one percent of the students believed their health classes to be "useful." Among parents surveyed, 78 percent be-lieved that comprehensive health education[3] is "very important;" an-other 20 percent believed such class work to be "somewhat important;" 84 percent also believed it was important for their child's school to get involved in teaching about good health habits. However, only 36 percent of the teachers interviewed through the Harris survey believed that their schools supported the health education program "very strongly."

---

[3]The term "comprehensive health education" refers only to the educational program component and should not be confused with a "comprehensive school health program," which involves *all* components.

In 1994, the American Cancer Society (ACS) commissioned a survey by the Gallup Organization entitled *Values and Opinions of Comprehensive School Health Education in U.S. Public Schools: Adolescents, Parents, and School District Administrators* (American Cancer Society, 1994). Its results proved very similar to the Harris survey. The ACS report states that "parents of adolescents clearly see comprehensive school health education as a very important part of their children's education. More than four in five parents (82 percent) feel comprehensive school health education is either more important than (40 percent) or as important as (42 percent) other things taught in school." The survey indicated that 55 percent of adolescents would like the amount of time devoted to health education increased, and an additional 25 percent think the time devoted to health education should be at least equal the time devoted to other subjects. Of particular interest in this survey was the administrators' belief that the same amount of time (41 percent) or more time (27 percent) should be devoted to health education compared to other subjects.

The ACS survey provided perceptions of both students and administrators regarding the teaching of health. The majority of administrators (56 percent) did not believe that teachers are adequately prepared to teach a comprehensive health education program. Adolescents were ambivalent about the quality of the health teaching they had experienced. Sixty-five percent valued their instruction as either good (41 percent) or excellent (24 percent), but that implies that slightly more than one-third of the students felt the quality of their health instruction to be only fair or poor. Of particular interest in the ACS survey is that adolescents, parents, and administrators all ranked problem-solving and decisionmaking skills related to health as an especially important area. These skills were ranked as "very important" by 60 percent of the adolescents, 65 percent of the parents, and 69 percent of the administrators.

The executive vice-president of the American Cancer Society concluded, "The results of this Gallup Poll should render moot any protestations that we don't have the time or support to teach comprehensive school health education. The change in public attitude tells us the time is right to push ahead in this area, to take up leadership that is necessary to bring better health to all Americans" (Joint Committee on National Health Education Standards, 1995).

In summary, these surveys provide a profile of support for school health education instructional programs. Health education is valued, and parents and students would like to see it placed on an equal basis with other school subjects. Both students and administrators indicate a need for teachers to have more knowledge and skills in delivering health education programs, a feeling that probably results from the large numbers of teachers assigned to teach health education with insufficient preparation in the field.

The Integration[4] of Health Across the Curriculum

The historical separation of health education from other aspects of the curriculum is the result of factors that were largely logistical and political—the compartmentalization of the curriculum and restrictive requirements for teacher certification, to name a few—not of conceptual differences between health and other subjects. This gulf should be bridged because students now must understand the scientific, social, political, and economic dimensions of modern morbidity and mortality.

Given that most major health problems facing students have a multifactorial etiology, it seems reasonable to assume that health messages delivered by a single teacher—perhaps for one semester sometime in middle school and again in secondary school—are not as effective as multiple messages delivered more frequently from different perspectives. Consistent and repeated messages delivered by many teachers, school staff, peers, and parents may be more likely to be effective in promoting changes in expectations, norms, and behavior.[5]

An integrated curriculum is one approach to linking the variety of messages delivered to students in segmented, 45-minute sessions throughout the academic day. An integrated, interdisciplinary curriculum is one in which teachers of various subjects build coherent cross-cutting themes. As an example, the "planning wheel" shown in Figure 3-1, illustrates how teachers developed an integrated curriculum on smoking that made learning more meaningful for students (Palmer, 1991). In this approach, faculty met in cross-disciplinary groups and developed a strategy that allowed for each discipline's core instruction to remain central, while the integration of the health topic flowed logically across disciplines.

Health Information in Other Disciplines

The following discussion reviews further the possibilities for curricular integration and connections between health and other subjects.

Health-related information is an integral part of a wide variety of disciplines, including biology and other sciences, physical education, home economics, psychology, and even social studies and language arts. Given the interdisciplinary nature of contemporary health problems, it can be asserted that health issues should have a place in virtually all other

---

[4] The term "integration" as used in this section refers to planned and deliberate efforts to address common content in separate but related courses. Some use the term "correlation" to describe this process.

[5] Although such statements appear reasonable, the committee acknowledges that research has not been carried out and no data exist to support these assumptions.

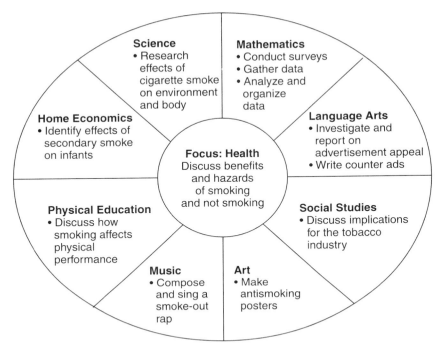

FIGURE 3-1 Planning wheel. SOURCE: Adapted from Palmer, J.M. 1991. Planning wheels turn curriculum around. Educational Leadership 49(2):58.

school subjects. However, health issues are sometimes addressed only indirectly or superficially in other subjects, which means that an opportunity to increase student awareness is lost. In other cases, didactic instruction may impart factual knowledge—for example, information about the structure and functioning of the human reproductive system—but such knowledge does not necessarily translate into desired behaviors in reproductive matters. If a CSHP can attune all curricular areas to providing consistent and relevant health messages at all possible opportunities, the resulting impact on students is likely to be intensified. However, the inclusion of health topics in other courses is not a substitute for a dedicated health education course; the integrated approach should augment, not replace, a stand-alone curriculum in health education.

Two levels of interaction between health issues and other subjects are immediately obvious. The first concerns those disciplines where there is a direct connection to health: science, physical education, and home economics. The second level of interaction—in courses such as social studies, mathematics, or language arts—is somewhat more diffuse, although progress in integration has been made in this area.

Subjects with Direct Connections to Health

Science. Science and health overlap most directly in the life sciences or biology curriculum, where there are obvious connections in traditional topics such as immunology, anatomy and physiology, genetics, and ecology. Although these topics embrace issues of personal and community health, the health-related treatment is often cursory. Most high school biology textbooks, for example, include information about genetic disorders and might even discuss the mechanisms for prenatal detection of selected genetic disorders. The primary focus, however, is on the mechanisms of inheritance and on the basic science of DNA, not on the ever-growing understanding of genotype–environment interaction in helping to explain the leading causes of mortality and morbidity in developed countries. Similarly, instruction about immunology details the components of the immune system and the steps in the immune response, but generally provides only superficial treatment of the importance of immunization in the control of communicable disease.

Although a focus on basic science is appropriate in a biology course, the basic science can provide an opportunity to consider the roles of biology, life-style, and personal decisions in the development of chronic, multifactorial disorders. As long ago as 1974, geneticist Barton Childs (Childs, 1974) highlighted the natural relationship between genetics and heath education, explaining that the objectives of health promotion and disease prevention are congruent with a genetic view of human disease, which holds that much morbidity results from genetic factors expressed in environments that precipitate disease. For example, susceptibility to certain types of cancer has been shown to be genetic; environmental and behavioral factors can influence how and when this susceptibility is expressed. This view has grown in power in the past two decades and, in fact, is at the heart of the assumptions that drive the Human Genome Project, which has as its goal the mapping of all human genes—the complete set of chemical instructions used by cells to make a human being.

Increasingly, health education and science education converge in terms of content and pedagogical approaches—for example, a focus on inquiry, decisionmaking, and problem-solving. They diverge to some extent in their treatments of the affective dimensions of health, although this distinction is receding. For example, issues related to health care now are finding their way into the biology curriculum in the form of ethical, legal, and social issues related to progress in biomedicine. These issues provide opportunities for health educators and biology educators to work together to provide a broad picture of the nature of health problems worldwide—their biological bases and their social and political dimensions.

Health also has direct connections in the physical sciences. Chemistry, for example, addresses a host of environmental issues, such as water quality and air pollution; the basic science of chemistry can be made more relevant in discussing the molecular basis for nutrition, disease, and substance addiction. Physics instruction introduces students to the science that underlies the many powerful imaging technologies that are used in health care, and basic laws of physics are important in understanding safety measures—for example, the optimal design of a bicycle helmet or why doubling the speed of a car quadruples the braking distance. The study of earth science and space science can introduce such issues as the public health effects of global warming and ozone depletion, air and water pollution, and natural disasters such as earthquakes and tornadoes.

Physical Education. As discussed earlier in this chapter, physical education is an integral curricular component of a CSHP, connecting directly to health education (and also to biology) by serving as a laboratory for demonstrating the relationship between physical fitness and health and between human biology and physical performance. The physical education curriculum should support classroom health education instruction by emphasizing lifelong physical fitness, proper nutrition, good health habits, and self-discipline and respect.

Home Economics. Courses previously known as "home economics" are expanding their emphasis and frequently acquiring new titles such as "family and consumer studies" or "work and family management." Whatever the nomenclature, these kinds of courses can reinforce health education through such topics as parenting, human development, infant and child care, nutrition and meal planning, household safety and environmental quality, and insurance and related financial matters. Through such courses, students can learn to become responsible and informed consumers of health products and health systems and can acquire critical thinking and decisionmaking skills in gathering and using health-related information.

Connections Between Health Education and Other Subjects

The connections between health education and disciplines, such as social studies, literature, or mathematics are not as remote as might be imagined. Disease and medicine, for example, have helped to influence the course of human history and have shaped the human population itself, and debates about the equitable provision of health care now dominate the political landscape in America. Health and disease also have figured prominently in great literature throughout the ages, and mathematics—particularly in statistical analysis and epidemiology—has been indispensable to humanity's progress against morbidity and early death.

Models and approaches for connecting health with supposedly unrelated disciplines have been developed. Several authors have identified how literature may be used in language arts classes to provide health content (Manna and Wolford, 1992; Rubin, 1993; Rubin and Brodie, 1992), and the State of Texas has developed a K–12 curriculum guide to infuse health education content in substance abuse prevention, nutrition promotion, and STD prevention into language arts, science, mathematics, social studies, and home economics (Texas Education Agency, 1992). Substantive integration of health education into some of these other disciplines will call for creative thinking and interdisciplinary collaboration, but many more connections will undoubtedly surface as teachers examine their own subjects for connections to health.

Connections Between National Standards in Science Education and the National Health Education Standards

The recent development of national standards in both science and health education provides excellent conceptual and practical guidance for the mutual reinforcement of health and scientific understanding across the two disciplines. Standards and recommendations from the National Research Council (1996), the American Association for the Advancement of Science (1989, 1993), and the Joint Committee on National Health Education Standards (1995) all provide support for the type of integrated education to promote health that should be found in a comprehensive school health program. The following excerpts from documents published by each of these groups, illustrate areas in common and possibilities of integration between science and health.

- **National Science Education Standards** (National Research Council, 1996):

> Hazards and the potential for accidents exist. Regardless of the environment, the possibility of injury, illness, disability, or death may be present. Humans have a variety of mechanisms—sensory, motor, emotional, social and technological—that can reduce and modify hazards.
>
> The severity of disease symptoms is dependent on many factors, such as human resistance and the virulence of the disease-producing organism. Many diseases can be prevented, controlled, or cured. Some diseases, such as cancer, result from specific body dysfunctions and cannot be transmitted.

Personal choice concerning fitness and health involves multiple factors. Personal goals, peer and social pressures, ethnic and religious beliefs, and understanding of biological consequences, can all influence decisions about health practices.

An individual's mood and behavior may be modified by substances. Students should understand that drug use can result in physical dependence and can increase the risk of injury, accidents, and death.

Selection of foods and eating patterns determine nutritional balance. Nutritional balance has a direct effect on growth and development and personal well-being. Personal and social factors—such as habits, family income, ethnic heritage, body size, advertising, and peer pressure—influence nutritional choices.

Family systems serve basic health needs, especially for young children. Regardless of the family structure, individuals have a variety of physical, mental, and social relationships that influence the maintenance and improvement of health.

Sexuality is basic to the physical, mental, and social development of humans. Students should understand that human sexuality involves biological functions, psychological motives, and cultural, ethnic, religious, and technological influences. Sex is a basic and powerful force that has consequences to individuals' health and to society. Students should understand various methods of controlling the reproduction process and that each method has a different type of effectiveness and different health and social consequences.

• **Science for All Americans** (American Association for the Advancement of Science, 1989):

To stay in good operating condition, the human body requires a variety of foods and experiences.

Regular exercise is important for maintaining a healthy heart/lung system, muscle tone, and for keeping bones from becoming brittle.

Good health depends on the avoidance of excessive exposure to substances that interfere with the body's operation. Chief among those that each individual can control are tobacco, addictive drugs, and excessive amounts of alcohol.

Biological abnormalities, such as brain injuries or chemical imbalances, can cause or increase susceptibility to psychological disturbances. Conversely, intense emotional states have some distinct biochemical effects.

Ideas about what constitutes good mental health and proper treatment for abnormal mental states vary from one culture to another and from one time period to another.

Individuals differ greatly in their ability to cope with stressful environments. Stresses are especially difficult for children to deal with and may have long-lasting effects.

Prolonged disturbance of behavior may result in strong reactions from families, work supervisors, and civic authorities that add to the stress on the individual.

• **National Health Education Standards** (Joint Committee on National Health Education Standards, 1995):

Standard 1: Students will comprehend concepts related to health promotion and disease prevention. Rationale: Basic to health education is a foundation of knowledge about the interrelationship of behavior and health, interactions within the human body, and the prevention of diseases and other health problems. Comprehension of health promotion strategies and disease prevention concepts enables students to become health-literate, self-directed, learners which establishes a foundation for leading healthy and productive lives.

Standard 3: Students will demonstrate the ability to practice health-enhancing behaviors and reduce health risks. Rationale: Research confirms that many diseases and injuries can be prevented by reducing harmful and risk-taking behaviors. By accepting responsibility for personal health, students will have a foundation for living a healthy, productive life.

Standard 5: Students will demonstrate the ability to use interpersonal communication skills to enhance health. Rationale: Personal, family, and community health are enhanced through effective communication. A responsible individual will use verbal and nonverbal skills in developing and maintaining healthy personal relationships. Ability to organize and to convey information, beliefs, opinions, and feelings are skills which strengthen interactions and can reduce or avoid conflict. When communicating, individuals who are health-literate demonstrate care, consideration, and respect of self and others.

Although health education depends heavily on knowledge about and understanding of the basic science related to the functioning of the human body, it should be emphasized that such studies in science should not substitute for health education. Health education goes beyond the mere acquisition of knowledge in linking such areas as biology and chemistry with the psychosocial domain, as students learn how their bodies function and then how they personally can and should behave in relationship to themselves, their friends, family, and community.

Needs in Health Education

Implementation of Effective Curricula

Curricular decisions represent local options that must follow broad state guidelines. These decisions may follow a local assessment to determine community-wide health and health education needs or may be based only on the perceptions of the curriculum committee. Communities may use commercially available materials in their curriculum or may develop their own. Many health education curricula exist, but most have not been evaluated as to their effectiveness. Curricula evaluated as effective are the most likely to assist in the attainment of the third National Health Education Standard, which calls for the demonstration of health-enhancing behaviors to reduce health risks. The number of schools using evaluated, effective curricula is unknown. Further, the efficacy of some evaluated curricula in naturalistic settings has not been established. Although it is known that numerous schools have adopted such research-based curricula as *Know Your Body*, *Growing Healthy*, and *Teenage Health Teaching Modules*, it is not known if these schools have achieved the same results in day-to-day implementation as were achieved in the experimental trials.

For health education to achieve the public health goals of influencing the adoption of health-enhancing behaviors, not only should schools adopt or adapt curricula shown to be effective, but the curriculum must also allot sufficient time to the priority health areas identified by the CDC—sexual behaviors that result in HIV infection, other STDs, and unintended pregnancy; alcohol and other drug use; behaviors that result in unintentional and intentional injuries; tobacco use; dietary patterns that result in disease; and sedentary life-style. For example, the leading cause of premature adult mortality and morbidity is cigarette smoking. Yet, according to SHPPS, only 53 percent of health education teachers spent more than one class period discussing the topic, and only 29 percent of infused classroom teachers allotted more than one class period to this topic (Table 3-9). Whether this is the fault of the curriculum or teachers' implementation of the curriculum is not clear.

In addition to health content, it has been recognized that quality of instruction and practice in social skills are important elements in health curricula if the goal is to affect health behaviors. Although a majority of regular and infused class health teachers say they have taught risk reduction skills (see Table 3-12), the figures no doubt overstate the proportion of teachers providing high-quality, effective instruction. Students cannot learn and become proficient in behavioral skills without practice, and an indicator of instructional quality is whether teachers provide opportunities for students to practice skills. Such opportunities were provided by a

TABLE 3-12 Percentage of Health Education Classroom Teachers and Infused Classroom Teachers Teaching Risk Reduction Skills and Having Students Practice Skills—by Skill[a]

Skill	Health Education Classroom Teachers (%)		Infused Classroom Teachers (%)	
	Teaching Skill	Have Students Practice Skill	Teaching Skill	Have Students Practice Skill
Communication	86.6	62.8	72.3	53.8
Decision-making	90.2	76.9	81.9	60.2
Goal-setting	79.9	59.1	72.3	45.3
Non-violent conflict resolution	72.5	44.2	64.9	34.4
Resisting social pressure for unhealthy behaviors	89.6	60.8	73.9	40.2
Stress management	82.2	52.2	60.3	27.3

[a]School Health Policies and Programs Study, 1994

SOURCE: Collins et al., 1995.

smaller proportion of regular and infused teachers, perhaps due to lack of emphasis on skills practice in curricular packages or teachers' lack of comfort with skills practice.

Improved Professional Preparation

Although behavioral scientists from various disciplines are beginning to reach a consensus about what works to prevent high-risk behaviors (Allensworth and Wolford, 1989; American Public Health Association, 1975; Benard, 1986; Elders, 1991; Perry, 1991; Tobler, 1986), most schools have not adopted these concepts (Bartlett, 1981; Bremberg, 1991; National Commission on the Role of the School and the Community in Improving Adolescent Health, 1989; Seffrin, 1990). Policymakers, administrators, health professionals, and educators are asking for "a new kind of health education—a sophisticated, multifaceted program that goes light years beyond present lectures about personal hygiene or the four basic food groups" (National Commission on the Role of the School and the Community in Improving Adolescent Health, 1989). These new approaches require the leadership and skills of a new type of health educator, but inadequate teacher preparation is a major obstacle to the implementation of today's new programs.

As mentioned earlier in this chapter, only 5 percent of health teachers in the secondary classroom majored in health education. Whether the topic is HIV or AIDS, pregnancy prevention, tobacco avoidance, substance abuse, or violence prevention, the majority of students receive instruction from teachers who did not have formal training in teaching these areas during their college preservice program (English, 1994). Both preservice and inservice preparation of health education teachers has not utilized to maximum advantage the most effective means of preventing youth from engaging in high-risk activity (Gingiss, 1992; Gingiss et al., 1991; Holtzman et al., 1992; National Commission on AIDS, 1993). More emphasis should be placed on hiring new health education teachers who have had the proper preservice preparation, and improved professional development for current staff should be the norm. There is a need for inservice programs that assist health education teachers to understand the problems facing students, the principles of prevention, and the key concepts for implementing primary health care and health promotion programs that are effective (Tobler, 1986). Confronted with the risks and dangers of modern society, young people need access to properly prepared teachers who can implement state-of-the-art curricula and address student health needs and concerns.

In some school districts, it is traditional for physical education teachers to teach health education. Because physical education teachers have extensive health science training (biology, anatomy, physiology, and so forth), they are well grounded in health facts. Many science teachers also are called upon to teach health education, for they may have training and sensitivity in and about health facts. However, health education today is a discipline that goes far beyond health facts. Teachers who specialize in health education have additional training in health pedagogy and behavioral psychology, which are critical to the understanding of factors that influence or change health behaviors. While it is important for physical education and science teachers to provide knowledge that impacts health and to encourage or reinforce healthful behaviors, it is equally important that a separate health class be taught by teachers specifically prepared to teach today's health education.

Beyond providing continuing staff development to health educators, there is a need to provide all teachers, regardless of subject area, with expert information on how they can participate in promoting the health and well-being of students, especially students at risk. Staff development can occur in a variety of ways—course work for college credit, local or regional seminars and workshops, continuing education via correspondence courses, technical assistance, and computer networking. Community health and medical professionals can play an active role in the process.

Improved Environment

An improved environment is needed that supports and affirms the value of the new generation of health education. Administrators, other educators, parents, and students should understand the relevance and potential of health education and consider it an integral part of the curriculum. Policies regarding teacher qualifications, available resources, and required courses and assessment in health education should reflect the importance placed on this essential subject.

Further Research

Although much has been learned over the past several decades about the development and delivery of health education, many research questions remain unresolved. For example, research is needed to determine the optimal content, approach, frequency, and timing of the health education curriculum. Because health education is expected to justify its position in the curriculum, a better understanding of what outcomes can reasonably be expected and measured is essential. Since categorical programs that address a single problem, such as tobacco avoidance, require a considerable amount of instructional time to effect behavior change, questions arise about how schools can find time to address the entire spectrum of health-threatening behaviors. Identifying effective approaches for integrating health education with other school- and community-based health and social programs is also important. Chapter 6 further examines some of these priority research areas.

Recent Recommendations of Other Groups to Strengthen Health Education

During recent years, several highly visible national initiatives have developed recommendations for health education that cover the essential issues discussed in this chapter. The most notable of these initiatives include the National Action Plan for Comprehensive School Health Education, the National Health Education Standards, and recommendations emanating from the SHPPS analysis of health education. There is considerable commonality and synergism among these sets of recommendations, and the committee believes that these collective recommendations provide a strong foundation and direction for health education in the future. The highlights of these three sets of recommendations are described below.

The National Action Plan for Comprehensive School Health Education

In 1992, the American Cancer Society organized a consensus conference of almost 40 national health and education organizations to develop a national agenda for school health education (ACS, 1993). Representatives developed a practical collaborative plan to institutionalize comprehensive school health education that presented action steps to overcome barriers and meet identified needs. The plan is divided into six areas: (1) policy; (2) public awareness; (3) professional preparation and practice; (4) parent, family, and community involvement; (5) educational outcomes and standards; and (6) resources. For each area, the plan describes the scope and definition of the issues, the needs and the justification of these needs, research that should be conducted, desired outcomes, and specific actions to achieve the desired outcomes. The following policy needs identified by the plan serve as overarching recommendations:

• Foster leadership that will articulate, at all levels of government, the needs of children and the rights of children to lead healthy and productive lives.
• Build a broad consensus about the effectiveness of health education as a strategy to improve the health and education of the nation's children.
• Establish goals for health education that guide and direct program development and the standards-setting process and that serve as a means of assessment.

National Health Education Standards

As described earlier, the National Health Education Standards describe what students should know and be able to do and provide indicators to measure student performance (Joint Committee on National Health Education Standards, 1995). The developers of these standards realized that health education is sometimes criticized because health problems among children and youth are not changed or eliminated after health instruction occurs, but that the effectiveness of health education is often compromised by deficiencies in the delivery system. To address this problem, the National Health Education Standards include a section on Opportunity-to-Learn Standards for local and state education agencies, communities, state health agencies, institutions of higher education, and national organizations. These standards address the conditions that need to be developed and/or organized and supported for successful health education program delivery. According to these Opportunity-to-Learn Standards the following measures are necessary.

Local Education Agency. The local education agency needs to

1. implement collaborative planning among school personnel, students, families, related community agencies, and business organizations to design and assess health instruction,
2. employ elementary and secondary teachers professionally prepared to teach health education,
3. implement school policies that create a climate which promotes health literacy, and
4. coordinate the comprehensive health education curriculum, including assessment, materials, and professional development.

Community. The community needs to

1. create community awareness and support for school health instruction,
2. provide learning opportunities at home and in the community that enhance and reinforce student achievement of the National Health Education Standards,
3. participate in planning with school personnel, students, governmental units, and business organizations to design, implement, and assess health instruction, and
4. foster community programs that create a climate to promote child and adolescent health and health literacy.

State Education and Health Agencies. These agencies need to

1. support planning and policies at the state and local levels to achieve quality health instruction in schools,
2. establish health education as a core academic subject with a state plan, budget, and specified instructional time,
3. provide technical assistance by professional health educators to local education agencies and communities,
4. require adequate preservice preparation of elementary and middle school teachers to prepare them to deliver quality health education instruction,
5. require that secondary health instruction be taught by professionally prepared school health educators, and
6. adopt public policies and social marketing programs advocating health literacy.

Institutions for Higher Education. These institutions need to

1. prepare future school health educators in a manner consistent with the National Commission on Health Education Credentialing, Inc.,
2. provide health instruction preservice programs taught by qualified and experienced school health education faculty,
3. prepare future teachers to make health education connections across the curriculum,
4. prepare future teachers to be able to assess student achievement of the National Health Education Standards,
5. prepare future teachers to deal effectively with the health needs, interests, and strengths of culturally diverse populations, and
6. prepare administrators and other key school personnel to implement health education within schools.

National Organizations. These organizations need to

1. support implementation of the National Health Education Standards and health education as a core subject,
2. foster public policies advocating health literacy for all children and youth, and
3. support research in health education.

School Health Policies and Programs Study Recommendations

As a result of its analysis of the current condition of health education in this country, the School Health Policies and Programs Study developed the following recommendations (Collins et al., 1995):

- Increase the number of states that include health education content as part of their state assessment requirements.
- Increase the number of districts that appoint an individual responsible for coordinating health education.
- Increase the number of health education teachers who major in health education.
- Increase the number of schools that require more than one course devoted primarily to health education issues.
- Increase coverage of priority health issues for youth including pregnancy prevention, STD prevention, violence prevention, and injury prevention.
- Use infused classes as an adjunct to, instead of a substitute for, a planned course of study in health education.
- Increase the number of schools and districts with school health

advisory councils that involve key constituents in planning and implementing school health education.

SUMMARY OF FINDINGS AND CONCLUSIONS

As mentioned earlier in this chapter, the status of the two curricular components of a comprehensive school health program—physical education and health education—is sometimes questioned because they were not originally mentioned in the National Education Goals as "core subjects" in which students should demonstrate competence. However, with each update report, the National Education Goals Panel has added language emphasizing the importance of physical education and health education, affirming that these two subjects should be an integral part of the school curriculum.

Physical Education: Research has confirmed a direct relationship between a physically active life-style and improved long-term health status, and the new generation of physical education programs is shifting emphasis from competitive sports to physical activity and fitness. Three recent documents—the National Standards for Physical Education, the School Health Programs and Policies Study,[6] and the CDC Guidelines for School and Community Health Programs to Promote Physical Activity Among Youth—emphasize the new priorities and recommendations in physical education and collectively provide a sound basis for quality physical education programs in the future. **The committee supports these recommendations.**

Health Education: The traditional health education curriculum has been based on 10 conceptual areas identified by the School Health Education Study of the 1960s: community health, consumer health, environmental health, family life, mental and emotional health, injury prevention and safety, nutrition, personal health, prevention and control of disease, and substance use and abuse. Recently, the CDC has recommended that the six major contributors to adolescent mortality and morbidity, mentioned earlier, be priority areas of emphasis for health education, since these problems are based in behaviors that can be prevented or changed. The overarching goal of the recently-released National Health Education Standards is the development of health literacy—the capacity to obtain,

---

[6]The School Health Policies and Programs Study was conducted in 1994 by the Centers for Disease Control and Prevention to examine policies and programs across multiple components of school health programs at the state, district, school, and classroom levels.

interpret, and understand basic health information and services, and the competence to use such information and services to enhance health.

Research has shown that specific health education curricula are effective, for example, those focused on specific categorical problems such as tobacco avoidance. Studies have shown that in order for health education to produce behavior change, effective strategies, considerable instructional time, and well-prepared teachers are required. Students' behavioral decisions are also heavily influenced by environmental variables—peers, family, schools, community, and the media. A recent cost–benefit analysis shows that school health education is cost-effective, and several recent national surveys indicate that parents and students overwhelmingly consider health education to be very important and useful.

In spite of the potential effectiveness and favorable perception of health education, SHPPS found a considerable gap between desired practice and actual current practice. Typically, only one semester of health education is required at the middle or junior high level and one semester at the high school level, and the attention given to certain priority topics falls considerably short of recommended goals. Although most teachers of health education have not majored in the field, there is not an overwhelming demand for staff development, perhaps due to a lack of awareness on the part of teachers and administrators of the potential and complexities of health education or the fact that teachers with majors in other fields prefer to teach in those fields and see no value in improving their skills in health education.

RECOMMENDATIONS

The committee believes that three recently released documents—the National Action Plan for Comprehensive School Health Education, the National Health Education Standards, and the SHPPS report—collectively provide comprehensive recommendations and a strong framework to move health education forward in the future. Several areas merit further emphasis and discussion.

The committee believes that the period prior to high school is the most crucial for shaping attitudes and behaviors. By the time students reach high school, many are already engaging in risky behaviors or at least have formed accepting attitudes toward these behaviors.

The committee recommends that all students receive sequential, age-appropriate health education every year during the elementary and middle or junior high grades.

At all grade levels, instruction should focus on achieving the performance indicators outlined in the National Health Education Standards. Early years might focus on such topics as nutrition and safety, but beginning at the late elementary or early middle school grades, instruction should shift focus to an intensive, age-appropriate emphasis on the CDC priority behaviors and be provided by teachers who understand early adolescents and are especially prepared to deal with these sensitive and difficult topics.

The committee recommends that a one-semester health education course at the secondary level immediately become a minimum requirement for high school graduation. Instruction should follow the National Health Education Standards, use effective up-to-date curricula, be provided by qualified health education teachers interested in teaching the subject, and emphasize the six priority behavioral areas identified by the CDC.

According to SHPPS, 83.9 percent of all senior high schools already require at least one semester of health education, and the CDC topics are emphasized in a large majority of schools. Thus, such an immediate requirement is not unrealistic. *Additional courses or electives in health education at the high school level would be preferable to a single semester.*

The committee debated how to reconcile the call for students to receive health education every year, K–12, with the reality of the crowded curriculum at the secondary level and decided that the critical issue should be whether high school students achieve the performance indicators described in the National Health Education Standards, not the amount of "seat time." Thus, the committee recommends that the seat time be a minimum of at least one semester but that student health knowledge and understanding be assessed at the end of this course. If a community finds its young people falling short on this assessment, then the existing course must be improved or additional courses instituted. The committee believes that some form of health education must occur every year at the secondary level but that some of this education can take place through alternative approaches, such as "booster" sessions, health modules in other courses, field trips, assemblies, school-wide campaigns, after-school peer discussion groups, and one-on-one or small group counseling for students with identified needs.

Effective elementary health education is the foundation for the future critical middle school years, and well-prepared elementary teachers are the key for providing this education.

The committee recommends that all elementary teachers receive substantive preparation in health education content and methodology during their preservice college training. This preparation should give elementary generalist teachers strategies for infusing health instruction into the curriculum and prepare upper elementary teachers to lay the groundwork for the intensive middle or junior high health education program.

REFERENCES

Advertising Age. 1990. Special supplement: Marketing to Hispanics.

Allensworth, D.D. 1994. The research base for innovative practices in school health education at the secondary level. *Journal of School Health* 64(5):80–186.

Allensworth, D.D., and Wolford, C. 1989. A theoretical approach to HIV prevention. *Journal of School Health* 59(2):56–65.

American Alliance for Health, Physical Education, Recreation, and Dance. 1995. *AAHE/NCATE Guidelines Review Book.* Reston, Va.: Association for the Advancement of Health Education.

American Association for the Advancement of Science. 1989. *Project 2061: Science for All Americans.* Washington, D.C.: American Association for the Advancement of Science.

American Association for the Advancement of Science. 1993. *Benchmarks for Science Literacy.* New York: Oxford University Press.

American Cancer Society. 1993. National action plan for comprehensive school health education. *Journal of School Health* 63(1):46–66.

American Cancer Society. 1994. *Values and Opinions of Comprehensive School Health Education in U.S. Public Schools: Adolescents, Parents, and School District Administrators.* Atlanta, Ga.: American Cancer Society.

American Public Health Association. 1975. Resolutions and position papers: Education for health in the community setting. *American Journal of Public Health* 65(2):201–202.

Bartlett, E. 1981. The contribution of school health education to community health promotion: What can we reasonably expect? *American Journal of Public Health* 71:1384–1391.

Benard, B. 1986. Characteristics of effective prevention programs. *Network* 3:6–8.

Bennett, B.B. 1987. The Effectiveness of Staff Development Training Practices: A Meta-Analysis. Ann Arbor, Mich.: Doctoral Dissertation No. 8721226.

Berkowitz, R.I., Agras, W.S., Korner, A.F., Kraement, H.C., and Zeanah, C.H. 1985. Physical activity and adiposity: A longitudinal study from birth to childhood. *Journal of Pediatrics* 106:734–738.

Berlin, J.A., and Colditz, G.A. 1990. A meta-analysis of physical activity in the prevention of coronary heart disease. *American Journal of Epidemiology* 132:253–287.

Bertera, R.L., and Cuthie, J.C. 1984. Blood pressure self-monitoring in the workplace. *Journal of Occupational Medicine* 26:183–188.

Blair, S.N., Kohl, H.W. III, Paffenbarger, R.S., Clark, D.G., Cooper, K.H., and Gibbons, L.W. 1989. Physical fitness and all-cause mortality. *Journal of the American Medical Association* 262:2395–2401.

Botvin, G.J., and Eng, A. 1982. The efficacy of a multicomponent approach to the prevention of cigarette smoking. *Preventive Medicine* 11:199–211.

Boyer, E.L. 1983. *High School: A Report on Secondary Education in America.* New York: Carnegie Foundation for the Advancement of Teaching.

Bremberg, S. 1991. Does school health education affect the health of students? Pp. 89–107. In *Youth Health Promotion: From Theory to Practice in School and Community*, D. Nutbeam, B. Haglund, P. Farley, and P. Tillgren, eds. London: Forbes Publications.

Broadhead, W.E., Gehlcah, S.H., DeGruy, F.V., and Kaplan, B.H. 1989. Functional versus structural social support and health care utilization in a family medicine outpatient practice. *Medical Care* 27:221–233.

Bruce, C., and Emshoff, J. 1992. The SUPER II Program: An early intervention program. *Journal of Community Psychology* (OSAP Special Issue):310–321.

Bush, P.J., Zuckerman, A.E., Taggert, V.S., Theiss, P.K., Peleg, E.O., and Smith, S.A. 1989a. Cardiovascular risk factor prevention in black school children: The "Know Your Body" evaluation project. *Health Education Quarterly* 16(2):215–227.

Bush, P.J., Zuckerman, A.E., Theiss, P.K., Taggert, V.S., Horowitz, C., Sheridan, M.J., and Walter, H.J. 1989b. Cardiovascular risk factor prevention in black school children: Two-year results of the "Know Your Body" program. *American Journal of Epidemiology* 129(3):466–482.

Cale, L., and Harris, J. 1993. Exercise recommendations for children and young people. *Physical Education Review* 16:89–98.

Centers for Disease Control and Prevention. 1997. Guidelines for school and community health programs to promote physical activity among youth. *Morbidity and Mortality Weekly Report* 46(Rr-6):1–36.

Childs, B. 1974. A place for genetics in health education, and vice versa. *American Journal of Human Genetics* 26:120–134.

Coates, T.J., Jeffery, R.W., and Slinkard, L.A. 1981. Heart healthy eating and exercise: Introducing and maintaining changes in health behaviors. *American Journal of Public Health* 71(1):15–23.

Collins, J.L., Small, M.G., Kann, L., Pateman, B.C., Gold, R.S., and Kolbe, L.J. 1995. School health education. *Journal of School Health* 65(8):302–311.

Collins, M. 1991. Promoting healthy body image through the comprehensive school health program. *Journal of Health Education* 22(5):297–302.

Connell, D.P., Turner, R.R., and Mason, E.F. 1985. Summary of findings of the school health education evaluation: Health promotion effectiveness, implementation, and costs. *Journal of School Health* 55(8):316–334.

Conner, J.L., and Conner, C.N. 1992. Effects of primary prevention on attitudes and alcohol and other drug use with at-risk American-Indian youth. In *Working with Youth in High-Risk Environments: Experience in Prevention,* C.E. Marcus and J.D. Swisher, eds. OSAP Prevention Monograph 12. DHHS Publication No. (ADM)92–1815. Rockville, Md.: U.S. Department of Health and Human Services.

Cortese, P.A. 1993. Accomplishments in comprehensive school health education. *Journal of School Health* 63(1):21–23.

Council of Chief State School Officers. 1994. *SCASS Health Education Project.* Washington, D.C.: Council of Chief State School Officers.

Crockett, S., Mullis, R., Perry, C.L., and Luepker, R.V. 1989. Parent education in youth-directed nutrition interventions. *Preventive Medicine* 18(4):475–491.

Cummings, S.R., Kelsey, J.L., Nevitt, M.C., and Dowd, K.J. 1985. Epidemiology of osteoporosis and osteoporotic fractures. *Epidemiology Review* 7:178–207.

Davis, K.E., Jackson, K.L., Dronenfeld, J.J., and Blair, S.N. 1987. Determinants of participation in worksite health promotion activities. *Health Education Quarterly* 17:18–22.

Decker, M.D., Graitcer, P.L., and Schaffner, W. 1988. Reduction in motor vehicle fatalities associated with an increase in the minimum drinking age. *Journal of the American Medical Association* 260:3604–3610.

DeGraw, C. 1994. A community-based school health system: Parameters for developing a comprehensive student health promotion program. *Journal of School Health* 64(5):192–195.

DeMarsh, J., and Kumpfer, K.L. 1986. Family-oriented interventions for prevention of chemical dependency in children and adolescents. In *Childhood and Chemical Abuse: Prevention and Intervention*, S. Griswold-Ezekoye, K. Kumpfer, and W. Bukoski, eds. New York: Haworth Press.

Devine, C.M., Olson, D.M., and Frongillo, E.A. 1992. Impact of the "Nutrition for Life" program on junior high students in New York State. *Journal of School Health* 62(8):381–385.

DiClemente, R.J., Pies, C.A., Stoller, E.J., Straits, C., Olivia, G.E., Haskin, J., and Rutherford, G.W. 1989. Evaluation of school-based AIDS education curricula in San Francisco. *Journal of Sex Research* 26(2):188–198.

Duncan, B., Burris, W.T., Itami, R. and Puffenbarger, N. 1983. A controlled trial of a physical fitness program for fifth grade students. *Journal of School Health* 53:467–471.

Durant, R.J., Linder, D., and Mahoney, O. 1983. Relationship between habitual physical activity and serum lipoprotein levels in white male adolescents. *Journal of Adolescent Health Care* 4(4):235–239.

Dwyer, T., Coonan, W.E., Leitch, D.R., Hetzel, B.S., and Baghurst, R.A. 1983. An investigation of the effects of daily physical activity on the health of primary school students in South Australia. *International Journal of Epidemiology* 12:308–312.

Dwyer, T., Viney, R., and Jones, M. 1991. Assessing school health education programs. *International Journal of Technology Assessment and Health Care* 7(3):286–295.

Elders, J.P. 1991. From experimentation to dissemination: Strategies for maximizing the impact and spread of school health education. In *Youth Health Promotion: From Theory to Practice in School and Community*, D. Nutbeam, B. Haglund, P. Farley, and P. Tillgren, eds. London: Forbes Publications.

Elders, J.P., Sallis, J.F., Woodruff, S.I., and Wildey, M.B. 1993. Tobacco-refusal skills and tobacco use among high-risk adolescents. *Journal of Behavioral Medicine* 16:629–642.

English, J. 1994. Innovative practices in comprehensive health education programs for elementary schools. *Journal of School Health* 64(5):188–191.

Errecart, M.T., Walberg, H.J., Ross, J.G., Gold, R.S., Fiedler, J.L., and Kolbe, L.J. 1991. Effectiveness of teenage health teaching modules. *Journal of School Health* 61(1):26–30.

Faucette, N., McKenzie, T.L., and Patterson, P. 1990. Descriptive analysis of nonspecialist elementary physical education teachers' curricular choices and class organization. *Journal of Teaching in Physical Education* 9:284–298.

Flay, B.R. 1985. What we know about the social influences to smoking prevention: Review and recommendations. In *Prevention Research: Deterring Drug Abuse Among Children and Adolescents*, C. Bell and R. Battjes, eds. NIDA Research Monograph 63, DHHS Publication No. (ADM) 87–1334. Rockville, Md.: National Institute on Drug Abuse.

Freedman, M. 1988. *Partners in Growth: Elder Mentors and At-Risk Youth*. Philadelphia: Public/Private Ventures.

Gans, K.M., Levin, S., Lasater, T.M., Sennett, L.L., Maroni, A., Ronan, A., and Carleton, R.A. 1990. Heart healthy cook-offs in home economics classes: An evaluation with junior high school students. *Journal of School Health* 60(3):99–102.

Gingiss, P.L. 1992. Enhancing program implementation and maintenance through a multiphase approach to peer-based staff development. *Journal of School Health* 62(5):161–166.

Gingiss, P.L., Smith, D.W., and Buckner, W.P. 1991. After the conference is over: Future directions for school health programs. *Journal of Health Education* 22(5):325–327.

Glider, P., Kressler, H., and McGrew, G. 1992. Prevention and early intervention through peer support retreats. In *Working with Youth in High-Risk Environments: Experiences in Prevention*, C.E. Marcus and J.D. Swisher, eds. OSAP Prevention Monograph 12. DHHS

Publication No. (ADM) 92–1815. Rockville, Md.: U.S. Department of Health and Human Services.

Glynn, T.J. 1989. Essential elements of school-based smoking prevention programs. *Journal of School Health* 59(5):181–188.

Gold, R.S. 1994. The science base for comprehensive health education. In *The Comprehensive School Health Challenge: Promoting Health Through Education*, P. Cortese and K. Middleton, eds. Santa Cruz, Calif.: Education, Training, and Research Associates.

Gold, R.S., Parcel, G.S., Walberg, H.J., Luepker, R.V., Portnoy, B., and Stone, E.J. 1991. Summary and conclusions of the Teenage Health Teaching Modules evaluation: The expert work group perspective. *Journal of School Health* 61(1):39–42.

Hahn, R.A., Teutsch, S.M., Rothenberg, R.B., and Marks, J.S. 1986. Excess deaths from nine chronic diseases in the United States. *Journal of the American Medical Association* 264:2654–2659.

Hall, P.A., and Reyes, M.B. 1992. Evaluation of alcohol and other drug use prevention programs with Mexican-American youth. In *Working with Youth in High-Risk Environments: Experiences in Prevention*, C.E. Marcus and J.D. Swisher, eds. OSAP Prevention Monograph 12. DHHS Publication No. (ADM) 92–1815. Rockville, Md.: U.S. Department of Health and Human Services.

Hamburg, M.V. 1994. School health education: What are the possibilities? In *The Comprehensive School Health Challenge*, P. Cortese, and K. Middleton, eds. Santa Cruz, Calif.: Education, Training, and Research Associates.

Hansen, W.B., and Graham, J.W. 1991. Preventing alcohol, marijuana, and cigarette use among adolescents: Peer pressure resistance training versus establishing conservative norms. *Preventive Medicine* 20:414–430.

Hansen, W.B., Johnson, C.A., Flay, B.R., Graham, J.W., et al. 1988. Affective and social influences approaches to the prevention of multiple substance abuse among seventh grade students. Results from Project SMART. *Preventive Medicine* 17:135–154.

Harris, L. 1988. *Health: You've Got to Be Taught: An Evaluation of Comprehensive Health Education in American Public Schools.* New York: Metropolitan Life Foundation.

Hawkins, J., Lishner, R., Catalano, R., and Howard, M. 1986. Childhood predictors of adolescent substance abuse: Toward an empirically grounded theory, pp. 11–48. In *Childhood and Chemical Abuse: Prevention and Intervention*, S. Griswold-Ezekoye, K. Kumpfer, and W. Bukoski, eds. New York: Haworth Press.

Hoadley, J.F., Fuchs, B.C., and Holder, H.D. 1984. The effect of alcohol beverage restrictions on consumption: A 25-year longitudinal analysis. *American Journal of Drug and Alcohol Abuse* 10:375–401.

Hofman, A., Walter, H.J., Connelly, P.A., and Vaughan, R.D. 1987. Blood pressure and physical fitness in children. *Hypertension* 9:188–191.

Holloway, R.L., Spivey, R.N., Zismer, D., and Withington, A.M. 1988. Aptitude x treatment interaction: Implications for patient education research. *Health Education Quarterly* 15:241–259.

Holtzman, D., Green, B., Ingraham, G., Daily, L., and Kolbe, L. 1992. HIV education and health education in the United States: A national survey of local school district policies and practices. *Journal of School Health* 62(9):421–427.

Howard, M., and McCabe, J.B. 1990. Helping teenagers postpone sexual involvement. *Family Planning Perspectives* 22(1):21–26.

Ireland, D.F. 1990. New attitude/new look: An African-American adolescent health education program. *Pediatric Nursing* 16(2):175–178, 205.

Isikoff, M. 1989. Anti-drug ad campaign directed at blacks. *Washington Post*, November.

Iverson, D.C., Colonge, B.N., Main, D., and Holcomb, S. 1989. BP American fitness center evaluation: Final report. Denver: University of Colorado Health Sciences Center, Department of Family Medicine.

LIVERPOOL JOHN MOORES UNIVERSITY
LEARNING SERVICES

Jackson, S.A. 1994. Comprehensive school health education programs: Innovative practices and issues in standard setting. *Journal of School Health* 64(5):177–179.

Jarvik, M.E., and Schneider, N.G. 1984. Degree of addiction and effectiveness of nicotine gum therapy for smoking. *American Journal of Psychiatry* 141:790–791.

Johnson, C.A., Hansen, W.B., Collins, L.M., and Graham, J.W. 1986. High school smoking prevention: Results of a three-year longitudinal study. *Journal of Behavioral Medicine* 9:439–452.

Johnson, E.M. 1992. *Signs of Effectiveness. The High-Risk Youth Demonstration Grants.* Rockville, Md.: U.S. Department of Health and Human Services, Office of Substance Abuse Prevention.

Joint Committee on Health Education Terminology. 1991. Report of the 1990 Joint Committee on Health Education Terminology. *Journal of Health Education* 22(2):97–108.

Joint Committee on National Health Education Standards. 1995. *National Health Education Standards: Achieving Health Literacy.* Atlanta, Ga.: American Cancer Society.

Jones, R., McCullough, L., and Dewoody, M. 1992. The child welfare challenge in meeting developmental needs. In *Identifying the Needs of Drug-Affected Children: Public Policy Issues.* OSAP Prevention Monograph 11. DHHS Publication No. (ADM)92–1814. Rockville, Md.: U.S. Department of Health and Human Services.

Kann, L., Collins, J.L., Pateman, B.C., Small, M.L., Russ, J.G., and Kolbe, L.J. 1995. The School Health Policies and Programs Study (SHPPS): Rationale for a nationwide status report on school health programs. *Journal of School Health* 65(8):291–294.

Kelder, S.H., Perry, C.L., and Klepp, K.I. 1993. Community-wide youth exercise promotion: Long-term outcomes of the Minnesota Heart Health Program of the Class of 1989 study. *Journal of School Health* 63:218–223.

Killen, J.D., Telch, M.J., Robinson, T.N., Macoby, N., Taylor, B., and Farquhar, J.W. 1988. Cardiovascular disease risk reduction for tenth graders. *Journal of the American Medical Association* 260(23):1728–1733.

Killen, J.D., Robinson, T.N., Telch, M.J., Saylor, K.E., Maron, D.J., Rich, T., and Bryson, S. 1989. The Stanford Adolescent Heart Health Program. *Health Education Quarterly* 16(2):263–283.

King, A.C., and Tribble, D.L. 1991. The role of exercise in weight regulation in non-athletes. *Sports Medicine* 11(5):331–349.

King, A.C., Taylor, C.B., Haskell, W.L., and Debusk, R.R. 1988. Strategies for increasing early adherence to and long-term maintenance of home-based exercise training in health of middle-aged men and women. *American Journal of Cardiology* 61:628–632.

Kirby, D., Barth, R.P., Leland, N., and Fetro, J.V. 1991. Reducing the risk: Impact of a new curriculum on sexual risk taking. *Family Planning Perspectives* 23(6):253–262.

Klesges, R.C., Brown, K., Pascale, R.W., Murphy, M., et al. 1988. Factors associated with participation, attrition, and outcome in a smoking cessation program at the workplace. *Health Psychology* 7(6):575-589.

Knight, C.M. 1991. Educational policy issues in serving infants and toddlers born toxic-positive to drugs. In *Identifying the Needs of Drug-Affected Children: Public Policy Issues.* OSAP Prevention Monograph 11. DHHS Publication No. (ADM)92–1814. Rockville, Md.: U.S. Department of Health and Human Services.

Koegel, L.K., Koegel, R.L., and Ingham, J.C. 1986. Programming rapid generalization of correct articulation through self-monitoring procedures. *Journal of Speech and Hearing Disorders* 51:24–32.

Koenig, L. 1992. Training teachers to integrate prevention concepts into the primary curriculum. In *Working with Youth in High-Risk Environments: Experiences in Prevention.* C.E. Marcus and J.D. Swisher, eds. OSAP Prevention Monograph 12. DHHS Publication No. (ADM) 92–1815. Rockville, Md.: U.S. Department of Health and Human Services.

Kohl, H.W., LaPorte, R.E., and Blair, S.N. 1988. Physical activity and cancer: An epidemiological perspective. *Sports Medicine* 6:222–237.

Kottke, T.E., Puska, P., Salonen, J.T., Tuomilehto, J., et al. 1985. Projected effects of a high-risk vs. population-based prevention strategies in coronary heart disease. *American Journal of Epidemiology* 121:697–704.

Kumpfer, K.L. 1987. Etiology and prevention of vulnerability to chemical dependency in children of substance abusers. In *Youth at High Risk for Substance Abuse.* B.S. Brown and A.R. Mills, eds. Rockville, Md.: National Institute on Drug Abuse.

Lee, I., Paffenbarger, R.S., and Hsieh, C. 1992. Physical activity and risk of prostatic cancer among college alumni. *American Journal of Epidemiology* 135:169–179.

Lefbvre, R.C., Lasater, T.M., Carleton, R.A., and Peterson, G. 1987. Theory and delivery of health programming in the community: The Pawtucket heart health program. *Preventive Medicine* 16:80–95.

Leon, A.S. 1989. *Effects of Physical Fitness and Physical Activity in Population-Based Surveys.* DHHS Publication No. (PHS) 89–1253. Hyattsville, Md.: U.S. Department of Health and Human Services.

Leon, A.S., Connett, J., Jacobs, D.R., and Raurama, R. 1987. Leisure-time physical activity levels and risk of coronary heart disease and death: The multiple risk factor intervention trail. *Journal of the American Medical Association* 258(17):2388–2395.

Lewis, C., Battistich, V., and Schaps, E. 1990. School-based primary prevention: What is an effective program? *New Directions in Child Development* 50:35–59.

Lorion, R.P., and Ross, J.G., 1992. Programs for changes: A realistic look at the nation's potential for preventing substance involvement among high-risk youth. *Journal of Community Psychology* (OSAP Special Issue):3–9.

Luepker, R.V., Perry, C.L., McKinlay, S.M., Nader, P.R., Parcel, G.S., Stone, E.J., Webber, L.S., Elder, J.P., Feldman, H.A., Johnson, C.C., Kelder, S.H., and Wu, M. 1996. Outcomes of a field trial to improve children's dietary patterns and physical activity: The Child and Adolescent Trial for Cardiovascular Health (CATCH). *Journal of the American Medical Association* 275(10):768-776.

Mahon, A.D., and Vaccaro, P. 1989. Ventilatory threshold and VO_2 max changes in children following endurance training. *Medicine and Science in Sports* 21:425–431.

Manna, T., and Wolford, C. 1992. *Children's Literature for Health Awareness.* Metuchen, N.J.: Scarecrow Press.

Marburger, E.A., and Friedel, B. 1987. Seat belt legislation and seat belt effectiveness in the Federal Republic of Germany. *Journal of Trauma* 27:703–705.

Marin, G., and Marin, B.V. 1991. Research with Hispanic populations. *Applied Social Research Methods Series,* Volume 23, Beverly Hills, Calif.: Sage Publications.

Mayer, J.A., Heins, J.M., Vogel, J.M., Morrison, D.C., et al. 1986. Promoting low-fat entree choices in a public cafeteria. *Journal of Applied Behavioral Analysis* 19:397–402.

Maynard, E.J., Coonan, W.E., Worsley, A., Dwyer, T., and Baghurst, P.A. 1987. The development of the life-style education program in Australia. In *Cardiovascular Risk Factors in Children: Epidemiology and Prevention,* B.S. Hetzel and G.S. Berenson, eds. Amsterdam: Elsevier.

McCaul, K.D., and Glasgow, R.E. 1985. Preventing adolescent smoking: What have we learned about treatment construct validity? *Health Psychology* 4:361–387.

McGinnis, J.M. 1992. The public health burden of a sedentary life-style. *Medical Science Sports Exercise* 24 (Suppl.):S196–S200.

McGinnis, J.M., Kanner, L., and DeGraw, C. 1991. Physical education's role in achieving national health objectives. *Research Quarterly for Exercise and Sport* 62(2):138–142.

McKenzie, T.L., Sallis, J.F., and Nader, P.R. 1992. SOFIT: System for observing fitness instruction time. *Journal of Teaching in Physical Education* 11:18–22.

McKenzie, T.L., Sallis, J.F., Faucette, N., Roby, J.J., and Kolody, B. 1993. Effects of a curriculum and inservice program on the quantity and quality of elementary physical education classes. *Research Quarterly for Exercise and Sport* 64(2):178–187.

Means, R.K. 1975. *Historical Perspectives on School Health.* Thorofare, N.J.: Charles B. Slack.

Morisky, D.E., DeMuth, N.M., Field-Fass, M., Green, L.W., et al. 1985. Evaluation of family health education to build social support for long-term control of high blood pressure. *Health Education Quarterly* 12:35–50.

Murray, D.M., Richards, P.S., Luepker, R.V., and Johnson, C.A. 1987. The prevention of cigarette smoking in children: Two- and three-year follow-up comparisons for four prevention strategies. *Journal of Behavioral Medicine* 10:595–611.

Nader, P.R. 1990. The concept of "comprehensiveness" in the design and implementation of school health programs. *Journal of School Health* 60(4):133–138.

National Association for Sport and Physical Education. 1992. *Outcomes of Quality Physical Education Programs.* Reston, Va.: National Association for Sport and Physical Education.

National Association for Sport and Physical Education. 1994. *Guidelines for Elementary School Physical Education.* Reston, Va.: National Association for Sport and Physical Education.

National Association for Sport and Physical Education. 1995. *Moving into the Future: National Standards for Physical Education: A Guide to Content and Assessment.* St. Louis, Mo.: Mosby.

National Commission on AIDS. 1993. *Preventing HIV/AIDS in Adolescents.* Washington, D.C.: National Commission on AIDS.

National Commission on the Role of the School and the Community in Improving Adolescent Health. 1989. *Code Blue: Uniting for Healthier Youth.* Alexandria, Va.: National Association of State Boards of Education.

National Education Goals Panel. 1994. *The National Education Goals Report: Building a Nation of Learners.* Washington, D.C.: U.S. Government Printing Office.

National Research Council. 1996. *National Science Education Standards.* Washington, D.C.: National Academy Press.

National School Boards Association. 1991. *School Health: Helping Children Learn.* Alexandria, Va.: National School Boards Association.

Nelson, G.D., Cross, F.S., and Kolbe, L.J. 1991. Introduction: Teenage Health Teaching Modules evaluation. *Journal of School Health* 61(1):20.

Ounce of Prevention Fund. 1990. *Success for Every Teen: Programs That Help Adolescents Avoid Pregnancy, Gangs, Drug Abuse, and School Drop-Out.* Chicago, Ill.: Ounce of Prevention Fund.

Owen, S.L., Kirkpatrick, M.A., Lavery, S.W., Gosner, H.L., Nelson, S.R., Kavis, R.L., Mason, E.R., and Connell, D.B. 1985. Selecting and recruiting health programs for the school health education evaluation. *Journal of School Health* 55(8):305–308.

Oyemade, U.J., and Brandon-Monye, D.B. 1990. *Ecology of Alcohol and Other Drug Use: Helping Black High-Risk Youth.* OSAP Prevention Monograph 7. DHHS Publication No. (ADM) 90–1672. Rockville, Md.: U.S. Department of Health and Human Services.

Paffenbarger, R.S., Hyde, R.T., Wing, A.L., and Hsieh, C. 1986. Physical activity, all-cause mortality, and longevity of college alumni. *New England Journal of Medicine* 314:605–613.

Palmer, J.M. 1991. Planning wheels turn curriculum around. *Education Leadership* 42(2):57–60.

Panico, S., Celentano, E., Krogh, V., Jossa, F., Farinaro, I., Trevisan, M., and Mancini, M. 1987. Physical activity and its relationship to blood pressure in school children. *Journal of Chronic Diseases* 40 (10): 925–930.

Parcel, G.S., Simons-Morton, B.G., O'Hara, N.M., Baranowsky, T., Kolbe, L.J., and Bee, D.E. 1987. School promotion of healthful diet and exercise behavior: An integration of organizational change and social learning theory interventions. *Journal of School Health* 57:150–156.

Parcel, G.S., Simons-Morton, B., O'Hara, N.M., Baranowski, T., and Wilson, B. 1989. School promotion of healthful diet and physical activity: Impact on learning outcomes and self–reported behavior. *Health Education Quarterly* 16(2):181–199.

Pate, R.R., and Ward, D.S. 1990. Endurance exercise trainability in children and youth. In *Advances in Sports Medicine and Fitness*, Volume 3, W.A. Grana, ed. Chicago, Ill.: Year Book Medical Publishers.

Pate, R.R., Small, M.L., Ross, J.G., Young, J.C., Flint, K.H., and Warren, C.W. 1995. School physical education. *Journal of School Health* 65(8):312–318.

Pentz, M.A., Dwyer, J.D., MacKinnon, D.P., Flay, B.R., Hansen, W.B., Wang, E.Y., and Johnson, C.S. 1989. A multicommunity trial for primary prevention of adolescent drug abuse: Effects on drug use prevalence. *Journal of the American Medical Association* 261:3259–3266.

Perry, C.L. 1991. Conceptualizing community-wide youth health promotion programs. In *Youth Health Promotion: From Theory to Practice in School and Community*, D. Nutbeam, B. Haglund, P. Farley, and P. Tillgren, eds. London: Forbes Publications.

Perry, C.L., Luepker, R.V., Murray, D.M., Hearn, M.D., Halper, A., Dudovitz, B., Maile, M.C., and Smyth, M. 1989. Parent involvement with children's health promotion: A one-year follow-up of the Minnesota home team. *Health Education Quarterly* 16(2):171–180.

Perry, C.L., Murray, D.M., and Griffin, G. 1990. Evaluating the statewide dissemination of smoking prevention curricula: Factors in teacher compliance. *Journal of School Health* 60:(10):501–504.

Perry, C.L., Kelder, S.H., Murray, D.M., and Klepp, K. 1992. Community-wide smoking prevention: Long-term outcomes of the Minnesota Heart Health Program of the Class of 1989 study. *American Journal of Public Health* 82:1210–1216.

Powell, K.E., Thompson, P.D., Caspersen, C.J., and Kendrick, J.S. 1987. Physical activity and the incidence of coronary heart disease. *Annual Review of Public Health* 8:253–287.

Powell, K.E., Caspersen, C.J., Koplan, J.P., and Ford, E.S. 1989. Physical activity and chronic disease. *American Health and Clinical Nutrition* 49:999–1006.

Puska, P.A., McAllister, A., Pekkola, J., and Koskela, K. 1981. Television in health promotion: Evaluation of a national programme in Finland. *International Journal of Health Education* 24:2–14.

Puska, P.A., Nissinen, J. Tuomilehto, J., Salonen, T., et al. 1988. The community-based strategy to prevent coronary heart disease: Conclusion from the ten years of the North Karelia project. *Annual Review of Public Health* 6:147–193.

Rana, S.R., Knasel, A.L., and Haddy, T.B. 1992. Cancer knowledge and attitudes of African-American and white adolescents: A comparison of two secondary schools. *Journal of the Association of the Academy of Minority Physicians* 3(1):13–16.

Resnicow, K., and Botvin, G. 1993. On the effects of school health education programs: Why do they decay? *Preventive Medicine* 22:484–490.

Resnicow, K., Orlandi, M.A., Vaccaro, D., and Wynder, E.L. 1989. Implementation of a pilot school-site cholesterol reduction intervention. *Journal of School Health* 29(2):74–78.

Resnicow, K., Ross, D., and Wynder, E.L. 1991. The role of comprehensive school-based interventions: The results of four "Know Your Body" studies. *Annals of the New York Academy of Sciences* (April 12):285–298.

Resnicow, K., Cohn, L., Reinhardt, J., Cross, D., Futterman, R., Kirschner, E., Wynder, E.L., and Allegrante, J. 1992. A three-year evaluation of the "Know Your Body" program in minority school children. *Health Education Quarterly* 19:463–480.

Resnicow, K., Cherry, J., and Cross, D. 1993a. Ten unanswered questions regarding comprehensive school health promotion. *Journal of School Health* 63(4):171–175.

Resnicow, K., Cross, D., Lacosse, J., and Nichols, P. 1993b. Evaluation of a school-site cardiovascular risk factor screening program. *Preventive Medicine* 22:838–856.

Resnicow, K., Cross, D., and Wynder, E.L. 1993c. The "Know Your Body" program: A review of evaluation studies. *Bulletin of the New York Academy of Medicine* 70(3):188–207.

Rohrbach, L.A., Graham, J.W., and Hansen, W.B. 1993. Diffusion of a school-based substance abuse prevention program: Predictors of program implementation. *Preventive Medicine* 22(2):237–260.

Ross, J.G., and Gilbert, G.G. 1985. National Children and Youth Fitness Study: A summary of findings. *Journal of Physical Education, Recreation, and Dance* 56(1):45–50.

Ross, J.G., and Pate, R.R. 1987. National Children and Youth Fitness Study II: A summary of findings. *Journal of Physical Education, Recreation, and Dance* 58(1):50–96.

Ross, J.G., Errecart, M.T., Fieldler, J.A., and Lavin, A.T. 1989. Draft final report: Teenage Health Teaching Modules Evaluation. CDC Contract No. 200–86–3932. Silver Spring, Md.: Macro International.

Ross, J.G., Nelson, G.D., and Kolbe, L.J., eds. 1991. A special insert. Teenage Health Teaching Modules evaluation. *Journal of School Health* 61(1):19–20.

Ross, J.G., Saavedra, P.J., Shur, G.H., Winters, F., and Felner, R.D. 1992. The effectiveness of an after-school program for primary grade latchkey students on precursors of substance abuse. *Journal of Community Psychology* (OSAP Special Issue):22–38.

Rothman, M.L., Ehreth, J.L., Palmer, C.S., Collins, J., Reblando, J.A., and Luce, B.R. 1993. The potential benefits and costs of a comprehensive school health education program. Paper presented at the Annual Meeting of the American Public Health Association, San Francisco, Calif., October 24-28.

Rubin, M.A. 1993. Promoting books and media: Healthy attitudes. *School Library Media Activities Monthly* 10(11):65–66.

Rubin, M.A., and Brodie, C.S. 1992. Promoting books and media: Healthy picture books. *School Library Media Activities Monthly* 9(9):43–44.

Ruch-Ross, H.S. 1992. The child and family options program: Primary drug and alcohol prevention for young children. *Journal of Community Psychology* (OSAP Special Issue):39–54.

Sallis, J.F., and McKenzie, T.L. 1991. Physical education's role in public health. *Research Quarterly for Exercise and Sport* 62(2):124–137.

Sallis, J.F., Haskell, W.L., Fortmann, S.P., Wood, P.D., and Uranizan, K.M. 1986. Moderate-intensity physical activity and cardiovascular risk factors: The Stanford five-city project. *Preventive Medicine* 15:561–568.

Saris, W.H., Binkhorst, R., Cramwinckel, A., van Waesberghe, F., and van der Veen-Hezemans, A. 1980. The relationship between working performance, daily physical activity, fatness, blood lipids, and nutrition in school children. In *Children and Exercise IX*, K. Berg and B. Erikssen, eds. Baltimore: University Park Press.

Sasaki, J., Shindo, M., Tanaka, H., Ando, M., and Arakawa, K. 1987. A long-term aerobic exercise program decreases the obesity index and increases the high density lipoprotein cholesterol concentration in obese children. *International Journal of Obesity* 11:339–345.

Schinke, S.P., Gilchrist, L.D., and Snow, W.H. 1985. Skills intervention to prevent cigarette smoking among adolescents. *American Journal of Public Health* 75:665–667.

Seekins, T.S., Fawcett, B., Choen, S.H., Elder, J.P., et al. 1988. Experimental evaluation of public policy: The case of state legislation for child passenger safety. *Journal of Applied Behavioral Analysis* 21:233–243.

Seffrin, J.R. 1990. The comprehensive school health curriculum: Closing the gaps between the state-of-the-art and the state-of-the-practice. *Journal of School Health* 60(4):151–156.

Shane, V.T., and Kaplan, B.J. 1988. AIDS education for adolescents. *Youth and Society* 20(2):180–208.

Shannon, B., and Chen, A.N. 1988. A three-year school-based nutrition education study. *Journal of Nutrition Education* 20(3):114–124.

Shephard, R.J., Volle, M., Lavallee, H., LaBarre, R., Jequier, J.C., and Rajic, M. 1984. Required physical activity and academic grades: A controlled study. In *Children and Sport: Paediatric Work Physiology*, J. Ilmarinen and I. Vaelimaeki, eds. Berlin, Germany: Springer-Verlag.

Siegel, K.A., and Manfrede, T.G. 1984. Effects of a ten-month fitness program on children. *The Physician and Sports Medicine* 12:91–97.

Simons-Morton, B.G., Parcel, G.S., O'Hara, N.M., Blair, S.N., and Pate, R.R. 1988. Health-related physical fitness in childhood: Status and recommendations. *Annual Review of Public Health* 9:403–425.

Simons-Morton, B.G., Parcel, G.S., Baronowski, T., Forthofer, L., and O'Hara, N.M. 1991. Promoting healthful diet and physical activity among children: Results of a school-based intervention study. *American Journal of Public Health* 81(8):886–991.

Sliepcevich, E. 1964. *School Health Education Study: A Summary Report*. Washington, D.C.: School Health Education Study.

Smith, I.E. 1992. An ecological perspective: The impact of culture and social environment on drug-exposed children. In *Identifying the Needs of Drug-Affected Children: Public Policy Issues*. OSAP Prevention Monograph 11. DHHS Publication No. (ADM) 92–1814. Rockville, Md.: U.S. Department of Health and Human Services.

Sparks, G. 1986. The effectiveness of alternative training activities in changing teaching practices. *American Education Research Journal* 23(2):217–225.

Springer, J.F., Phillips, J.L., Phillips, L., Cannady, P., and Kerst-Harris, E. 1992. CODA: A creative therapy program for children in families affected by abuse of alcohol and other drugs. *Journal of Community Psychology* (OSAP Special Issue):55–74.

Starfield, B. 1989. Preventive interventions in the health and health-related sections with potential relevance for youth suicide. In *ADAMHA: Report of the Secretary's Task Force on Youth Suicide*, Volume 4: *Strategies for the Prevention of Youth Suicide*. DHHS Publication No. (ADM) 89–1624. Washington, D.C.:U.S. Government Printing Office.

Stone, E.J., Perry, C.L., and Luepker, R.V. 1989. Synthesis of cardiovascular behavioral research for youth health promotion. *Health Education Quarterly* 16(2):155–169.

Sussman, S., Dent, C.W., Stacy, A.W., Sun, P., Craig, S., Simon, T.R., Burton, D., and Flay, B.R. 1993. Project towards no tobacco use, one-year behavior outcomes. *American Journal of Public Health* 83(9):1245–1250.

Taggart, V.S., Bush, P.J., Zuckerman, A.E., and Theiss, P.K. 1990. A process of evaluation of the District of Columbia "Know Your Body" project. *Journal of School Health* 60:60–66.

Terry, J.P., Silka, L., and Terry, L. 1992. Designing evaluation models to assess primary prevention and cultural changes: An evaluation report of the Leadership Project. In *Working with Youth In High-Risk Environments: Experiences in Prevention*. C.E. Marcus, and J.D. Swisher, eds. OSAP Prevention Monograph 12. DHHS Publication No. (ADM) 92–1815. Rockville, Md.: U.S. Department of Health and Human Services.

Texas Education Agency. 1992. Prevention of HIV/AIDS and other communicable diseases; Prevention of drug use; Nutrition education. *Education for Self Responsibility (ESR)*. Austin: Texas Education Agency.

Thomas, S.M., Fick, A.C., and Henderson, J.A. 1992. Meeting the needs of special populations: A formative evaluation of a school-based smoking prevention program. *Journal
of the Louisiana State Medical Society* 144(4):157–161.

Tobler, N. 1986. Meta-analysis of 143 adolescent drug prevention programs: Quantitative
outcome results of program participants compared to a control or comparison group.
Journal of Drug Issues 16:537–567.

Tortu, S., and Botvin, G.J. 1989. School-based smoking prevention: The teacher training
process. *Preventive Medicine* 18(2):280–289.

U.S. Department of Health and Human Services, Public Health Service. 1979. *Healthy People:
Surgeon General's Report on Health Promotion and Disease Prevention.* Washington, D.C.:
U.S. Government Printing Office.

U.S. Department of Health and Human Services, Public Health Service. 1991. *Healthy People
2000: National Health Promotion and Disease Prevention Objectives.* DHHS Publication
No. (PHS) 91-50213 Washington, D.C.: U.S. Government Printing Office.

U.S. Department of Health and Human Services, Public Health Service. 1993. *School Health:
Findings from Evaluated Programs.* Washington, D.C.: U.S. Government Printing Office.

Vaillant, G.E. 1988. What can long-term follow-up teach us about relapse and prevention of
relapse in addiction? *British Journal of Addiction* 83:1147–1157.

Wagner, J.L., and Winnett, R.A. 1988. Prompting one low-fat, high-fiber selection in a fast-
food restaurant. *Journal of Applied Behavioral Analysis* 21:179–185.

Walter, H.J. 1989. Primary prevention of chronic disease among children: The school-based
"Know Your Body" intervention trials. *Health Education Quarterly* 16(2):201–214.

Walter, H.J., and Wynder, E.L. 1989. The development, implementation, evaluation, and
future directions of a chronic disease prevention program for children: The "Know
Your Body" studies. *Preventive Medicine* 18(1):59–71.

Walter, H.J., Vaughan, R.D., and Wynder, E.L. 1989. Primary prevention of cancer among
children: Changes in cigarette smoking and diet after six years of intervention. *Journal
of the National Cancer Institute* 31(13):995–999.

Williams, C., Carter, B., and Wynder, E. 1983. Prevalence of selected cardiovascular and
cancer risk factors in a pediatric population: The "Know Your Body" project. *Preventive Medicine* 10:235–50.

Wynne, E.A. 1989. Preventing youth suicide through education. In *ADAMHA: Report of the
Secretary's Task Force on Youth Suicide,* Volume 4, *Strategies for the Prevention of Youth
Suicide.* DHHS Publication No. (ADM) 89–1624. Washington, D.C.: U.S. Government
Printing Office.

4

School Health Services

INTRODUCTION

Common Elements of School Health Services

Although a universally accepted definition of the term "school health services" has not been adopted, the School Health Policies and Programs Study (SHPPS) has described school health services as a "coordinated system that ensures a continuum of care from school to home to community health care provider and back" (Small et al., 1995). The goals and program elements of school health services vary at the state, community, school district, and individual school levels. Some of the factors that contribute to these variations include student needs, community resources for health care, available funding, local preference, leadership for providers of school health services, and the view of health services held by school administrators and other key decisionmakers in the school systems.

There is similarity, however, in the types of services offered from one school system to the next, which is likely the result of several factors. A majority of states have state school nurse consultants, many of whom have distributed sample policy and procedure manuals from their state department of health or education or both, to guide the development and delivery of health services in local settings. The National Association of School Nurses has defined roles and standards for school nurses (Proctor et al., 1993) and provides a system for disseminating information and training to nurses who practice in schools. The American School Food Service Association has recently released standards for school foodservice and nutrition practices (American School Food Service Association, 1995). Similarly, organizations such as the National Association of School Psychologists, the American School Counselor Association, and the National Association of Social Workers have published position statements and standards for their professions. The American School Health Association (ASHA), through its interdisciplinary committees, has studied the advantages and disadvantages of different services, the organization and delivery of services, and the roles of various school health service providers. Subsequently, ASHA publications have brought this information to the attention of state and local health and education agencies. The American Academy of Pediatrics, working closely with national representatives of the school health services sector as well as the community health system, periodically updates a school health manual, *School Health: Policy and Practice*, that serves both as another unifying force and as an informal mechanism for ensuring local program quality (American Academy of Pediatrics, 1993). Within this document are the following seven goals of a school health program:

Goal 1 Ensure access to primary health care.[1]
Goal 2 Provide a system for dealing with crisis medical situations.
Goal 3 Provide mandated screening and immunization monitoring.
Goal 4 Provide systems for identification and solution of students' health and educational problems.
Goal 5 Provide comprehensive and appropriate health education.
Goal 6 Provide a healthful and safe school environment that facilitates learning.

---

[1] It should be noted that the IOM (IOM) Committee on the Future of Primary Care has distinguished between the terms "primary care" and "primary health care" (Institute of Medicine, 1994). According to its definition, "primary care" refers to personal health services, whereas "primary health care," as originally described by the World Health Organization, goes beyond personal health services to include such public health measures as sanitation and ensuring clean water for populations. This report attempts to be consistent with this distinction, but other sources—particularly those that appeared before 1994—may use the two terms interchangeably. The IOM Committee on Comprehensive School Health Programs in Grades K–12 assumes that in Goal 1, the American Academy of Pediatrics is referring to personal health services, or "primary care" as recently defined. Consistent with the view of the IOM Committee on the Future of Primary Care, primary care should include screening and referral for oral health problems, and treatment of and, if appropriate, referral for mental health problems.

Goal 7 Provide a system of evaluation of the effectiveness of the school health program.

Goals 1–4 and 7 are of particular relevance to school health services.

Recently, findings from national surveys conducted by the Division of Adolescent and School Health (DASH) of the Centers for Disease Control and Prevention (CDC), the Office of School Health at the University of Colorado Health Sciences Center in Denver, and other groups show that most schools do provide some type of school health services and that a degree of consistency does exist in the kinds of services delivered from one school system to the next. According to SHPPS (Small et al., 1995), 86 percent of all middle or junior high and senior high schools provide some type of school health services (first aid, screening, medication administration), although 32 percent of all middle/junior and senior high schools do not have a dedicated health services facility, such as a separate health room or clinic. SHPPS reports that most school districts require screening and follow-up in at least one grade, with vision (96 percent), hearing (95.4 percent), and scoliosis (88.2 percent) being the most common of the required screenings. Almost all districts keep student health records on file and monitor student immunization status, and most districts also keep student medical emergency and medical information forms on file.

The University of Colorado Health Sciences Center's survey, entitled *A Closer Look*, examined a systematic random sample of public school districts nationwide for the 1993–1994 school year (Davis et al., 1995). One goal of the survey was to determine the type of health services provided in schools, types of school health services personnel, methods of governance and financing, organizational structures for the delivery of services in and outside of school, and barriers to services. The *Closer Look* survey provided the profile of the types of school health services currently delivered across the country, as shown in Table 4-1.

According to *A Closer Look*, two health services appear to be provided almost universally by school districts, first aid (98.7 percent) and administration of medications (97.1 percent). Other commonly provided services include such health screenings as height, weight, vision, and hearing (86.8 percent); child abuse evaluations and follow-up (82.8 percent); and evaluation of emotional or behavioral problems (80 percent). The three next most commonly provided services are for children with special needs: monitoring of vital signs (77.7 percent), application and cleaning of dressings (76.8 percent), and development of the health component of the Individualized Education Plan (75.6 percent). In view of the health problems cited in earlier chapters of this report, it is interesting to note that only slightly more than half of the districts were found to provide mental health counseling and nutrition counseling, and less than 40 percent con-

TABLE 4-1 Health Services Provided in the Schools

Type of Service	Percentage of Districts Providing Service
Administer first aid	98.7
Administer medication	97.1
Provide screening (height/weight) vision, hearing	86.8
Child abuse evaluation and follow-up	82.8
Evaluate emotional or behavioral problems	80.0
Monitor vital signs	77.7
Clean and change dressings	76.8
Health component of Individualized Education Plan (IEP)	75.6
Case management for chronic health problems	58.1
Provide nutritional counseling	57.5
Provide mental health counseling	56.2
Conduct cardiovascular screenings	49.6
Provide complex nursing care to students with special needs	49.6
Employee wellness programs	48.6
Physical fitness screenings	45.2
Perform urinary catheterizations	40.2
Conduct health risk appraisals to determine life-style practices	35.7
Process worker's compensation claims	33.4
Provide immunizations at school	33.3
Physical exams	33.1
Provide family counseling	31.8
Tube feedings	28.1
Irrigations	25.3
Perform dental services	24.3
Conduct alcohol and drug screenings	23.9
Health component of Individualized Family Service Plan (IFSP)	21.4
Administer or monitor oxygen	20.7
Provide alcohol and drug treatment	16.3
Provide physicals, other primary health care services for school employees	14.4
Provide prenatal care	10.4
Collect and test blood samples	9.3
Throat cultures	6.6
Provide prenatal testing	4.6
Other	16.6

SOURCE: From Davis et al., 1995.

duct health risk appraisal to determine life-style practices. The committee has not attempted to reconcile these figures with those reported by SHPPS, which states that 89.2 percent of senior high schools and 84.4 percent of middle or junior high schools provide individual counseling. The latter figures could refer to counseling with primarily an academic focus, which schools may be more inclined to offer, although there is certainly overlap between academic and mental health problems. Data from *A Closer Look* indicate that the types of services available to students do not appear to vary substantially by the size of the school district.

The Need for School Health Services

Since schools bring large numbers of students and staff together, prudence dictates that—as in any workplace—a system must be in place to deal with such issues as first aid, medical emergencies, and detection of contagious conditions that could spread a group situation. Unlike other workplaces, however, a system must also be established in schools to provide routine administration of medications, since students—especially young students—may not be able to assume this responsibility themselves, and concern for substance abuse has led to policies in most schools that prohibit older students from administrating their own medication. Laws pertaining to special education students[2] require that schools provide the services necessary for these students to receive an appropriate education. Such services might include monitoring vital signs, changing dressings, catheterization, tube feeding, or administering oxygen. The school must also provide services to non-special education students with chronic health problems—such as asthma, diabetes, and seizures—in order that they can be educated. Schools have little or no choice in providing such services, for they are dictated either by legislative mandate or by precautions pertaining to risks and liability.

Services such as screenings and immunizations are also widely accepted as belonging in the schools, with the motivation having to do more with access, efficiency, and economies of scale than with liability. Since schools are where children spend a significant portion of their time, schools are seen by many observers as the logical site for services that are based on public health principles of population-based prevention. There is some debate, however, about the relative benefits and disadvantages of a population-based versus a selective high-risk approach, which targets

---

[2]"Special education" students are those with a wide range of disabilities, including mental retardation; hearing, visual, and speech impairment; serious emotional disturbances; orthopedic impairments; and learning disabilities (Walker, 1992).

preventive services only toward children at high risk. The population-based approach has the advantage of producing a large potential impact on the population as a whole, but a major disadvantage is that the benefits are frequently very small for the individual. Another potential disadvantage is that all interventions have a finite risk of unintended adverse side effects, which are also amplified along with benefits in the population-based approach, possibly resulting in an unfavorable benefit-risk ratio. Depending on the health issue, one approach may be superior to the other, or a combination of the two may be appropriate. For example, the National Cholesterol Education program recommends a population-based approach for implementing dietary guidelines for children, combined with a high-risk approach to blood lipid screening targeted only at children considered at risk based on family history (Starfield and Vivier, 1995).

Further, schools are strategically positioned to serve in the public health battle against the resurgence of infectious diseases, such as tuberculosis and hepatitis. Another feature of school health services—one that is often overlooked—is its potential for expanding the knowledge base. School health services can be a rich source of data for studying the relation between health status and learning capacity, and for assessing unmet needs and monitoring the health status of children and adolescents.

Given the above needs and benefits, a basic health services program must be in place in all schools. The issues currently generating much discussion and debate, however, are the role of the school in providing access to primary care, the appropriate lead agency for the more traditional basic school health services, the advantages and disadvantages of a population-focused versus a high-risk approach to the delivery of health services in schools, and the need to develop an integrated system of school health services.

The role of the school in providing access to primary care is a particularly difficult and critical issue. Since schools are a public system whereas health care is predominately private, there appears to be a fundamental mismatch between the two systems. Many students already have their own source of primary care, but a significant and growing segment of the student population does not. Those students without access to primary care are usually poor and are often at greatest risk of academic failure.

Special Needs Due to Poverty

Chapter 1 of this report documents some of the major problems facing children and adolescents in this country—the new social morbidities, changing family structures, limited access to health care, and lack of health

TABLE 4-2 Relative Frequency of Health Problems in Low-Income Children Compared with Other Children

Health Problem	Relative Frequency in Low-Income Children
Low birthweight	Double
Delayed immunization	Triple
Asthma	Higher
Bacterial meningitis	Double
Rheumatic fever	Double–triple
Lead poisoning	Triple
Neonatal mortality	1.5 times
Postneonatal mortality	Double–triple
Child deaths due to accidents	Double–triple
Child deaths due to disease	Triple–quadruple
Complications of appendicitis	Double–triple
Diabetic ketoacidosis	Double–triple
Complications of bacterial meningitis	Double–triple
Percentage with conditions limiting school activity	Double–triple
Lost school days	40 percent more
Severely impaired vision	Double–triple
Severe iron-deficiency anemia	Double

SOURCE: Starfield, 1982, 1992.

insurance. Poverty is the common denominator among many of these problems.

Research has identified an explicable link between poverty and health outcomes. Children in poverty are much less likely than their affluent peers to receive an excellent or very good health rating, and they visit their health care provider fewer times in a year. Low-income families, facing routine pediatric care costs that consume a large fraction of their annual income, may decide they cannot afford health care until their children's treatment leads to unnecessary hospitalization and valuable days lost from school (see Table 4-2). For example, preventable hospitalizations for pneumonia, asthma, and ear, nose, and throat infections are up to four times higher for poor children than for who are not poor children (Center for Health Economics Research, 1993). Poor children are also more likely to be limited in school or play activities by chronic health problems and to suffer more severe consequences than their more affluent peers when afflicted by the same illness (Newacheck et al., 1995).

Relative Frequency of Health Problems in Low-Income Children Compared with Other Children

It is estimated that as many as 12 million children under the age of 18 have no health insurance, or approximately 17 percent of all children in that population (American Medical Association Council on Scientific Affairs, 1990). Millions more have inadequate plans that fail to cover even basic preventive services, such as immunizations (National Health Education Consortium, 1992). Although progress has been made in establishing publicly financed community health centers in inner cities and rural areas, school-age youth rarely visit these facilities until their health problems reach crisis stage. Although Medicaid is intended to provide services for poor children, variations in state Medicaid policies have left almost 40 percent of children who live in poverty without access to basic primary and preventive care (Solloway and Budetti, 1995). Possible changes in the system imply even greater uncertainty about the role Medicaid will play in providing universal coverage for poor children and adolescents (Newacheck et al., 1995).

Absenteeism among students is clearly associated with school failure (Wolfe, 1985). Research has shown that students who miss more than 10 days of school in a 90-day semester have trouble remaining at their grade level (Klerman, 1988). In particular, children who are poor are two to three times more likely to miss school due to their illnesses (Starfield, 1982). Indeed, children with health problems are disproportionately poor students on the verge of academic failure. Youth frequently must miss valuable class time in order to get care for their illnesses during the regular office hours of public and private health professionals. In fact, a recent study found that students utilizing public clinics missed entire days of school per appointment (Kornguth, 1990). Thus, "health-related risk factors often set in motion a cycle of absenteeism and school failure" (Lewis and Lewis, 1990). Studies have also found that people living in poverty are twice as likely to have mental health problems; hence, low-income children are especially affected by the absence of accessible mental health care (Starfield, 1982).

Given these findings, it appears that the lack of accessible primary care has a high cost, in terms of both health and education outcomes. Providing primary care to needy students at the school site has been proposed to be efficient and cost-effective in the long run, in order to improve academic performance and detect health problems early before they require more expensive treatment. Then the difficult question naturally follows: Would all students, not only those in poverty, benefit from availability of convenient, accessible basic primary care services at school, provided by professionals specially trained to deal with their age level? In their studies of school-based health centers (SBHCs) in northern California, Brindis and coworkers found that a higher proportion of students who already had conventional private insurance or health maintenance organization (HMO) coverage utilized the SBHC than those without other coverage, suggesting that ease of access and an understanding staff are perhaps more important factors in utilization than the mere lack of other source of care (Brindis et al., 1995). (The surprisingly greater rate of utilization for students who already have insurance may possibly be attributed to their greater awareness of the importance of health care, parental encouragement, or understanding how to access the system.) Also, many working parents apparently appreciate the convenience of their children being able to receive basic health care at school (U.S. General Accounting Office, 1994b). If the school is seen as the most effective site for providing a set of basic primary services, how can these services be organized? Who will pay? How will these services be connected with the traditional "core" services of the school? These are questions without easy answers—or possibly, with different answers depending on the community. Some of these issues are considered in greater depth later in this chapter.

OVERVIEW OF BASIC SCHOOL SERVICES

The following section provides a summary of typical services found in the school setting. These services tend to be the most common and basic, although many schools may not provide all of the services described in this section. For the sake of organization, services have been divided into three categories: health care services, mental health or pupil services, and nutrition and foodservice. It should be emphasized that boundaries between categories are not sharp, and considerable overlap and interaction among services exist.

For each category, there is a description of the service, information about the personnel who provide the service, and a review of some of the important issues in that field. Much of the material in this section came from the discussion at the committee's third meeting and was contributed by representatives of various professional organizations who served on a panel on services at that meeting. The committee has not attempted to assess the professional standards, recommended student-professional ratios, or other issues in this section for validity or adequacy; instead, this section is intended simply to transmit the contributed information. For further details, the professional organizations can be contacted directly.[3]

---

[3]Participants in the panel discussion on services at the committee's third meeting included representatives from the National Association of School Nurses, American Acad-

Additional information may also be obtained from the University of Colorado School Health Resource Services project, which maintains an extensive reference collection of profiles of school health services programs from school districts throughout the country.

Health Care Services

Nurses and Nurse Practitioners

Services Provided. School nurses are the traditional "backbone" of school health services and are often the only health care providers at the school site on a regular basis. As mentioned earlier in this chapter, standards for school nursing have been established by the National Association of School Nurses. The school nurse typically provides population-based primary prevention and health care services, including

- physical and mental health assessment and referral for care;
- development and implementation of health care plans for students with special health care needs;
- health counseling;
- mandated screenings, such as vision, hearing, and immunization status;
- monitoring the presence of infectious conditions among students and enforcing public health precautions to prevent spread of infections and infestations;
- skilled nursing services for students with complex health care needs;
- case management of students with chronic and special health care needs;
- outreach to students and their families;
- interpretation of the health care needs of students to school personnel;
- development and implementation of emergency care plans and provision of emergency care and first aid;
- serving as liaison for the school, parents, and community health agencies;
- collaboration with other school professionals—particularly counselors, psychologists, and social workers—to address the health, developmental, and educational needs of students; and

emy of Pediatrics, National Association of School Psychologists, American School Counselor Association, National Association of Social Workers, and American School Food Service Association.

• for nurse practitioners only, the provision of primary care, including prescribing medications when allowed under the State Nurse Practice Act.

The traditional model for school nursing provides for a school nurse, typically in an office or health room, with or without an aide. The National Association of School Nurses and other organizations in the National Nursing Coalition for School Health have prepared and distributed standards of nursing practice that guide the services nurses deliver in schools (Proctor et al., 1993). A single nurse may also be shared among several schools. In *School Health: Policy and Practice,* the American Academy of Pediatrics has analyzed the various nurse staffing patterns which are listed in Table 4-3.

Personnel. The professional training required for school nurses varies, depending on location and changing economic conditions. The American Academy of Pediatrics (1993) reported in 1993 that only 38 states required school nurses to be registered nurses, and only 19 required the attainment of specific school nurse certification. SHPPS found that although only 8 percent of all states required school nurses to be certified through the American Nurses Association or the National Association of School Nurses, 62 percent of states offered their own certification for school nurses. Of those states offering certification, 66 percent required it for employment as a school nurse. Health aides are employed in 76 percent of states, but only 8 percent of these states required prior technical training for health aides (Small et al., 1995). The *Closer Look* investigation reports similar findings.

In some school districts, school nurses are employees of the school system; in others, school nurses are provided by the local health department or another agency. The National Association of School Nurses recommends a ratio of one school nurse per 750 students. In recent years, there has been interest in expanding the school nursing function through the use of nurse practitioners, nurses with additional training (generally at the master's level) who are certified by state laws to provide a range of primary care services. School-based nurse practitioners can perform physical examinations, prescribe certain medications with physician protocols, and frequently serve as the anchor provider in school-based clinics. The drive for independence from physicians has characterized the nurse practitioner movement (Clawson and Osterweis, 1993); however, school-based nurse practitioners usually have a backup relationship with a licensed physician in the community. Other graduate programs prepare school nurses for administrative and management roles, as well as for mental health positions in schools.

TABLE 4-3 Nursing Staffing Patterns for School Health Services

Model	Advantages	Disadvantages
Nurse aide alone	Cost: with appropriate backup, systems might be able to meet basic and required needs (e.g., immunization records and first aid)	Requires outside resources; special education needs will not be met
Aide with nurse	Frees nurse to meet more important needs	Increases costs if ratio is too "rich"
Nurse-teacher	Potential for increasing integration of health services and health education	Costs may be difficult to justify; half of job is usually sacrificed
School nurse	Readily available resource for children, teachers, parents	Costs for services may be difficult to justify in traditional programs
Public health nurse	Costs to district may be lower than district-supplied nurses	Services to schools diluted by other tasks
Nurse practitioner	Costs for services obtained may be cost-effective; meets more special education needs on-site (potentially decreases unnecessary referrals); better problem definition; potential for generating income for services provided	Should have some form of physician backup (may increase costs); role change difficult; requires time and training; expanded services may conflict with existing sources of care

SOURCE: Adapted from Nader, 1993. Reprinted with permission from Pediatrics in Review.

Important Issues. The emergence of the nurse practitioner role has broadened the possible functions of school nurses. However, budget constraints have led to the elimination of school nursing in some school districts. In other districts, a single nurse is shared among several schools, with health aides, clerical staff, or volunteers serving when the nurse is not available. Concern has been raised that the absence of a trained health care provider on-site could lead to unfortunate consequences in an emergency situation or in the supervision of students with special health care needs.

Burdens and responsibilities of school nurses are expanding as the increasing numbers of students with special needs and students without adequate health care and health insurance increase. School nurses must keep up with changing practices and procedures, but sometimes education in the specialty of school nursing is not readily available. In 1995, the Southern Council on Collegiate Education for Nursing, an affiliate of the Southern Regional Education Board (SREB), conducted a survey of 450 institutions with college-based nursing programs in SREB states[4] to examine the programs of study available for school nursing. Less than 5 percent of respondents offered such programs, and less than 1 percent of faculty have school nurse practitioner credentials (Strickland, 1995).

Another issue of importance to school nursing is the linkage of nursing services to other school health providers in order to form an integrated services team. Continued examination is also needed of the relative value of such primary prevention efforts as appropriate screenings for vision, hearing, growth, and eating disorders; early identification of individual students at risk for physical and mental health problems; development and implementation of safety programs; and case management of students with chronic diseases. Finally, of special concern to school nurses is the tailoring of school health services to local community needs through the formation of school or community planning councils and the use of needs assessments to guide planning efforts. These concerns and other priority issues were the topic of an invitational conference on school nursing in 1994, which called for more appropriate and greater access to educational opportunities for school nurses, the support of additional outcomes-based research, and the need for further policy development regarding the role of the school nurse in supervising unlicensed assistive personnel in the care of students (National Nursing Coalition for School Health, 1995).

Physicians

Services Provided. While the number and role of "school physicians," per se have declined over the years, physicians have increasingly been assuming roles as consultants and advocates. Physicians are involved in schools and school health programs from many vantage points, including

---

[4]SREB states are Alabama, Arkansas, Florida, Georgia, Kentucky, Louisiana, Maryland, Mississippi, North Carolina, Oklahoma, South Carolina, Tennessee, Texas, Virginia, and West Virginia.

serving as public health officials to university teachers and researchers and as generalist and specialist providers of direct patient services. The services they provide include consultation on health policy, health curricula, and evaluation of programs and services; direct consultation regarding individual patients or groups of patients; and participation in provision of health services at the school site. Asthma specialists have set up asthma education programs, orthopedic surgeons have set up scoliosis screening and sports medicine programs, and pediatricians have advocated for and helped to develop sexuality education and health education programs. With the recent emphasis on education for all students with disabilities, the diagnosis of conditions and review of programs for these students have become additional responsibilities. Community primary care physicians (pediatricians and family physicians) frequently interact with the schools' health programs as linkages to ancillary services for their patients' medical, learning, and behavioral problems. They also assist with assessing community health needs and resources and devising mechanisms to coordinate school and community services.

Personnel. The training and certification of physicians who interact with the schools depends on their own discipline and specialty rather than standards of the school health program. Many pediatric residencies now offer community pediatrics experiences that often include school health. New residency requirements, which were put into effect in 1996, specify a defined community pediatrics experience in order for a program to meet American Academy of Pediatrics Board requirements. Physicians are typically not employees of the school system; instead, their services are usually provided by contractual agreements with hospitals, universities, clinics, and HMOs. Insurance and malpractice issues usually dictate that their source of employment be able to handle such coverage for physician activities routinely.

Important Issues. As described in Chapter 2, physicians have been active in school health programs to varying degrees since the mid-nineteenth century. The boundaries between private medical practice and school health programs, which arose during the period of the National Education Association–American Medical Association alliance from the 1920s to the 1960s, are now beginning to disappear, and schools are receiving increased attention as strategic sites for health promotion and access points for primary care. In order to meet these demands, expanded and improved education in school health is needed in the medical and residency education of physicians. In addition, mechanisms and incentives are needed for effectively involving community providers of primary and secondary health care with school programs, both in direct provision of care and in consultative roles.

Innui (1992) has pointed out that there is a social contract between the public and the medical field; optimal medical practice and research should not be thought of as ends in themselves but rather as means to sustaining the health of the population. Physicians, especially pediatricians, meet this social contract by working in the societal domain outside the usual practice setting; work in or for schools is a prime example. There is a strong subset among those concerned with the future of the medical field who believe that it is an increasingly important responsibility of medicine to prepare physicians to work in the social domain, including schools (Elias et al., 1994).

Dentists

Earlier in this century, many schools had established dental clinics, but in recent years schools have typically provided only a low level of dental services. Still, dental health needs are pressing. Dental services often are not covered by insurance, and families postpone seeking preventive treatment until more expensive services are necessary. Many children and young people, especially in disadvantaged and rural areas, have no access to a family dentist. As a result, a few school-based clinics have added dental services to their protocols.

A 1992 survey of 87 school districts selected as exemplary models for school health programs, conducted by the National School Boards Association, revealed that about one-half provided some type of dental services (Poehlman and Manager, 1992). A follow-up survey (with a 35 percent response rate) showed that most of the activity was located in elementary schools. Three-fourths of the schools with dental services provided screening at the school, about one-fourth also offered teeth cleaning, and one in ten gave fluoride rinses or sealants for the prevention of tooth decay. Actual treatment was provided in more than one-third of the schools with dental programs, while education for dental health was offered in two-thirds. In some schools, toothbrushes and toothpaste were distributed. In others, local dentists gave presentations, contributed their services at schools, or accepted referrals with low or no fee. In some communities, a local service club was active in providing funds for school dental services.

Although from a national perspective the oral health of children has probably never been better, it is estimated that about 80 percent of dental caries of school-age children exist in approximately 20 percent of the population—most of whom are lower-income subgroups (National Institute of Dental Research, 1995). Health examination surveys conducted by the National Center for Health Statistics found that the most significant problems detected among U.S. children were "dental problems" (Starfield, 1992). The National Institute of Dental Research of the National Institutes of Health conducts a variety of research and demonstration studies and carries out periodic surveys concerning the oral health of school children. However, there do not appear to be dedicated, coherent funding streams for school dental services; rather, dental services, if they exist at all, are typically provided on a local ad hoc basis, often involving volunteers and donated or reduced-cost services.

Services for Students with Special Needs

In 1975, Congress enacted the landmark Education of the Handicapped Act, which in 1990 was renamed the Individuals with Disabilities Education Act (IDEA). The act requires free and appropriate education for all children with disabilities, including those with physical or mental disorders, in the least restrictive setting from birth through age 21.

Federal law holds all state and local education agencies responsible for formulating Individualized Education Plans for all students with disabilities and for providing the special education and related services they require. These services include everything from physical and speech therapy and psychological services to intensive nursing care and case management. Congress annually appropriates funds to help state and local education agencies carry out this mandate, but many of the costs for special education services must be financed from state and local government revenues.

Examples of professionals providing these specialized services, in addition to school nurses, consulting physicians, and dietitians include the following:

- **Physical therapists** emphasize the remediation of, or compensation for, mobility, gait, muscle strength, and postural deficits. According to the American Physical Therapy Association, 3 percent of the association's members work in schools.
- **Occupational therapists** focus on remediation of or compensation for perceptual, sensory, visual motor, fine motor, and self-care deficits. More than one-third of the membership of the American Occupational Therapy Association work in the schools.
- **Speech, language, and hearing therapists** provide special education and related services and work closely with teachers and parents to help children overcome communication problems. More than one-half of the members of the American Speech, Language, and Hearing Association work in schools. Speech, language and hearing problems represent

25 percent of children's primary disabilities in schools; another 50 percent of children with other primary disabilities have speech, language, and hearing problems as additional disabilities.

• **Audiologists** are certified professionals who specialize in the identification and management of children's hearing impairments in the school setting. According to the Education Audiology Association, approximately 1,000 audiologists are employed by school districts across the country.

An issue of general concern in special services is the lack of trained professionals who are interested in working in the schools, for often case loads are greater and salaries lower than in other health care settings. As a result, these services sometimes are provided by paraprofessionals and assistants, under the supervision of a professional. Another issue is that eligibility of students for these services is determined by the state and/or local school system, based on recommendations of a team that may or may not include professionals in the special services fields. Further, although the special education law appears to be an entitlement, in fact, not all students with disabilities are served. Those with emotional disturbances are neglected; among those identified, less than one-third received social work, psychological, or other counseling services. Knitzer (1989) estimated that only 19 percent of students with serious emotional problems are being served.

Mental Health or Pupil Services

These services typically include school psychology, counseling, and social work, as well as the health services personnel (e.g., physicians and nurses) previously described. There is considerable overlap and collaboration among these fields, with their mutual emphasis on maximizing students' potential and addressing students' academic, psychological, and social problems. School psychologists tend to focus on special learning and behavior problems, school counselors on academic and career-related guidance, and school social workers on family and community factors that influence learning. In today's climate of limited resources, lack of funding has sometimes resulted in extremely high ratios of students to providers, making these services not fully available or accessible.

School Psychologists

Services Provided. Services provided by school psychologists can be categorized as follows:

- **Consultation:** Collaborate with teachers, parents, and other school personnel about learning, social, emotional, and behavioral problems.
- **Education:** Provide educational programs on classroom management strategies, parenting skills, substance abuse, and teaching and learning strategies.
- **Research:** Evaluate the effectiveness of academic programs, behavior management procedures, and other services provided in the school setting.
- **Assessment:** Work closely with parents and teachers, using a variety of techniques, to evaluate academic skills, social skills, self-help skills, and personality and emotional development.
- **Intervention:** Work directly with students and families to help solve conflicts related to learning and adjustment. Provide psychological counseling, social skills training, behavior management, and other interventions.

School psychological services are one of the related services designated by the Individuals with Disabilities Education Act to be available to students with disabilities who are in need of special education. School psychologists also work with other targeted school-related groups, such as Head Start.

Personnel. School psychologists are found in all 15,000 local education agencies in all states and territories, as well as in U.S. Department of Defense schools. Most are employed by the local education agency; cooperatives are also found in rural areas and areas that have many small school systems. The National Association of School Psychologists (NASP) recommends a ratio of one school psychologist for every 1,000 students, but the actual national average is closer to 1:2,100. Funding often comes from a combination of streams, including such federal sources as IDEA, the Elementary and Secondary Education Act (ESEA), and Head Start. Medicaid can be used to fund school psychological services for Medicaid-eligible children with disabilities. All school psychologists are required to be certified and/or licensed by the state in which services are provided, and requirements vary from state to state. NASP offers a national certification that requires a master's or higher degree in school psychology, an extensive internship in a school setting, a passing score on the National School Psychology exam, and continuing professional education. The ESEA legislation of 1994 defined school psychology standards.

Important Issues. School psychology has long been perceived as a marginal, special education assessment service rather than as a full system of mental health or education services for the mainstream, although this situation appears to be changing. Policymakers are beginning to recognize that education reform requires attention to the social-emotional barriers to learning. School psychologists maintain that increased expertise is necessary to deal with greater cultural diversity and educational demands of a technological workplace, as well as interdisciplinary teamwork. However, retraining and professional development are often supported inadequately within state and local budgets. Although gains have been made in the understanding and practice of school psychology, there is currently no office or program within the U.S. Department of Education, or any other federal agency, to support ongoing research in this area. Much remains to be learned about the relationship between psychological and other student-related services and student academic performance or other outcomes.

School Counselors

Services Provided. School counselors are specialists who assist students, school staff, parents, and community members in problem-solving and decisionmaking on issues involving learning, development, and human relations. Counseling can take place in individual, small group, or large group settings. Counselors provide services, from one-on-one counseling on a student's individual problems to large group sessions with teachers to explore effective cooperative learning strategies. Traditionally, school counseling has been associated with career and vocational guidance. School counselors typically advise students in course selections, career options, college application procedures, and school-to-work programs. School counselors are increasingly called upon to work on interdisciplinary teams with school nurses, psychologists, social workers, and other school staff.

Personnel. Counselors are usually employed by the school district. They typically have an education background with additional training in the behavioral sciences, counseling, theory, and skills related to the school setting. Through the American School Counselor Association, which has 13,000 members, standards and ethics have been developed for the profession. Each state has its individual certification requirements and laws pertaining to the practice of school counseling. Many states prescribe a ratio of one counselor for every 500 students, although the ratio is much higher, more than 1:1,000 in some states. School counselors are found at levels K–12, but they are less prevalent at the elementary level.

Important Issues. There is a perception among school counselors that they are underutilized and have been stereotyped by the fact that the school counseling movement originated with vocational guidance as its focus. Given schools counselors' background in human behavior and human relations, their role is likely to continue to expand and overlap with those of other pupil services personnel. Another issue for school counselors is the balance between providing help to children from difficult family situations while at the same time respecting private family matters.

School Social Workers

Services Provided. School social workers consider themselves the link among the home, school, and community. Although school social workers and school counselors frequently perform similar tasks, the counselor's focus tends to be inward on the internal functions and programs of the school, whereas the social worker's focus tends to be outward on the family and community context. Social workers regularly deal with discipline and attendance problems, child abuse and neglect, divorce and family separation, substance abuse, and issues involving pregnancy and parenting, suicide, and even family finances. Services provided by school social workers include the following:

- individual and group counseling;
- support groups for students and parents;
- crisis prevention and intervention;
- home visits;
- social-developmental assessments;
- parent education and training;
- professional case management;
- information and referral;
- collaboration with other pupil services personnel and with community agencies;
- advocacy for students, parents, and the school system;
- coordination of programs such as Head Start, mentoring, and peer counseling; and
- school staff development and policy development, such as discipline and attendance policies.

Social work is also considered a "related service" that students are entitled to under IDEA. ESEA recognized school social workers as part of pupil services teams serving students in Title I programs, Even Start, Safe and Drug-Free Schools, and related legislated programs.

Personnel. The National Association of Social Workers (NASW) estimates that nationwide there are at least 13,000 school social workers. Most of them are employed by the educational system, although some are employed by community agencies. Funding is at least partially provided by ESEA Title I and IDEA funds in most districts. School social workers typically possess a master's degree in social work. As of June 1995, more than 30 states require school social work certification by their educational agency, and some states also require licensure by their social work licensing board. The National Teachers Examination contains a section on school social work, and the NASW has developed a voluntary school social work specialist credential for those with advanced training and experience.

Important Issues. Coordination of social work services provided by outside community agencies with those provided by the school is an important matter. School social workers believe they are better attuned to address situations involving the educational goals of the schools, since they are located within the system. As with other pupil services personnel, school social work is often threatened by budget cuts during a time of financial constraints. Another issue is the challenge of interpreting to educators how social work services can contribute to improving the educational performance of students.

Mechanisms for Providing Mental Health and Pupil Services

Pupil Personnel Teams. This term typically refers to a team composed of the school social worker, guidance counselor, nurse, and psychologist. The team meets with the principal and selected teachers to review "cases" and ensure that everyone is working together to address the needs of students and their families. The major pupil personnel agencies have joined together to form the National Alliance of Pupil Services Organizations, whose mission is to promote interdisciplinary approaches to their professions and to support integrated service delivery processes (National Alliance of Pupil Services Organizations, 1992). The group's policy statement spells out the roles for its 2.5 million professional constituents: "School-based pupil services personnel, who are responsible for delivering education, health, mental health, and social services within school systems, comprise a critical element which forms a natural bridge between educators and community personnel who enter schools to provide services . . . . They can serve to mediate, interpret, and negotiate between other school personnel and persons entering the school from the outside."

Adelman and Taylor (1997) promote the creation of a Resource Coordinating Team, which would focus on identifying resources rather than individual cases. This team "provides a necessary mechanism for enhancing systems for coordination, integration, and development of intervention . . . ensures that effective referral and case management systems are in place, [works on] communication among school staff and with the home . . . [and] explores ways to develop additional resources." The Resource Coordinating Team includes, in addition to pupil personnel team members, special education and bilingual teachers, dropout counselors, and representatives from relevant community agencies.

As mentioned previously, budget cuts have forced many school systems to cut back on pupil personnel staff, particularly in disadvantaged communities. Social workers and psychologists are often shared between schools, which increases demands on their time and prevents their working in teams. An approach that has been tried in some needy areas is for outside agencies, with funding separate from the school budget, to put together teams and locate them in schools.

Student Assistance Programs. Many schools have Student Assistance Programs that were developed initially to help students who were abusing alcohol or other drugs. These programs, funded through the Drug Free Schools Act, are modeled after the successful Employee Assistance Programs in industry that were established to assist workers with alcohol problems. Just as the employee programs have steadily enlarged their range of services, the Student Assistance Programs movement has also expanded its scope to address the variety of problems that interfere with student learning. Students exhibiting problems might be referred to external mental health professionals or to internal support groups and counseling organized by the school. Problems addressed include such divergent topics as substance abuse, absenteeism, weight management, reentry to school after treatment in a detoxification center, and the difficulties of being a child of alcoholics or divorced parents.

Nutrition and Foodservice

Services Provided. School food and nutrition services vary significantly from school to school depending on the perceived needs, resources, and priorities of schools and communities. School food- and nutrition services can be categorized as follows:

- federally supported, nonprofit school lunches, breakfasts, and snacks, including those for students with special health care needs;
- for-profit food programs, including snack bars, school stores, vending machines, á la carte items sold in school cafeterias, and special functions for students or staff;
- nutrition education activities integrated with classroom instruction;

- nutrition screening, assessments, and referral; and
- foodservice provided for nonschool populations, including child care, Head Start, elderly feeding, summer feeding, and contract services that meet the needs of local communities.

The National School Lunch Act established the National School Lunch Program (NSLP) in 1946, both to prevent the malnutrition that was discovered in army recruits and to provide an outlet for farm surpluses. In 1970, Congress established uniform national income guidelines for free and reduced-price meals. The School Breakfast Program (SBP) was authorized as a pilot in 1966 and made permanent in 1975. All lunches and breakfasts served under the NSLP and SBP are subsidized by the U.S. Department of Agriculture (USDA) in the form of cash reimbursements and commodities. All students are eligible to participate, although varying prices are charged based on the student's income and family size. Students whose family incomes are 130 or percent less of the poverty level qualify for free meals, whereas students with family incomes between 130 and 185 percent of the poverty level qualify for reduced-price meals. The price for paid meals is established by the local school district. There is no federal mandate for schools to provide these school lunch or school breakfast programs, although a few states have legislation requiring schools to make lunch and/or breakfast available to students.

Nationwide, almost 60 percent of students eat the school lunch and about 15 percent eat the school breakfast (Food Research and Action Center, 1996). In announcing its "Healthy Kids: Nutrition Objectives for School Meals" initiative in June 1994, the USDA stated that the National School Lunch Program is available in 95 percent of public schools, which are attended by 97 percent of public school children, and that about 59 percent of all public school children participate (USDA, 1994). A 1993 U.S. General Accounting Office (GAO) study reported that 6,400 private schools, about 30 percent of the total, also offer the NSLP (U.S. GAO, 1993b). There are major differences among states in the percentage of students who eat school meals. USDA data for school year 1993 show a high of 80.5 percent of Louisiana students eating the school lunch and a low of 40.1 percent of New Jersey students doing so (USDA, 1994). In New Jersey, 53.2 percent of school lunches were served free to students, while 63.1 percent were served free in Louisiana. The average of 26 million school lunches served each day is about 1 million less than the participation rate in 1979, prior to major federal funding cuts in the 1980s.

More than 6.5 million students in almost 65,000 schools participate in the SBP, a number that has grown consistently (Food Research and Action Center, 1996). The SBP may never achieve the same level of participation as the NSLP, since almost 60 percent of students report eating breakfast at home (Burghardt and Devaney, 1993). However, many students who do not eat at home do not have access to the SBP either because it is not offered at their school or because transportation and class schedules do not allow time to eat. Studies confirm that on any given day, 12 to 26 percent of students come to school without having eaten anything (Burghardt and Devaney, 1993; Sampson et al., 1995). A significantly greater proportion of students skipping breakfast failed to achieve dietary adequacy for nearly every nutrient studied, compared to students who ate breakfast (Sampson et al., 1995). Schools that are not yet offering the SBP or those in which transportation or other problems hinder participation may want to reexamine their needs and how difficulties might be overcome.

Many school cafeterias offer individual food items that students may purchase in addition to or instead of the school lunch or breakfast. These foods are described as á la carte options. Other foodservice options, such as vending machines, school stores, and snack bars, are often made available. These are sometimes operated by the school nutrition and foodservice department but are most often operated by the school principal or a school organization designated by the principal. Foods sold outside the reimbursable school lunch and school breakfast are not subject to USDA nutrition standards, with the exception that no carbonated beverages, water ices, hard candies, or chewing gum may be sold in the foodservice area (USDA, 1986). These restrictions do not apply to other areas of the school.

The use of the school cafeteria as a "laboratory" in which students can learn about foods and nutrition and practice decisionmaking skills learned in the classroom was called for by Congress in the Nutrition Education and Training (NET) Program. The NET Program was designed to "teach children, through a positive daily lunchroom experience and appropriate classroom reinforcement, the value of a nutritionally balanced diet, and to develop curricula and materials for training teachers and school foodservice staff to carry out this task" (P.L. 95-166, Child Nutrition Act as amended November 10, 1977). The provision of healthful meals in an environment that promotes healthy eating enhances the ability of the health education curriculum to achieve several of the performance indicators called for by the National Health Education Standards—including indicator 3, "to demonstrate the ability to practice health-enhancing behaviors and reduce health risks," and indicator 6, "to demonstrate the ability to use goal setting and decision-making skills to enhance health."

Consensus on the importance of integrating nutrition screening, counseling, and referral as integral components of health services is growing. At this time, few school nutrition and foodservice departments have adequate staff to provide these services. Other school health service providers (on-site or contracted) may be responsible for screening students for nutrition problems, making referrals to qualified nutrition professionals, and providing support and reinforcement for the nutrition care provided (American Dietetic Association et al., 1995).

Meals for students with special health care needs are an increasing aspect of school foodservice and nutrition programs. Although the cost of food is similar to that in regular programs, labor and administrative expenses make these meals more costly. If nutrition goals are part of an Individualized Education Plan, special education funds may be provided for costly food products and counseling. Medicaid is another potential source of funds. The family may not be charged for additional costs of meeting the dietary requirements of students with special needs.

The foodservice operation in many schools is responding to community needs, forging new partnerships, and generating new revenue by providing services for populations outside the school. Using existing space, equipment, and personnel, schools can often provide meals for elderly feeding, summer feeding, child and adult day care, and other community groups. Some schools have even developed large catering operations for public events.

Personnel. As early as the 1930s, major teacher training institutions established a curriculum in school foodservice. When the National School Lunch Act was passed in 1946 and school foodservice and nutrition emerged as a profession, dietitians and home economists were the early leaders (Frank et al., 1987). At the present time, USDA has no specific requirements for school foodservice and nutrition program directors or managers. A 1993 survey by the National Food Service Management Institute found that 2.6 percent of directors had less than a high school education, 38.8 percent had a high school diploma, 19.9 percent had taken some college courses, 23.3 percent had a college degree, and 15.5 percent had earned a graduate degree (Sneed and White, 1993). According to SHPPS, few states or local school districts have established standards for school foodservice directors, and only 2.8 percent of directors are registered dietitians (Pateman et al., 1995). If nutrition screening, assessments, and counseling are provided by the school, consulting dietitians, nurses, or public health staff are often used.

Important Issues. There is consensus today that school nutrition and foodservices are important to learning readiness, health promotion, and disease prevention (National Research Council, 1989; U.S. Department of Health and Human Services, 1988, 1991). The *Healthy People 2000* goals call for at least 90 percent of school lunch and breakfast services to be consistent with the Dietary Guidelines for Americans and for at least 75 percent of schools to provide nutrition education from preschool through grade 12 (U.S. Department of Health and Human Services, 1991). School nutrition can also have an effect on the goal to reduce the incidence of being overweight to a prevalence of no more than 15 percent among adolescents and on the goal to increase calcium intake so that at least 50 percent of youth and young adults consume three or more servings daily of calcium-rich foods.

Children's cognitive, behavioral, and physical performance is impaired by poor nutrition (Center on Hunger, Poverty, and Nutrition Policy, 1993; Centers for Disease Control, 1996; Meyers et al., 1989). Awareness of these findings is important for school administrators and teachers, who are likely to view nutrition as a priority only to the extent that it facilitates their primary mission—education (American Dietetic Association et al., 1995).

However, despite the clear connection of nutrition to health and of health to education, there is a wide variance in the priority placed on school nutrition and foodservice across the country. Students today have increasing food options at school. The School Nutrition Dietary Assessment study found that the most prevalent option was still a lunch brought from home, although vending machines, school stores, snack bars, and á la carte food items offered in addition to the school meal are increasingly available. Some of these choices contained as little as 20 percent of the recommended dietary allowances (RDAs) for certain nutrients, and none was equal in nutritional value to school lunches that met the USDA-mandated goals of one-third of the RDAs for key nutrients. School lunch participants ate more fruits and vegetables and drank more milk than did nonparticipants and were more likely to get their carbohydrates from grain and grain mixtures than were nonparticipants, whose carbohydrate sources were more likely to be sweetened beverages and salty snacks (Gordon and McKinney, 1995).

The USDA has published regulations requiring schools to plan menus with the goal of having no more than 30 percent of calories from fat and 10 percent of calories from saturated fat in the average meal selected by all students over a week. These standards will not apply to á la carte foods served in the cafeteria or to foods sold in snack bars, school stores, or vending machines. The regulations became effective in the 1996–1997 school year. Prior to the issuing of the USDA's recommendations, the School Nutrition Dietary Assessment study found that in 44 percent of school lunch programs, students had at least one menu option with no more than 30 percent of its calories from fat, but in only 1 percent of schools did all available school lunch menus have this low fat level.

Many intervention studies have focused on environmental changes and have shown promising results in lowering the fat content of meals selected by students (Ellison et al., 1989; Nicklas et al., 1989; Simons-Morton et al., 1991; Snyder et al., 1994; Whitaker et al., 1993). The Child and Adolescent Trial for Cardiovascular Health (CATCH), a multicenter school-based health promotion program funded by the National Heart, Lung, and Blood Institute, tested the effectiveness of the Eat Smart School Nutrition Program in four states in 96 public elementary schools with more than 5,000 students (Perry et al., 1990). Data collected on this baseline measurement cohort during the period 1991 to 1994 show that in intervention school lunches, the percentage of calories from fat decreased significantly more (38.7 to 31.9 percent) than in controls (38.9 to 36.2 percent). The level of student self-reported daily energy intake from fat also was significantly reduced in intervention schools (32.7 to 30.3 percent) compared to controls (32.6 percent to 32.2 percent) (Luepker et al., 1996).

Policy decisions are important to maximizing program influence on current and future eating behaviors of students. Among the policies that local schools and communities must address in order to achieve a school nutrition and foodservice program that meets national goals are those that relate not only to nutrition standards but also to consideration of student preferences, purchasing practices, production methods, professional development of school nutrition staff, team building for school staff and community members, development of eating environments that provide optimum time, space, support for healthful choices, positive supervision, and role modeling (American School Food Service Association, 1994). Policies are also necessary to guard against such problems as those that recently arose in the New York City schools, where foodservice management was reorganized after criticism that it approved shipments of outdated meat and covered up outbreaks of food poisoning (Rousseau, 1995).

Funding for school meals also has major implications for program outcomes. Private funds raised by the community financed the first programs in the late 1800s and early 1900s. Local boards of education later added the program to their budgets, and limited federal support, primarily through work programs in the 1930s, provided subsidies that encouraged schools to provide school lunches. The first specific federal legislation was the National School Lunch Act of 1946, which provided an incentive to local schools to operate nutritionally sound programs. It was not until the 1960s that additional funding was provided for schools with large numbers of low-income children.

In the 1980s, federal support for school nutrition programs declined significantly. Adjusted for inflation, federal funding for school lunch is only 58 percent of its initial 1946 level (Citizens' Commission on School Nutrition, 1990). Local and state funding has also declined, and school nutrition and foodservice programs in many communities are expected to operate as businesses with no local support. SHPPS reported that 29 percent of all middle or junior and senior high schools were expected to generate funds beyond the costs of the program.

Profit-making has become pervasive in the school nutrition and food-service environment. SHPPS reported that more than one-third (37.2 percent) of schools reported that they have been contacted by a fast-food company interested in providing food for students, and foodservice management companies have increased their focus on the school market. Operating in such an environment, school nutrition programs are under great pressure to attract student customers even if it means compromising the nutrition integrity of meals or á la carte offerings. Decisions on food offerings often are based on the food item's profit margin rather than on its nutritional profile. Some observers maintain that such decisions send the message that it is acceptable to compromise health for financial reasons, a message inconsistent with classroom education (American Dietetic Association, 1991). The degree to which students' nutritional intake and lifelong eating behaviors are influenced by this environment and by the local, state, and federal policies that impact the environment merits further study.

Policies that promote universal access to healthful meals are widely viewed as important to the health of children and youth (American Dietetic Association et al., 1995; National Health Education Consortium, 1993; Nestle, 1992). However, the increase in for-profit options in schools has not only encouraged students to make selections that are not covered by nutritional standards, but also emphasized the social distinctions between students with unlimited dollars to spend on for-profit foods of their choice and students receiving free or reduced-price meals or those from working poor families who can afford only the price of the paid meal. A USDA study identified 4.1 million eligible low-income students who did not apply for free or reduced-price meals; stigma has been cited as a possible reason (Abt Associates, 1990).

Children's recognition of the importance of healthful eating is increasing. A 1994 Gallup survey of students between the ages of 9 and 15 found that 97 percent agreed that a balanced diet is very important for good health, 96 percent liked eating different types of foods, and 87 percent agreed that eating smaller amounts of a variety of foods is better than eating large amounts of only a few. Yet one-half the respondents (51 percent) said they skip breakfast and 28 percent skip lunch (International Food Information Council, 1995).

The dynamic nature of school nutrition and foodservice requires directors and managers with strong skills in financial and program management that include the ability to provide services for students with special health care needs, to coordinate the instructional component with health educators and teachers, and to serve as an effective member of the school–community health team. Strong inservice programs for food-service assistants are critical to successful implementation.

Increased understanding by school administrators and other community leaders of the relationship between the school nutrition and food-service program and children's health and education will lead schools and communities to establish expectations consistent with community values and resources and to implement policies that maximize outcomes.

EXTENDED SERVICES

The term "extended services" is used here to refer to the rapidly growing area of services that go beyond traditional basic school health services. Extended services often target individual students with limited access to services and students at risk, are usually supported with funds from outside the educational budget, and typically involve collaboration between the school and personnel from community agencies. The design of extended services programs often relies on research related to the prevention and/or management of high-risk behaviors of children and youth (e.g., the importance of individual attention, on-site diagnosis and treatment, confidentiality, and effectiveness of therapeutic protocols). Much of the information in this section is adapted from a paper on extended services that can be found in Appendix D.

Questions are sometimes raised about whether extended services go beyond the basic mission of the schools. The committee believes that these services should not be the sole—or even major—responsibility of the schools but require leadership and cooperation from other community agencies and providers. In examples described in this section and in Appendix D, extended services are not another responsibility that must be shouldered by the school; instead, the school is considered by community agencies and providers as a partner and an effective site for provision of needed services—services that will ultimately advance the primary academic mission of the school. This view is consistent with that of a recent report from the Committee for Economic Development (1994), which states:

> Schools are not social service institutions; they should not be asked to solve all our nation's social ills and cultural conflicts. States and communities must lift the burden of addressing children's health and social needs from the backs of educators. They must, of course, arrange needed services for children and their families, often in collaboration with the schools. But other state and community agencies should pay for and provide these services so that schools can concentrate on their primary mission: learning and academic achievement.

School-Based Health Centers

School-based health centers—also called school-based clinics—are a response to the growing health needs and decreasing access to health services of many students. There are now about 650 SBHCs in almost all parts of the country, and the number continues to grow rapidly. SBHCs are most frequently located in inner city high schools, but they are also increasingly found in middle and elementary schools. According to SHPPS, at least one SBHC exists in 11.5 percent of all school districts (Small et al., 1995).

An SBHC consists of one or more rooms within a school building or on the property of the school that are designated as a place where students can go to receive primary health services. An SBHC is more than a school nursing station; students can receive on-site diagnosis and treatment services from one or more members of an interdisciplinary team of clinicians that may include physicians, nurse practitioners, nurses, social workers, health aides, and similar professionals. Examples of provided services include physical examinations, treatment for minor injuries and illnesses, screening for sexually transmitted diseases (STDs), pregnancy tests, and psychosocial counseling. Usually outside agencies—health departments, hospitals, medical schools, schools of nursing, or social service agencies—manage the SBHC and employ the practitioners; these agencies often keep the SBHC open or serve as backup after school hours and during weekends, summers, and other vacations. Service providers in SBHCs are typically selected—often self-selected—for their interest in working with children and young people in such a setting. Studies have shown that SBHCs remove barriers to care and are particularly suited to meet adolescents' needs for trust and confidentiality (U.S. General Accounting Office, 1994b).

For secondary schools with SBHCs, some of the most frequently provided services to students are listed in Table 4-4 (Santelli et al., 1995). Most SBHCs also provide health education and health promotion in the clinic, the classroom, for staff, and even for the community. A majority of SBHCs offer health education in classrooms in clinic schools, and most run group counseling sessions in reproductive health care, family problems, asthma control, dealing with depression, and other relevant subjects. It is not always clear how these services interface with the school and whether they complement or duplicate existing school programs.

In some communities, a school-based health services program provides care for more than one school. A mobile van is equipped to go from school to school to provide physical examinations, ambulatory services, immunizations, and referrals for more comprehensive medical and dental care. For example, Baltimore has a mobile van program operated by

TABLE 4-4 Services Offered by School Base
Health Centers to Students

Service	Percentage of Clinics Offering Service
Nutrition education	97
Injury treatment	94
Physicals	88
Sports physicals	83
Prescriptions	82
Pregnancy testing	81
Laboratory services	81
Immunizations	78
Gynecological exams	70
Medications dispensed	70
Social work services	69
Chronic illness management	68
Outreach	58
Job counseling	25
Day care for children of students	15
Street outreach	13

SOURCE: Adapted from Santelli et al., 1995.

the University of Maryland School of Nursing and supported through special project funds from the state governor's office.

The average expenditure reported by SBHCs in 1993 was approximately $150,000; approximately $30,000 more was reported spent from in-kind or matching funds (Hauser-McKinney and Peak, 1995). The total of both amounted to $163 per enrolled student and $64 per student visit. Sources of funding included Maternal and Child Health (MCH) Title V block grants, Medicaid, Title XX (social services), Drug-Free Schools, and Title X (family planning). The Robert Wood Johnson Foundation (RWJ) has been instrumental in providing support for SBHCs through its School-Based Adolescent Health Care and Making the Grade initiatives.

Instructive "case studies" of a collection of SBHCs—including discussions of clinic origin, staffing, facilities, services, costs, impact, and ongoing concerns for each SBHC—are found in *School-Based Clinics That Work* (U.S. Department of Health and Human Services, 1993b). *Healthy Caring*, a process evaluation of RWJ's School-Based Adolescent Health Care Program, also provides useful lessons for further SBHC initiatives (Marks and Marzke, 1993). The National Health and Education Consortium has prepared a report providing information about SBHCs at the elementary school level (Shearer and Holschneider, 1995) and a primer for community health professionals to use in establishing elementary school-linked health centers (Shearer, 1995).

Other Extended Services

Mental Health Centers

One of the most important unmet needs of young people is mental health counseling. In addition, mental health and behavioral problems are sometimes associated with or aggravated by underlying biomedical factors. The demand for mental health services has led to the development of school clinics that have a primary function of screening and treatment for psychosocial problems (Adelman and Taylor, 1991). In some communities, mental health services are provided in a school center by personnel employed by community mental health agencies. Such a center is usually not labeled a "mental health" facility but is presented as a place where students can go for all kinds of support and remediation. A number of universities also have collaborative arrangements for internship experiences in schools for preprofessional students preparing to enter mental health counseling.

A network of school-based mental health programs has been organized by the School Mental Health Project of the Department of Psychology at the University of California in Los Angeles, which is working closely with the Center for School Mental Health Assistance being developed at the University of Maryland at Baltimore. These groups are establishing a national clearinghouse for school mental health that will provide continuing education, research, and technical assistance to enhance local school mental health programs and improve practitioner competence.

Cities in Schools

Cities in Schools, a national nonprofit organization that operates in more than 100 communities, brings health, social, and employment services into schools to help high-risk youngsters (Cities in Schools, 1988; Leonard, 1992). Each local entity has its own version, but in general the program involves "brokering" community social service and juvenile corrections agencies in the provision of case management services within the school building. In most programs, a case manager is assigned to each high-risk child, and local businesses arrange for mentoring and apprenticeship experiences. A wide array of partnerships has been established through the Cities in Schools program, involving Boys Clubs of America, VISTA, United Way, and the Junior League.

School-Based Youth Service Centers

School-based youth service centers provide a wide range of activities—including health services, counseling, recreation, and educational remediation—to needy adolescent students. Some centers deliver services on-site whereas others focus on coordination and referral to other community agencies. In 1988, Kentucky's school reform initiative called for the development of youth service centers in high schools in which more than 20 percent of the students were eligible for free school meals. In New York City, the Beacons program, created by the city's youth agency, supports community-based agencies to develop "lighted school houses" that offer a wide range of activities for young people and are open from early morning until late at night, as well as during weekends and summers (Dryfoos, 1994a).

Family Resource Centers

Family Resource Centers deliver, either at the school site or by referral to community providers, a set of comprehensive services—including parent education, child care, counseling, health services, home visiting, and career training—to students of all ages and their families (Igoe and Giordano, 1992). Funds are provided through various federal and state programs and private sources, such as the United Way. Some centers are located in school buildings; others are based in the community. A few states have passed legislation that appropriates funds for Family Resource Centers, including California, Connecticut, Florida, Kentucky, North Carolina, and Wisconsin (Kagan, 1991). Kentucky's legislation mandates that every elementary school with more than 20 percent of its students eligible for free lunch must have a Family Service Center (Dryfoos, 1994a).

Comprehensive Multicomponent Programs: Full-Service Schools

A number of school-based interventions have been initiated that address an array of interrelated issues, based on the premise that prevention approaches must be more holistic if they are to be successful. Many of the extended services discussed above are integrated into these efforts. Examples of services include family counseling, case management, substance abuse counseling, student assistance, parenting education, before- and after-school activities, youth programs, health care, and career training. Programs are typically put together by an outside organization that provides a full-time coordinator and other services to the school in order to implement all the separate pieces of the package.

Sometimes the term "full-service school" is applied to the most comprehensive models, although the definition of what constitutes full-service varies from place to place. The vision of a full-service school calls for restructured academic programs integrated with parent involvement and a wide range of services for students and families—health centers, family resource rooms, after-school activities, cultural and community activities, and extended operating hours. The term full-service schools is more reflective of an overall philosophy than of a particular type of delivery model or system. Students and families need a variety of services located in a variety of settings, and the key is networking school and community services to form an easily navigated, user-friendly, accessible system. Full-service schools strive to become a "village hub," in which joint efforts of the school and community agencies create a rich and supportive environment for children and their families (Dryfoos, 1994a).

Regional Approaches for Small School Districts

Approximately 85 percent of local school districts receive assistance from regional cooperative agencies, thereby allowing them to pool resources for health services, staff development, care of students with special needs, purchase of supplies, and technical assistance. A 1993 report of an investigation of these agencies' involvement in school health indicated considerable interest and activity in the delivery of school health services, including primary care. In light of the fact that 76 percent of school districts have a total enrollment of 2,500 students or less, a regional approach to the delivery of school health-related services is needed in such areas and has already been established in some situations (Igoe and Stephens, 1994).

RESEARCH ON SCHOOL HEALTH SERVICES

Basic School Health Services

Over the past three decades, research on traditional basic school health services has focused on four primary areas:

1. workforce issues (Bachman, 1995; Basco, 1963; Chen, 1975; Crowley and Johnson, 1977; Dungy and Mullins, 1981; Forbes, 1965; Frels, 1985; Goodwin and Keefe, 1984; Hilmar and McAtee, 1973; Johnson et al., 1983; Kalisch et al., 1983; Lewis et al., 1974; Lowis, 1964; McKaig et al., 1984; Oda et al., 1979; Piessens et al., 1995; Thurber et al., 1991);
2. organization, governance, and financing (Davis et al., 1995; Eisner, 1970; Howell and Martin, 1978; Igoe and Giordano, 1992; Meeker et al., 1986; Miller and Shunk, 1972; Patterson, 1967; Ratchick, 1968; Risser et al., 1985; Russo et al., 1982; Rustia et al., 1984; Small et al., 1995; Thurber et al., 1991; Yankauer and Lawrence, 1961);
3. student health needs (Bricco, 1985; Bryan, 1970; Cauffman et al.,

1969; Center for Health Economics Research, 1993; Cook et al., 1985; Korup, 1985; O'Neil et al., 1985; Spollen and Davidson, 1978; Starfield, 1992; U.S. Department of Health and Human Services, 1993a,b); and

4. the effectiveness of various screening tests and other interventions (Appelboom, 1985; Bricco, 1985; Brown et al., 1985; Frerichs, 1969; Goldberg et al., 1995; Harrelson et al., 1969; Jenne, 1970; Lewis and Lewis, 1990; MacBriar et al., 1995; Marcinak and Yount, 1995; Oda et al., 1985; Proctor, 1986; Risser et al., 1985; Roberts et al., 1969; Tuthill et al., 1972; Yankauer and Lawrence, 1961).

By far, the largest area of basic school health services research has been related to workforce, organization, and governance issues, particularly to the role, functions, and relationships of school health personnel to school administrators, classroom personnel, and others. Although much of this work has concentrated on nursing services, research has also examined dentists, physicians, school health assistants, counselors, social workers, and psychologists. Until the 1975 passage of the Education of the Handicapped Act (later renamed the Individuals with Disabilities Education Act) and the introduction of school-based student health centers around the same time, school-employed health service personnel limited their services to case finding and referral. Diagnosis and treatment services were the purview of primary care providers located in community health facilities. Consequently, the established line of authority for school health services, which frequently had clinicians reporting to nonclinicians in the school's chain of command, was rarely problematic. However, as increasing numbers of students have come to school in need of primary care and/or with special health needs that require clinical nursing care, the importance of closer links to the established community health system, both private and public, has become more apparent. For example, at least 40 percent of respondents to a survey involving supervisors of school nurses reported that they had no clinical preparation in the delivery of health services although they were expected to supervise complex nursing care, including tracheal suctioning, administration of medications, nasogastric tube feedings, and dressing changes (Igoe and Campos, 1991).

A nationwide investigation of the experiences of students with special health care needs, *The Collaborative Study of Children with Special Needs,* funded by the Robert Wood Johnson Foundation in the 1980s, recommended greater involvement of health care professionals in the planning and implementation of services (Robert Wood Johnson Foundation, 1988). Another nationwide investigation of the needs of children and youth with chronic illness (Hobbs et al., 1983) addressed the need to establish policies that would improve the quality of health care available at school for these students. Policies covering the administration of medication and home-bound students were given particular attention.

Another organization and workforce issue concerns the need for integrated school health services in which nurse, social worker, foodservice personnel, and others work together collaboratively as a team. Linked to this issue is the continuing evidence that well-prepared school health assistants paired with school nurses can, under supervision, manage basic services, which frees up nurses for more complex care and responsibilities befitting their preparation (Fryer and Igoe, 1996; Russo et al., 1982).

Traditionally, school health services have been the responsibility of local districts. Given the large number of small- and medium-size school districts—76 percent of districts have a total student enrollment of 2,500 students or less—a regional plan may potentially even out some of the maldistribution of school health services from one district to the next in a state as well as among states (Igoe and Stephens, 1994). The feasibility of a regional approach to the organization and delivery of school health services has been investigated by Igoe and Stephens (1994). Educational Service Agencies (ESAs) are intermediate educational agencies that act as cooperatives in approximately 85 percent of the nation's school districts, servicing such needs as staff development, bulk purchasing, and delivery of related services to students with special health needs. In the study, ESA administrators were contacted to determine their involvement in school health. Although the response rate was only about 50 percent, administrators reported being involved in a wide variety of school health activities, including traditional basic school health services, and they predicted increasing involvement in years to come. Another interesting qualitative finding was that ESA directors had considerable skill in identifying and negotiating financing arrangements for a variety of school services from both state and local education agencies. Based on the finding, the investigators recommended that ESAs may have untapped potential for devising new plans for financing school health services.

The issue of financing for school health services received almost no attention until the introduction of nurse practitioners and primary care into schools in the 1970s. Current efforts in this regard are described later in this chapter. However, one national school health demonstration project conducted from 1980 to 1985 did investigate financing for school health and primary care in schools and deserves mention (DeAngelis, 1981). According to Meeker and colleagues (1986), most school health service programs have sole-source financing provided by either a health or an education agency. An alternative approach recommended by the investigators is multisource financing, which involves both health and education agencies as well as other organizations that provide such services as primary care.

Some of the traditional population-focused basic school health services (e.g., screenings) have come under scrutiny. Although there has been little debate about the value of school-based screenings for vision and hearing, the value of growth screenings is uncertain. Furthermore, there is increasing evidence to suggest that scoliosis screening fails to meet the general criteria for screenings and therefore should no longer be recommended (Berg, 1993; Goldberg et al., 1995). Remaining to be evaluated with respect to mass screenings are such issues as the market value of these services and the value of a population-based approach versus a high-risk approach in which only those students needing screenings receive them at school.

Although investigations of the outcomes of traditional basic services have been limited, some of this work was well designed for its day, and the findings have influenced the development and evolution of school health services. For example, Basco (1963) conducted the first large-scale evaluation of school nurse activities. That study's finding of the need to better utilize the nurse's clinical and managerial skills has been confirmed on numerous occasions. Roberts and colleagues (1969) studied absence and attendance patterns of 2,000 students and developed a statistical model to use in evaluating the effects of changes in nursing practice on the functional state of students. By 1972, the focus of school health services research became further focused on students, and Lewis et al. (1974) explored the outcomes in situations in which students were empowered to become active participants in their own care during encounters with school nurses.

During the 1970s and 1980s, one principal area of research had to do with the effectiveness of the school nurse as a primary care provider, and another area of research concerned students with special health care needs. Three large studies during this period yielded valuable results: the Brookline Project, which investigated the developmental readiness of children (Levine et al., 1977); the Collaborative Study of Children with Special Needs (Walker, 1992); and the Vanderbilt study (Hobbs et al., 1983), which investigated the needs of students with chronic diseases. The Vanderbilt study established universal recommendations about the needs of students with chronic health conditions related to the pain they experience, the persistent sense of uncertainty that accompanies chronic health conditions, and the need for appropriate homebound policies and proper medication administration in the schools. Building on this work, Palfrey et al. (1992) developed Project School Care, which provided a comprehensive set of resources for schools regarding the management of students with special health needs.

Research on School-Based Health Centers and
Other Extended Services

Since school-based health centers and other extended services are a relatively new phenomenon, research on and evaluation of these programs are in the early stages. Many of these initiatives are special demonstration projects in a limited number of schools scattered throughout the country. A more complete discussion of selected findings from these initiatives is found in the background paper in Appendix D.

Much of the research has focused on school-based health centers. Studies over the past decade have shown that SBHCs can be implemented successfully in schools, enrolling substantial percentages of students (Dryfoos, 1994b; Kirby, 1994). SBHC users were reported to have received adequate care in a cost-effective manner and to be very satisfied with both the quality of the services and the caregivers. Research has documented that the services are used by youth who need them the most. Studies have also described the organization and functioning of SBHCs, as well as the barriers encountered and strategies for overcoming them. More challenging has been the conduct of studies on the impacts of SBHCs in terms of reducing risky behavior and improving long-term health and educational outcomes. Also, since many findings pertain to specialized initiatives dealing with targeted groups, it is not clear how generalizable the findings are to other settings and populations. Methodological difficulties in conducting research on school health programs are discussed further in Chapter 6. In spite of these limitations, it is possible to glean some interesting insights from existing studies, as described in the following sections.

Utilization Studies

A basic measure of program utilization is the number and fraction of students in a school enrolled in the SBHC. Typically, enrollment involves the submission of a form indicating parental consent to use the SBHC. Nonenrolled students can be treated for emergencies but then must go through the enrollment process. A related measure is the percentage of enrollees who actually use the facility.

Advocates for Youth reports that in 1993, about two-thirds of the students in the schools that responded were enrolled in their SBHCs, and 75 percent of them utilized the program over the reporting year (Hauser-McKinney and Peak, 1995). A survey supported by the Robert Wood Johnson Foundation of 19 schools showed identical proportions (Kisker et al., 1994a, 1994b).

Clinics responding to the Advocates for Youth survey reported that about 60 percent of enrolled students were female. One-third of the enrollees were African American, one-third white, 20 percent Latino, and the rest Asian, Native American, and other. Most reports show that although clinic users tend to mirror the student population in regard to race or ethnicity, females are more likely to use clinics, especially if reproductive health care is offered.

A study of a sample of students from nine Baltimore school-based clinics compared enrollees with nonenrollees (Santelli et al., 1996). It found that those enrolled were significantly more likely to have had health problems, came from families on Medicaid, were in special education, and were African American. Those who did not enroll reported a variety of reasons for their decision, primarily being satisfied with their current provider.

Enrollees in SBHCs show very different patterns of use. In one school-based clinic in Los Angeles, within a year, 5 percent of enrollees had made no visits, 41 percent had visited once, 39 percent had made two to five visits, 8 percent made six to ten visits, and 6 percent had used the clinic more than ten times (Adelman et al., 1993). Users reported ease of access as the most important reason for using the facility in the school and perceived the care provided as helpful and confidential. Nonusers said they did not use the clinic because they did not need it or were concerned about lack of confidentiality. In this sample, frequent clinic users were more likely to score high on indices of psychological stress. The investigators concluded that "an on-campus clinic can attract a significant number of students who otherwise would not have sought out or received such help" (Adelman et al., 1993).

Students who report higher rates of high-risk behaviors, such as substance abuse and early initiation of sexual intercourse, appear to be more likely to use school-based clinics than are other students. A study of students in four schools in Oregon showed a consistent and significant association between number of clinic visits and number of preexisting high-risk health behaviors (Stout, 1991). Only one-third of those students who reported no risk behaviors used the clinics as compared to more than two-thirds of the highest-risk students. In a study in Delaware, frequent users (three or more times) of school wellness centers were more likely than nonusers to report having engaged in such high-risk behaviors as suicide attempts, substance abuse, unprotected sexual activity, and eating-related purging (National Adolescent Health Resource Center, 1993).

Users of Denver's three high school clinics made an average of three visits per year (Wolk and Kaplan, 1993). However, a small number of students (11 percent) made 15 or more visits per year, accounting for 40 percent of all patient visits. These frequent visitors were significantly more likely to be females and to have lower grade point averages. Some 23 percent of the frequent visitors were diagnosed with mental health problems at the time of their initial visit, compared to 4 percent of the average users. By the end of the school year, 61 percent of all visits by frequent users were for mental health-related issues compared to 10 percent of all visits by the average users. High-risk behaviors—particularly unprotected sexual activity and use of alcohol and drugs (but not tobacco)—were significantly more prevalent among frequent users. It is important that most of the frequent users initially sought help for acute medical problems, at which time they were identified as students in need of mental health counseling. Many practitioners believe that the provision of comprehensive services in SBHCs offers a means for troubled students to enter into counseling and treatment for psychosocial problems. Youth are concerned about the stigma of attending a program specifically labeled "mental health," but are willing to participate if the program deals with broader health concerns.

The RWJ evaluation reports on the characteristics of the population of students in schools with SBHCs (rather than of students who used the clinics) (Kisker et al., 1994a). In these 19 schools, 15 percent were non-Hispanic white, 44 percent Hispanic, and one-third African American. One-fourth of the youths stated that their parents had not completed high school, and another one-third of the students said their parents had no post-secondary education. One in five families was on welfare, and one-third received free or reduced-price school lunches. In the 1992 follow-up survey, 30 percent of the health center school students reported that their families had no health insurance, 20 percent were covered by Medicaid, 31 percent had private insurance or belonged to an HMO, and the remaining 19 percent did not know what type of coverage they had.

Outcome Data

In the early 1980s, the potential of using SBHCs clinics as an integral part of pregnancy prevention efforts was stimulated by the publication of data from a study in St. Paul, Minnesota, which showed a decline in pregnancy rates in schools with clinics (Edwards et al., 1980). However, a later examination of birth rates showed large year-to-year fluctuations and no impact of the clinics (Kirby et al., 1993). In fact, a review of the other earlier studies showed mixed results for an array of behavior impact measures (Kirby, 1994). The studies that found positive effects on high-risk behaviors were offset by those that found negative effects or, more likely, no effects.

In general, studies have confirmed that the presence of a clinic in a school has no effect on the rates of sexual intercourse and little effect on contraceptive use, unless the clinic offers a visible pregnancy prevention program. A study that compared two schools with clinics that dispensed contraceptives on-site with two schools in which contraceptives were prescribed but not dispensed found few differences in contraceptive use. The only significant variable related to use was the greater number of contacts the students had with the clinic staff (Brindis et al., 1994).

Some initiatives targeting sexual behaviors are showing promising results, however. For example, the first evaluation of the California Healthy Start initiative presented data on 40 different grantees, including, 8 youth service programs, 5 of which are school-based clinics. Adolescent clients of programs that had an explicit goal of reducing teen pregnancy were found to have initiated sexual activity much less often and to have used a reliable form of contraception much more often (Wagner et al., 1994). Among teenagers in pregnancy prevention programs, about 45 percent were found to be sexually active after six months, a significant decrease from the proportion at intake (77 percent).

One of the most systematic outcome studies of SBHCs to date—the outcomes evaluation of the RWJ School-Based Adolescent Health Care Program—showed that although SBHCs provided access to care and increased students' health knowledge significantly, no reduction in high-risk behaviors could be measured (Kisker et al., 1994b). The SBHC users showed little or no difference relative to the comparison sample in sexual activity or use of alcohol, tobacco, and marijuana. These results are consistent with other interventions to reduce high-risk behavior, which generally have found that increased knowledge has little effect unless the environment and perceived norms are changed. Further, since clients of SBHCs tend to be students with greater problems and higher rates of risky behaviors than other students, it may not be reasonable to expect that an occasional clinic visit would turn their lives around.

Although results are sometimes inconclusive, other studies have shown generally positive effects of SBHCs and other extended services on absenteeism, behavior, and academic performance and on the use of hospital emergency rooms (McCord et al., 1993; Santelli et al., 1996; Wagner et al., 1994). The findings of a GAO study of six programs targeted at students at high risk for school failure are summarized in Table 4-5 (U.S. GAO, 1993a).

Cost-Benefit Studies

Several studies have estimated the cost-benefit ratio for SBHCs. One study estimated that if young people in New York State received early preventive care through school clinics, $327 million could be saved annually in hospitalizations for delivery of teen pregnancies, low-birthweight babies, and such chronic diseases as asthma (New York State Department of Health, 1994). A cost-benefit analysis of three California school-based

TABLE 4-5 Illustrative School-Linked Services Outcomes

Name	Target Population	Services	Outcomes
Project Pride, Joliet, Ill.	Grades 9–12 girls from AFDC families	Preemployment training Tutoring Academic and personal counseling Linkage to primary health and social services	28.8% of group still in high school, compared to 25.6% of control group 44.1% of group completed high school, compared to 37.8% of control group Data on attendance not reported
Focus on Youth	Grades K–12	Case management Counseling for alcohol or drugs Mentoring Primary health care Teen pregnancy case work Parenting services Job training or placement Mental health counseling Legal aid Recreation Shelter	Dropout rates for students enrolled in program from two schools, 12.8 and 8.9% compared with state estimated dropout rates for those schools of 66.4 and 49.3%, respectively Grade point averages climbed more rapidly than non-focus students, but over time both maintained a "C" Absenteeism varied greatly, making conclusion difficult

NYC Drop-Out Prevention Initiative (DPI)	At-Risk Students	Attendance outreach Counseling Alternative education courses Primary health care Conflict resolution training	Dropout rate lower for DPI students DPI did not improve courses passed for program participation
Texas Communities in Schools	K–12 students at risk for dropping out	Tutoring or mentoring Individual and group counseling Preemployment and vocational skills training Referrals to health and social services Home visiting	Decrease in dropouts rates from state average of 10% down to 5% Absences down by 18% 44% of students failing math raised grades to passing 42% of students failing English raised grades to passing
Walbridge Caring Community, St. Louis	Grades K–6	Academic tutoring Primary health care Recreation Day care Preemployment skills training for parents Case management	Academic achievement improved 26% Absenteeism not improved Dropout rates not examined
Hillsdale County Elementary Success Program	Grades K–6	Case management Home visits Students and family referred to needed services	Achievement improved, but students still perform slightly worse than nonparticipants Dropout rate not examined Absenteeism not reported

NOTE: AFDC = Aid to Families with Dependent Children. SOURCE: GAO, 1993a.

clinics compared the costs for the school services with the estimated cost in the absence of the school clinic (Brindis et al., 1995). Variables used included reduced emergency room use, pregnancies avoided, early pregnancy detection, and detection and treatment of the common STD, chlamydia. The ratios of savings to costs ranged from $1.38 to $2.00 in savings per $1.00 in costs, suggesting that the school clinic services were a good investment.

Potential Strengths and Weaknesses of School-Based Health Centers

The Johns Hopkins University Child and Adolescent Health Policy Center has recently published a report that analyzes the existing research on SBHCs and summarizes their strengths and weaknesses in improving access to primary care for adolescents (Santelli et al., 1995). This report defines primary care as having the following characteristics: "first contact, continuous, comprehensive, coordinated, community-oriented, family-centered, and culturally competent." The potential strengths and weaknesses of SBHCs in providing primary care identified by the report are outlined in Table 4-6.[5]

Research Needs

Many fundamental questions remain unanswered about SBHCs and other extended services. One of the most basic regards the relative advantages and disadvantages (in terms of quality, cost, and effectiveness) of providing primary care and social services at schools compared to providing these services at other sites in the community— for example, private physicians offices, other managed care providers, community clinics, or youth centers—or compared to not providing these services at all, as a function of the needs and characteristics of students and the community. A related question has to do with how the quality and effectiveness of SBHCs and other extended services should be defined and measured.

If SBHCs are indeed found to be a promising approach for many communities, then a broad research agenda will be needed to examine the implementation and dissemination of effective models. Greater understanding is needed about the best strategies for managing, staffing, and integrating the SBHC with the overall school program. Questions that must be addressed include: How does this activity get off the ground?

---

[5]The report notes that the primary care perspective is only one possible framework in which to view SBHCs; the focus in some communities may be on other extended social and family services.

TABLE 4-6 Potential Strengths and Weaknesses of School-Based Health Centers

Type of Primary Care	Strengths	Weaknesses
First-contact care	This type eliminates many barriers to access, reaches underserved, low-income, and high-risk populations, and often is the sole source of care. Successful in serving males, usually a more difficult group to reach.	Tight budgets restrict operation hours and days, resulting in access problems.
Continuous care	Continuous care can serve as "health care homes."	High turnover of personnel prevents long-term relationships between students and staff. Coverage must be arranged during summer, other vacations, evenings, and weekends.
Comprehensive care	A wide range of essential health services are usually provided. A variety of services to meet the physical, mental, and social needs of adolescents are provided. Adolescents use them for a variety of needs.	Little research has evaluated the adequacy and quality of the apparently wide range of services provided against the actual needs of the populations served. The scope of provided services is largely a function of funding. Provider availability may dictate scope of services offered. Many SBHCs are unable to provide a full range of reproductive health care services on site. Many centers are not able to employ full-time providers.
Coordinated care	Data management information and outcome analysis systems are increasingly being used. Some programs have successfully coordinated services with managed care organizations.	Difficulties are faced in coordinating care with other community providers. Little coordination occurs with managed care organizations.

continued on next page

TABLE 4-6 Continued

Type of Primary Care	Strengths	Weaknesses
Community-oriented care	Integrating a community or population perspective can meet the needs of all children and adolescents, involve the community in planning and governance, and provide an impetus for community needs assessment and resource mapping.	Few are able to expand their services beyond the student population.
Family-centered care	This type meets health care needs without disrupting everyday family functions. Limited data suggest popularity with parents and families. Efforts made to respect both confidentiality of clients and right of the family to be informed. Creative ways of involving families are being developed.	This type usually does not provide care to the entire family, thus limiting the gathering of family information and the development of client management strategies.
Culturally competent care	Culturally competent care provides care for culturally diverse populations.	Few data exist to allow assessment of cultural competence. A shortage of adequately trained bilingual or bicultural providers exists.

SOURCE: Adapted from Santelli et al., 1995.

Who calls the initial meeting, and what should be the lead agency in managing the program? What is the most cost-efficient staffing mix? How can SBHCs and backup referral agencies coordinate scheduling and other arrangements? What are the implications of an SBHC for health programs and health services personnel already at the school?

Studying the impacts and outcomes of SBHCs will be a long-term process. To begin this effort, however, uniform data collection standards and protocols should be established as soon as possible, not just for SBHCs but for other school health services providers as well. This will facilitate further research and allow data from various sources to be compared or aggregated as appropriate. An example of data inconsistency is the definition of what constitutes a "visit" with a school health provider. Some may consider this to include even a brief, spontaneous "drop-in" encounter. Others limit the term to a formal scheduled appointment. Still others may attempt to describe and categorize the nature of the visit. Such lack of standardization in data collection makes research and evaluation, including studies of cost-effectiveness, difficult. The committee does not believe that the costs associated with uniform data management will be an issue. Software packages are becoming easily available for record-keeping in school health services. For example, an electronic management information system called *School Health Care Online!!!* is already widely used in SBHCs; this system produces routine reports on utilization of services and serves as a basis for internal quality control (see Table 4-7) (Kaplan, 1995). The system is designed to collect information about the physical and mental health, health screening, and risk behaviors of clients, as well as epidemiologic, administrative, billing, and program outcome data. The software is set up to produce more than 100 preprogrammed reports, including linked files listing referrals, follow-up information, and statistical reports on users, immunizations, case management, and health screening.

MATCHING LEVEL OF SERVICES TO NEEDS

The question arises, how can a community determine whether only basic services are needed at a school or whether the situation calls for school-based primary care for students and other family services? Some states are beginning to define specific levels of services and assist local districts in matching these levels to needs at individual schools.

Missouri has described three levels of services, beginning with a core set of generalized services for schools with only minimal needs (Missouri School Children's Health Services Committee, 1993). Each succeeding level includes the services of the previous level, along with additional necessary services. Figure 4-1 illustrates this model.

Connecticut has defined five levels of services, with recommendations for matching school and community characteristics to level of services. This model is outlined in Box 4-1. Appendix G-3 describes in detail levels II through V, those levels beyond basic school health services. The Connecticut State Department of Public Health and Addiction Services will work with local communities in assessing their existing services and needs and developing the most appropriate level of services.

Florida enacted the Funding for School Health Services Act in 1990. This legislation provides funds for joint projects between county public health units and local school districts, particularly in areas where there is

TABLE 4-7 School Health Care ONLINE!!! Data Collection and Management Capabilities

Demographics
    Student and parent demographics
    Usual source of acute, primary, and emergency care
Visit Statistics
    Type of service provided
    Diagnoses and procedure codes
    Laboratory tests
    Morbidity data
    Prescriptions and other treatments
    Follow-up and referral dates and comments
Productivity
    Provider mix
    Complexity of user mix
    Provider time
Follow-up or referral tracking
    Tickler system for follow-up
    Referral tracking and completion rates
Billing
    HCFA, Medicaid, private insurance billing
    Sliding scale and fixed fee
    Accounting modules
Medical Case Management
    Detailed problem-specific interdisciplinary tracking and follow-up
    Clinical status and outcome assessment
    Follow-up prioritization
Problem List
    Active, inactive, and resolved problems and status for problem resolution
Health Screening
    User-defined health screening criteria
    Reports of normal, abnormal, and follow-up
Immunizations
    Automated immunization capture and documentation
    Report of recommended and delinquent immunizations
Clinical Information
    Measurements: height, weight, blood pressure
    Past medical history, allergies
    Medications prescribed
    Other treatments
Utilities
    Imports and exports
    User-defined variables
    Research statistical package interface
Health Education
    Individual and group health
    Education interventions

NOTE: HCFA = Health Care Financing Administration.

SOURCE: Kaplan, 1995.

FIGURE 4-1 Missouri School Children's Health Services Model Programs Schematic. SOURCE: Missouri School Children's Health Services Committee, 1993.

BOX 4-1
Connecticut Models

Connecticut Statewide Plan for Ensuring Primary Health Care, Substance Abuse and Mental Health Services for *All* Students

I. PHILOSOPHY

Every child or adolescent should have access to high-quality primary health care, substance abuse, and mental health services in his or her school. The design of services delivered in the school will be based on student needs.

II. MODELS OF SERVICE DELIVERY

LEVEL I: Basic School Health Services

This model should be in place in each of Connecticut's 998 public school buildings and available to all 478,300 (estimated) students age 3–21 years. The model addresses mandated basic school health but is not an enhancement of services to youth in need.

- Bachelor's-level school nurse (RN): Performs screenings, nursing assessments, referrals, triage functions; maintains student health records; meets daily student health needs.
- Master's-level clinically trained social worker or psychologist: Performs psychosocial assessments; provides services to special education students; short-term individual, family, and group counseling; and crisis intervention (ratio of one full-time equivalent to each 450 students, which may vary based on the needs of the students and the climate in the school).
- A qualified school medical adviser (M.D.) for every district; amount of time needed will vary with district size.
- Part-time support staff to carry out nonclinical functions and allow professional team to devote its time to addressing student needs.

LEVEL II: Increased Basic School Health Services

The school's volume of need is greater than can be met in Level I. Additional staff, including local pediatricians, would be added to meet the identified needs of the student population. More of the same types of service would be provided as outlined in Level I.

LEVEL III: Enhanced Clinical Services

Services beyond Level I and II may include the following:

- regular "built-in" consultation (i.e. psychiatrist, M.D., APRN, MSRD, MSW, and/or) and/or;
- clinical "in-school" services.

- APRN to deliver a higher level of primary care including physical exams, medical diagnosis and treatment, limited on-site lab tests, with more complex lab work available off-site.
- Master's-level mental health professionals to provide more intense and longer term individual, family, and group therapy to greater numbers of students (not only those receiving special education services).

LEVEL IV: School-Based Health Center (SBHC) Satellite Services

This model is designed for schools with student populations under 500 in high-need areas; hours of operation would be part-time and based on student need.

Staff would have the same background as those described in Level V and would travel to smaller school sites to provide services. Administratively, staff would be connected to a larger school's full-time SBHC located in the same school district.

LEVEL V: School-Based Health Center

This model is a full-time licensed comprehensive primary health care facility located within or on the grounds of a school. It is staffed by a multidisciplinary team (nurse practitioner, M.D. backup, MSW social worker, administrator, support staff, and appropriate ancillary health professions) who have particular expertise in working with children and adolescents. It provides a wide range of primary health care, substance abuse, mental health, and social services and prevention activities. It is operated by a community-based agency and works in partnership with school services. This model is for schools with high need and a student population in excess of 500 students.

SOURCE: State of Connecticut Department of Public Health and Addiction Services.

a high incidence of medically underserved children, low-birthweight babies, infant mortality, or teenage pregnancy. The following three models are specified as eligible for funding; in addition to these models, funding may also be available for other locally developed programs comparable to these three but designed to meet the particular needs of the community:

1. A basic health care program for an elementary, middle, and high school feeder system, with trained school health aides in each school, a full-time nurse to supervise the aides in the elementary and middle schools, and one full-time nurse in the high school—emphasis is on screenings, assessment, record reviews, and coordinating health services for students with parents or guardians and other agencies in the community.
2. Student support services teams that include one half-time psy-

chologist, one full-time nurse, and one full-time social worker—three such teams are funded per grant, with one team working at each of an elementary, middle, and high school that are part of one feeder school system. Teams are to coordinate all activities with the school administrator and guidance counselor. Emphasis is on health, behavioral, and learning problems, with referrals made to community providers for serious problems or extended services, such as drug or alcohol abuse and STD treatment.

3. Full-service schools, in which personnel from the Department of Health and Rehabilitative Services provide services to students and families on school grounds—such services may include nutritional services, medical services, aid to dependent children, parenting skills, counseling for abused children, and education for the students' parents or guardians.

In summary, progress is being made on the process of describing various configurations of services and in suggesting how these might be matched to particular community characteristics, but more research is needed on the outcomes and effectiveness—including cost-effectiveness—of these arrangements. Further, local districts will continue to need technical assistance in assessing their needs and in selecting and designing a service delivery system appropriate for them.

CONFIDENTIALITY OF STUDENTS' HEALTH AND EDUCATION RECORDS

Providing health care in an educational setting requires consideration of separate and sometimes conflicting standards about clients' rights to obtain health care and requirements for educators and health care providers to protect the privacy of their clients' records. Moreover, since the student population includes both minors and those who have reached the age of majority, each group requires a different procedure in order for schools to comply with legal guidelines about access to health care and confidentiality of records. In most states, the age of majority is 18, but in a few it is 19 (English et al., 1995). These variables create a complex matrix of overlapping and contradictory requirements for health care providers in school settings who provide services to children and adolescents, some of whom have developmental delays that require guardianship past the age of majority (Larson, 1992).

Further adding to the complexity are varying state regulations regarding the age at which youth can obtain certain types of health care, such as preventive care, diagnosis and treatment of sexually related conditions, mental health services, and drug or alcohol treatment services. For example, some states have enacted statutes that specifically allow minors who have reached a designated age (ranging from 14 to 16) to authorize their own health care (Office of Technology Assessment, 1991). Most states allow minors, beginning at the age of 12 to 14, to obtain diagnostic and treatment services for specified sexually related conditions (such as sexually transmitted diseases) without parental consent. In addition, health care providers are mandated by varying state and professional legal requirements to disclose information about a student's intent to harm herself or himself or others and about various types of child abuse.

When schools provide health care, they often file health records as part of the students' cumulative educational records. This is particularly important and necessary to facilitate audits by official health agencies of school systems' compliance with immunization and other public health requirements and to allow orderly transfer of student records to other schools and colleges. However, the Family Educational Rights and Privacy Act of 1974 (Buckley Amendment) guarantees that parents and guardians will have access to school records. Further, to fulfill their responsibilities, teachers and guidance counselors may have access to students' educational records. Therefore, the privacy of records for students who may have the legal right to authorize their own health care and receive specified confidential services may be jeopardized if the health record becomes part of the educational record.

Electronic storage and transmission systems raise additional questions about the privacy of student health records and about sharing of information among individual schools, school districts, public health departments, social service agencies, and individual health care providers from both the public and the private sectors. New questions have also emerged since school systems have been authorized to bill Medicaid and private insurers. Insurance billing raises questions about the extent to which parent or guardian and age-of-majority client permission is needed to share information with departments of health and social services and with billing services in order to determine eligibility for benefits and provide documentation of insurance-reimbursable services provided at school.

Although client health and social service records may belong to the agency where the data are collected, the individual (parent or guardian, in the case of a minor) maintains the right of control over the information in the records. In most situations, parents and students who have the right to control their own medical records and authorize their own treatment are merely asked to sign a consent to share information between individual health care providers and between agencies. In both medical and educational cultures, this is a well-established and frequently used way to authorize the sharing of medical information so as to facilitate less fragmented care, prevent redundant diagnostic services, and avoid treatments that in combination are harmful. Further, broad-based sharing of information can be essential for assessing community needs, monitoring the provision of services, and evaluating programs (Soler et al., 1993). Although most parents and clients are willing to give permission to share health records, this may be problematic when there is an issue related to mental health, drug use, or a sexually related condition. Further, some parents and guardians express concern for the consequences if such information—or information about health problems discovered at the school, such as asthma or seizures—might be obtained by their insurer.

If health records stored at school and health records compiled by outside health care professionals providing school services have the same high level of access as educational records, the privacy of families and adolescents may be compromised. The committee therefore believes that when state law eliminates the parental consent requirement for making specified counseling and treatment accessible to students, access to related medical records at school needs to be held to the same standards of confidentiality observed in other health care settings in communities in that state. In other words, confidentiality of school health records should be given high priority. Confidential health records of students should be handled and shared in a manner that is consistent with the handling of health care records in nonschool health care settings in the state.

FINANCING OF SCHOOL HEALTH SERVICES

Overview

As emphasized throughout this report, schools provide a nearly universal access point to the school-age population, and some countries utilize schools as an integral part of the community's health care delivery system (World Health Organization, 1995). In the United States, however, education is a public system that is primarily under local control while the health care system operates in the private sector, making it difficult to integrate the two systems. Thus, the lack of a consistent funding base has been a barrier to establishing school-based services. Within the educational establishment, there is little ownership of the responsibility for students' health, except when health is a substantial barrier to school attendance and achievement. Establishing the links between health and learning is one way to increase the interest in funding health programs from educational dollars (Barrett et al., 1983; Hack et al., 1991; Lewit et al., 1995). However, there is little consensus within the educational community about the fate of school health services when hard choices must be made about appropriating limited resources. Thus, there is a need to look beyond the education budget for dependable support for school services.

Currently, there are sources of external funds for school-affiliated services, but many of these sources tend to be transient and categorical. External funds are often designated for establishing "model programs" that test the feasibility and effectiveness of interventions on small populations of students for short periods of time. Some external funds are for politically charged services such as family planning, diagnosis and treatment of sexually related conditions, and programs for teen parents. External funding to provide ongoing health services designed to address identified needs of the overall student population and to monitor student outcomes is rare. The result is a often patchwork of "here today and gone tomorrow" funding for short-term, problem-specific and/or population-specific services.

Some federal funds authorized by Congress are available for health services, some funds are entitlements; others require periodic reauthorization. Health care for eligible children living in poverty can be reimbursed by Title XIX (Medicaid's Early and Periodic Screening, Diagnostic, and Treatment Program [EPSDT]); maternal and child health services are financed by Title V; health care of educationally disadvantaged children is funded by Title I of the Elementary and Secondary Education Act; specialized health services for children with disabilities are mandated but only partially financed by the Individuals with Disabilities Education Act; services to prevent Human Immunodeficiency Virus (HIV) infections and hepatitis B infections are funded by cooperative agreements with the Centers for Disease Control and Prevention of the U.S. Department of Health and Human Services (DHHS); drug use can be addressed with funds from the Safe and Drug-Free Schools and Communities Act; and model comprehensive school health programs that may include health services may be supported by grants from the U.S. Department of Education.

States often funnel the federal funds to schools through state departments of health, human services, and/or education. State tax funds may be added to federal money or dispersed separately for health services. For example, some states provide financial support to schools for health screening, tobacco use prevention, health care for children and families living in poverty, dental health care, or models of integrated health and social services delivery. Various states have also developed special initiatives and funding for school services; examples include California's Healthy Start and Florida's Full-Service Schools (Dryfoos, 1994a; Schlitt et al., 1994; Shearer and Holschneider, 1995).

Locally, funds may be available from service clubs, volunteer health organizations (such as the American Cancer Society, March of Dimes, and the American Red Cross), and private providers of health care. Managed care systems are emerging and evolving as centerpieces of health care delivery in communities throughout the United States. Arrangements for sharing responsibility for the health care of students who are members of managed care systems are being negotiated locally in some areas (Zimmerman and Reif, 1995). The economy of providing services at school is being explored, and agreements are being created to share capitated rates, responsibilities, and records between personnel who provide school-affiliated services and providers of services within the managed care systems.

Numerous private foundations offer grants to study specific health problems of the school-age population or to provide health services for students. The grants may be given directly to school systems, public health systems, private health care agencies, colleges, universities, academic health centers, or a combination of agencies. As with funds from the various levels of government, the duration of funding is varied, problem specific, and undependable if needed to provide consistent staffing for health services.

A consistent and adequate funding base for school health services is needed in this atmosphere of fragmentation and uncertainty. Some possible strategies for achieving this are discussed below.

Medicaid

The Medicaid program, also known as Title XIX of the Social Security Act, has become the primary source of financing medical care for poor children. The program is administered by the Health Care Financing Administration within DHHS, in conjunction with state government agencies. Within broad federal guidelines and minimum eligibility standards, each state sets its own policies regarding benefits, eligibility, and health care provider reimbursement. Financing is also jointly shared by the federal and state governments, with the federal share ranging from 50 to nearly 80 percent, depending on the state's per capita income. In most states, schools receive only the federal share of reimbursement for health services for eligible students.

Historically, eligibility for the program was tied to requirements for receiving welfare (Aid to Families with Dependent Children or Supplemental Security Income for elderly and disabled). In 1989, however, Congress mandated that states cover low-income pregnant women and children under age 6 who live in families making less than 133 percent of the federal poverty level, an income level that is higher than regular Medicaid eligibility levels in nearly all states.

In 1990, Congress required states to provide Medicaid coverage to all children ages 6 to 19 living in families earning up to 100 percent of the poverty level. But federal law permits states to phase in coverage of these children on a year-by-year basis, which means that all poor adolescents will not be covered by Medicaid until the year 2002.

Currently, states have the option of providing Medicaid benefits to children from families with earnings that exceed the federal poverty level. Furthermore, children with disabilities from families with higher income levels than allowed by the individual states may qualify for Medicaid coverage when their medical costs are excessive. In calculations to establish Medicaid eligibility, the cost of medical services already incurred is subtracted from the family's income and resources, allowing families with high medical costs to be eligible for Medicaid when their incomes would otherwise exceed the eligibility limit.

As required in federal law, all state Medicaid programs cover hospitalization, physician services, laboratory and x-ray services, family planning, and Early Periodic Screening, Diagnostic, and Treatment services for children under the age of 21. In addition to the option of extending coverage to families above the poverty level, states can also provide such other services as prescribed drugs, dental services, inpatient psychiatric care, case management, and transportation.

The EPSDT component of Medicaid was originally designed to provide comprehensive health screening for poor children, as well as subsequent diagnosis and treatment services for conditions found during the screening exams. Comprehensive screening included not only basic health, vision, hearing, and dental components but "anticipatory guidance" that could include counseling services, case management, and health prevention. Although federal law mandated EPSDT services for Medicaid eligible children and adolescents, most states have not accomplished the goal of screening all who are eligible.

The potential of Medicaid as a funding source for school-based services is ambiguous. Standards for qualifying as a Medicaid provider are rigorous and billing procedures can be complex. The possibility that Medicaid will be transferred to the states in the form of block grants presents further challenges and opportunities, since states may have more flexibility but fewer dollars. In many states, Medicaid enrollees are being required to obtain coverage through managed care. Many HMOs and other managed care providers may not include preventive services, mental health services, and health screening as part of the package. In some places, school health service providers may have to negotiate with multiple managed care plans for students in their schools. One proposal has been to create "school health resource partnerships" among districts, health providers, and community agencies to address the financial viability of school health service programs in a managed care environment. (Brellochs, 1995). States would require that managed care plans participate as a condition of licensure.

Many of the services required by disabled children protected by IDEA are medically necessary, but state Medicaid and education agencies have not always agreed about the responsibility for paying for health services delivered to disabled Medicaid-eligible children in school settings. However, many state health and education officials are recognizing the financial benefits to be gained by charging Medicaid for health services provided during the school day, and more than half of the states have obtained waivers that allow school systems to bill Medicaid for services such as speech, occupational, and physical therapy; nursing services; psychological and counseling services; audiological services; and assessments, thus freeing up some special education funds for other uses.

School-Based Health Insurance

A major obstacle for many students in receiving health care is the fact that they lack health insurance but do not qualify for Medicaid assistance. A program in Florida is tackling this problem by providing health insurance for all school children. The School Enrollment-Based Health Insurance (SEBHI) concept was proposed in 1988 to provide low-cost, comprehensive health insurance to families who did not qualify for Medicaid and could not afford private insurance (Freedman et al., 1988). SEBHI represents an alternative to employer-based health insurance by using the school system to create large groups to negotiate health insurance policies. SEBHI contains several attractive features. First, families with school-aged children represent approximately 66 percent of the uninsured families (Sulvetta and Swartz, 1986). These families are targeted through the SEBHI model. Second, school districts can be used to create large pools of uninsured individuals who represent a significant market share in the group health insurance market. Third, school-based insurance coverage for children is more portable. Because the school district is the grouping mechanism, coverage will not be disrupted if a parent changes or loses his or her job.

Several factors served as impetus for the implementation of the SEBHI concept. As mentioned earlier in this chapter, between one-fifth and one-sixth of children under 18 have no health insurance. Nearly two-thirds of these children live in families with incomes above the federal poverty level, making some of them ineligible for government-sponsored health programs. Employee-based health insurance coverage, which covers approximately two-thirds of all children who have private insurance, declined from 71 to 63 percent in 1990. Only 55 percent of all United States jobs, and 35 percent of low-wage jobs, include health insurance benefits (Employee Benefit Research Institute, 1993).

A SEBHI demonstration program was implemented in Volusia

County, Florida, in 1991. Its purpose is to encourage children in low-income families to use pediatric primary care services by reducing financial barriers to care. The SEBHI benefit package includes well-child visits and immunizations with no copayment required. Other benefits with minimal copayments include inpatient care, maternity benefits, mental health services, prescriptions, physical therapy, and emergency services and transportation.

All children who are not eligible for Medicaid are eligible for participation in the demonstration. Subsidized premiums are offered so that financial concerns will not be a barrier to families who want to enroll their children. The National School Lunch Program is used as a method to verify family income for insurance premium subsidy. Subsidized premiums are based on family income so that families with incomes below 100 percent of the federal poverty level receive fully subsidized premiums; those with incomes between 101 and 135 percent of the poverty level pay $2.50 per child per month; those between 136 percent and 185 percent of the poverty level pay $13 per child per month; and those at 186 percent of the poverty level or above pay the full premium of $46 per child per month.

A key feature of the program is the provision of care through the private sector. The program is not intended to extend Medicaid coverage or to provide health care as a variation of the current Medicaid system for children in Florida. In the SEBHI demonstration, care is provided through a health maintenance organization using both staff physicians and contract physicians in private practice. Prior to implementing the demonstration, it was presumed that a generous benefit package, the provision of free or greatly reduced health insurance premiums, and the availability of care within a private HMO would result in more low-income children making primary care visits. The market penetration of the program among the targeted uninsured children has exceeded 50 percent. Health care services in the early stages of the demonstration were provided at other community sites, but the project directors are now working with the HMO to move a set of widely used services to the school site in order to widen participation.

Given the continued erosion of employer-based health insurance, the SEBHI concept is an interesting and relevant approach for providing health insurance to previously uninsured children. The large numbers of uninsured school-age children make the school a useful grouping mechanism that is not dependent on the parents' employment status. In addition, it is clear that financial barriers to health care use must be removed, and the SEBHI model addresses this factor through the provision of free or greatly reduced insurance premiums.

However, results of the SEBHI demonstration indicate that attention must also be paid to addressing nonfinancial barriers to health care use. Factors such as length of time of program enrollment, the child's age and gender, the premium amount, and the child's race and ethnicity influence both the likelihood of health care use and health care use rates after reducing or removing financial barriers to care (Shenkman et al., 1996).

Nonfinancial barriers to health care use are perhaps more complex than financial barriers. For example, some minorities experience deep sociopolitical disenfranchisement within our society. It is often argued that in the face of poverty, crisis, and feelings of alienation, some minority parents may not place a high priority on taking their children for primary and preventive care (Murray-Garcia, 1995). Moreover, minority parents often face the significant barrier of receiving health care within a system that they feel is not sensitive to their cultural needs. These issues are deeply rooted in our society and not easily addressed. However, future efforts at providing health services within a comprehensive school health program must combine innovative financing strategies like the SEBHI concept with strategies to break down cultural, nonfinancial barriers to health care to ensure that all children receive pediatric health care services.

Financing for School-Based Health Centers

Several recent reports have analyzed financial issues associated with school-based health centers (Brellochs and Fothergill, 1993; Perino and Brindis, 1994; Schlitt et al., 1994; U.S. Department of Health and Human Services, 1993a; U.S. GAO, 1994a, 1994b; Zimmerman and Reif, 1995). A recent policy paper from the Making the Grade project, the national SBHC initiative sponsored by the Robert Wood Johnson Foundation, reviews recent events that have had a major—and mostly negative—impact on funding for SBHCs (Rosenberg and Associates, 1995). The collapse of federal health care reform, which had included provisions for large-scale grants for SBHCs, and the election of a fiscally conservative Congress imply that states and local communities cannot rely on federal funds for expanding SBHCs. Although Medicaid had been a potential means of expanding support for SBHC services, this source is uncertain because of possible Medicaid spending caps and state control of the allocation of block grants. Further, states are responding to fiscal pressures by assigning Medicaid clients to managed care systems; SBHCs that learned how to implement Medicaid billing systems may now encounter difficulty in collecting reimbursement for students enrolled in a Medicaid managed care plan. Also, SBHCs have not been included in any federal or state definition of "essential community providers." Therefore, SBHCs are not entitled automatically to any special treatment given to "safety net" services, and other designated essential community providers, such as community health centers, are not required to interact with SBHCs.

The Making the Grade policy paper (Rosenberg and Associates, 1995) discusses possible funding strategies in the current restrictive political and fiscal climate. The paper suggests that since limited resources preclude the expansion of SBHCs into every community or school that might desire one, decisions and priority setting must occur, preferably at the state level. Decisions about where clinics should be located and supported might be based on a combination of factors including community income, insurance status, access to primary care, and age level of school. The paper considers several possible approaches to funding, but perhaps the most promising is the "pooled fund" approach in which the state assumes direct responsibility for the overall program and funds it through a global budget paid directly to each SBHC. The state determines each center's operating costs and provides support through funds pooled from a variety of sources, including Medicaid funds, Maternal and Child Health (Title V) funds, other federal funds, and state and private sector funds.

SBHCs increasingly are looking to managed care organizations as possible partners, not only to secure stable funding but also to move SBHCs into the health care mainstream and improve care coordination for children (Alpha Center, 1995). Partnering has its barriers, however, including demonstrating the quality and effectiveness of school-based services and instituting more sophisticated billing and information systems. Also, many of the services provided by SBHCs, such as mental health counseling or behavior modification aimed at preventing teen pregnancy or AIDS (Acquired Immunodeficiency Syndrome), have not been reimbursable medical procedures. Although managed care understands the value of such preventive services, students do not stay in plans long enough for a managed care organization to recoup the benefits. Still, SBHCs can market themselves to managed care organizations as being uniquely positioned to provide the convenient care that parents—particularly working parents—are seeking for their children and to help managed care meet Medicaid mandates to screen a certain percentage of adolescents. Likewise, managed care organizations need to consider the development of plans in which a combination of health and social support services are provided and to recognize the potential role that schools could play to improve health outcomes for health plan beneficiaries.

Nonprofit Intermediary for Contracting Services

Both public and private health care delivery systems in the United States are undergoing rapid changes. As a result of the development and consolidation of large managed care organizations, there are new business arrangements for individuals and groups of health practitioners, new service delivery systems, and renewed interest in more cost-effective sites for service delivery.

At the same time, there is increasing demand for health services for students during the school day. School systems have had to provide specialized physical health care procedures, physical and occupational therapy, speech and language therapy, audiological services, and mental health counseling as a result of the federal legislation requiring free public education for children with disabilities (P.L. 94-142, Education for All Handicapped Children Act, 1975). Initially, this legislation contained provisions for funding, but federal funding currently covers less than 10 percent of costs for mandated special education services. Since school districts continue to be mandated to provide these services, most costs are paid out of education funds; this is sometimes called the "encroachment" of special education costs into the general education budget.

Until recently, insurers (private insurers and Medicaid health coverage) have not been approached on a large scale to contribute to the cost of health care at school for their beneficiaries. A few school systems are now making claims to private insurers as well as to Medicaid. There is an opportunity to further explore "externalizing" school health personnel into a private corporate structure for the purpose of contracting health services at school sites to the school system or managed care organizations, or to both. For example, the Department of Pediatrics of the University of Texas Health Sciences Center at Galveston has formed a nonprofit corporation to address the problems of the city's low-income, high-risk children, youth, and families, which is funded by contractual arrangements with school systems, Medicaid, and other health insurance claims. A joint partnership venture was launched, stimulated by the private practicing community, that included a previously existing Teen Health Center managed by private practitioners, the health district, the school district, the state Department of Human Services, and a consultant from the University Health Sciences Center. The corporation employs nurses and nurse practitioners and serves as a clinical teaching site for medical students and residents in pediatrics (Barnett et al., 1992).

In making such contractual arrangements, several factors must be considered. If there is only one managed care organization in the area that has members who are also students in a coterminous school system, then school-affiliated health services and/or school-based clinics could be wholly contracted to that organization. In this way, care at school becomes part of the larger full-service health care system, and barriers to sharing health information would be less cumbersome. However, if there are multiple managed care organizations in the community served by the school, the contractual arrangements would be more complicated and would have to take into consideration changes in membership among the students during a given school year. The major obstacles appear to be establishing rates for services and cost allocation among managed care organizations and school systems. Differentiating health services from educational services is often difficult when a student's health status is interwoven with the necessity for costly and individualized educational services.

Both the consolidation of existing health professional staff into a non-profit corporate unit for contracting services and the negotiation of school-based health services delivery through managed care organizations could enhance revenues to school districts, first by offsetting the cost of currently employed health professional services by selling those services to managed care organizations and second by having the cost of school-based clinics borne by managed care organizations rather than schools.

Other Funding Strategies

In the recent report *How to Fund Public Health Activities*, the Partnership for Prevention[6] suggested three possible approaches for providing stable and adequate funding for public health services (Meyer and Regenstein, 1994). The report also analyzes the advantages and disadvantages of each approach. These approaches are also relevant for school health services. Adapted for school health, these approaches are as follows:

1. **A surcharge on health care payers**—including private employer and employee premium contributions, beneficiary contributions from Medicare and the Department of Veterans Affairs, and similar sources—could be put into a fund, either at the federal or state level, to be disbursed to community or school providers of school health services. It is estimated that a 1 percent surcharge would raise about $4 billion, a 2 percent surcharge would raise about $8 billion, and so on. This option offers the advantage of spreading costs broadly across society, and funding would keep pace with overall health care spending since it would reflect a percentage of insurance premiums. A disadvantage is that this approach would exacerbate the current cost shift in which those paying for insurance are subsidizing those without coverage.

---

[6]Partnership for Prevention is a private, nonprofit organization of leaders in medicine and public health that was established in 1991. Partnership is committed to coordinating and unifying the prevention-oriented efforts of federal health agencies, corporations, states, and other nonprofit groups to achieve the *Healthy People 2000* objectives and make prevention a fundamental component of America's health system.

2. **The addition of school health services to standard benefit packages**—under this option, both public and private insurance benefit packages would designate school health services as "covered services." The insurers themselves would not directly reimburse those who provide the services but would send the reimbursement to a fund set up for school health services. This option amounts to making school health services a "mandated benefit" for all health coverage. It is estimated that establishing the cost of this new benefit at 1 percent of premiums would raise nearly $9 billion. This approach would also spread the cost broadly; in addition, establishing school health services as a covered service should help insulate it from the uncertainties of the political and administrative processes. Disadvantages of this approach include the cost shift problem of option 1. In addition, if "school health" coverage were a fixed dollar amount, the approach would be regressive, consuming a greater proportion of the premium of a low-cost plan.

3. **Excise taxes and penalties** on products or processes that affect health might include taxes on alcohol and tobacco products, gasoline, and ammunition, as well as penalties on polluters. An advantage to this approach is that it accomplishes two goals—financing school services and discouraging the use of products and practices linked to health problems. A limitation of this approach is that the revenue base will shrink if the tax is successful in reducing consumption. In addition, excise taxes are not as broad and progressive as the system-wide health contribution described in options 1 and 2.

FIRST STEPS FOR A COMMUNITY IN ESTABLISHING SCHOOL SERVICES

In this section, the committee uses the American Academy of Pediatric's seven "goals" for school health programs, listed at the beginning of this chapter and repeated below, to organize the discussion of specific questions and actions that a community might consider in establishing an appropriate set of school health services within a comprehensive school health program.

Goal 1   Ensure access to primary health care.
Goal 2   Provide a system for dealing with crisis medical situations.
Goal 3   Provide mandated screening and immunization monitoring.
Goal 4   Provide systems for identification and solution of students' health and educational problems.
Goal 5   Provide comprehensive and appropriate health education.
Goal 6   Provide a healthful and safe school environment that facilitates learning.

Goal 7   Provide a system of evaluation of the effectiveness of the school health program.

Before examining the steps implied by each goal, the following basic premises should be emphasized. Regardless of program structure or community characteristics, programs should be based upon a thorough assessment of community needs and resources, and this assessment should involve all stakeholders who will be impacted by the program—parents, students, educators, health and social services providers, insurers, and business and political leaders.[7] Who should convene and administer this process—the school system, health department, or other community entity—will depend on the situation; the crucial requirement is strong and committed leadership in the convening organization. Programs and services should be preventively oriented and family centered, avoid duplication, and be based on best practices gained from research.

Although schools represent relatively barrier-free systems for reaching children and youth about health issues, communities should recognize that not all populations may be comfortable with the school setting and school personnel (Chaskin and Richman, 1992). If this is the case, then steps must be taken to interact with those populations in ways with which they are comfortable, either by utilizing a more neutral setting or by altering the school environment to provide a climate with more trust.

Ensure Access to Primary Health Care

The school health service should be considered an integral part of a community's preventive health system. Utilizing the school health service for screening and detection of problems, follow-up, and the coordination or provision of services can make the community's primary care system more efficient, effective, and accessible. Although the extent of services provided at the school site will differ from one community to another, mechanisms must be developed so that school health services are coordinated with the community's mainstream health services to ensure efficiency, continuity, and quality of care (American Academy of Pediatrics, 1994).

---

[7]Procedures and instruments for carrying out such assessments have been described and developed (see, for example, *School Health: Policy and Practice,* from the American Academy of Pediatrics [1993]. The National Adolescent Health Resource Center of the University of Minnesota, sponsored by the Maternal and Child Health Bureau of the U.S. Department of Health and Human Services, also provides resource materials and technical assistance for carrying out community needs assessments on adolescent health issues.)

The following are initial steps that a community might take to ensure student access to primary care:

1. Identify sources of health care in the community.
2. Identify needs of population and barriers to health care—are they geographic, financial, cultural, or other?
3. Determine where and for what reason students have utilized a health care facility in the past year.
4. Consider the range of school-affiliated services needed on or near a school site and how they might be provided and supported.
5. Set up communication systems between providers of care and the school health service (e.g., phone or fax for referrals, feedback, follow-up).[8]

Deal with Crisis Medical Situations

Every day in this country, medical crises occur at schools. A teacher may suffer a myocardial infarction, or a student may fall from playground or gym equipment, be burned in a lab fire, be lacerated by broken glass, or fall on a discarded needle in a schoolyard. The effects of community violence spread to schools; suicides, homicides, and intentional and non-intentional injuries affect school populations. In addition, children may have seizures, suffer acute attacks of asthma, develop complications from diabetes, be technically dependent on fragile medical devices, and be transported in wheelchairs on school buses on dangerous country roads or busy freeways.

Procedures must be in place to deal with such crisis situations, including awareness of 911 access to community emergency medical services, standing medical orders for triage and first aid, and guidelines for contacting parents. Broad training of school personnel and older students in cardiopulmonary resuscitation (CPR) and first aid procedures is necessary, as is implementing school accident prevention programs (American Academy of Pediatrics, 1993). The recent Institute of Medicine (IOM) report *Emergency Medical Services for Children* (IOM, 1993) calls for teachers, coaches, and day care workers, along with parents, to receive the highest

---

[8]The survey, *A Closer Look*, found that exchange of information between school and community providers was inadequate; one out of five referrals from school health personnel failed to produce any response or feedback from the community provider. A step in the right direction would be to institute a two-way written referral system wherein both parties are expected to respond.

priority in education and training for safety and accident prevention, CPR, and first aid, and use of the community emergency medical system.

The following are initial questions that a community can ask to ensure that a system is in place to deal with potential crisis medical situations:

1. Does a school-based emergency system or plan exist? What are its provisions?

2. Are school personnel informed of access to the emergency medical care system of the community?

3. Are school personnel trained in first aid and CPR?

4. What school accident prevention and accident reporting systems are in place? Who reviews these reports? How is information from these reports used to modify existing risks for students?

5. How are community providers of emergency medical care services involved in education and training of school-based health personnel and other school staff?

6. Are school medical consultants available for establishing triage, guidelines for need or immediacy of referrals, or standing orders as deemed necessary?

Carry Out Mandated Screening Programs

Screening is the process of using a relatively simple test to identify those who may have a particular problem. Unfortunately, screening programs are ineffective unless procedures are in place for ensuring follow-up of identified problems. Certain mandates for screenings are old and outdated, and statutory requirements should be reviewed for scientific validity.[9] In a climate where resources are scarce, a balance may have to be struck between population-based screenings and targeted interventions for high-risk groups, as mentioned earlier in this chapter (Starfield and Vivier, 1995).

Overviews of screening recommendations are found in such publications as *School Health: Policy and Practice* from the American Academy of Pediatrics (1993) and *Principles and Practices of Student Health, Volume II* (Wallace et al., 1992b). The value of any screening program must be based on criteria outlined in Box 4-2.

As mentioned previously, Medicaid reimbursement for school-based

---

[9]Scoliosis screening, for example, is still mandated in many localities, but its scientific validity is questionable (American Academy of Pediatrics, 1993; Berg, 1993; Goldberg et al., 1995; Wallace et al., 1992b).

BOX 4-2
Criteria for a Useful and Effective Screening Program

Disease Undetected cases of the disease must be common (high prevalence), or new cases must occur frequently (high incidence). The disease must be associated with adverse consequences, either physical or psychological (morbidity).

Treatment Treatment must be available that will effectively prevent or reduce morbidity from the disease. There must be some benefit from this treatment before the disease would have become obvious without screening; that is, there must be an early intervention benefit.

Screening Test The ideal test detects all subjects who have the disease (high sensitivity) and correctly identifies all who do not (high specificity). Low sensitivity results in missed cases (false-negative results), and low specificity yields many false-positive results. Another measure of effectiveness is its positive predictive value, or the number of true-positive results divided by the total number who fail the test. A good test is simple, brief, and acceptable to the person being screened. The test must be reliable, that is, repeat testing will yield the same results.

Screener The screener must be well trained; experience is important, particularly if judgments must be made.

Target Population To reduce inefficiency, the screening should be focused on groups in which the undetected disease is most prevalent or in which early intervention will be most beneficial.

Referral and Treatment All of those with a positive screening test must receive a more definitive evaluation and, if indicated, appropriate treatment. The ultimate measure of effectiveness is a reduction in morbidity from early intervention among those with positive screening test results. This depends on the successful treatment of those in need.

Cost–Benefit Ratio Cost includes all expenses of screening, referral, and treatment, including administrative costs and the cost plus anxiety that result from false-positive results. The benefit is the reduction in morbidity from early intervention among those with true-positive results who are in need of treatment. This benefit is hard to quantify in dollars and may vary among communities. Greater efficiency at any level will improve this ratio.

Program Maintenance The need for improvements in program efficiency is determined by periodic review of research on the value of each screening program and an assessment of program effectiveness within the community. Local review also allows community leaders to make reasonable decisions as to the allocation of limited resources for screening. Local politicians can also be influenced to increase these resources when it can be shown that monies are being spent wisely.

SOURCE: Adapted from American Academy of Pediatrics, 1993.

Early and Periodic Screening, Diagnosis, and Treatment services is a possible means for expanding resources to provide screening programs for all students. However, Medicaid reimbursement is not an easy process, and possible changes in the system make Medicaid an uncertain future source of funding for screenings.

The following initial questions should be raised in establishing effective screening programs:

1. What screening programs are mandated, and what are the outcomes?

2. Are screening practices aligned with current research, knowledge, and technology? (Consider frequency of procedure and any gender-specific procedures.)

3. What mechanisms exist to ensure that identified problems are followed up and treated?

4. Do other sources—private health care, health fairs—duplicate school screening efforts? How is information, both positive and negative results, shared among systems? How is confidentiality maintained?

Provide Systems for Identification and Solution of Students' Health and Educational Problems

The school alone cannot identify and solve all problems that affect its students. However, a team approach utilizing the many resources within the school and community can lead to greater progress than will be achieved by separate, isolated efforts. Methods of problem identification from both within and outside the school, tracking of student problem resolution strategies, and suggested categories of classification of problem resolution have been described by the American Academy of Pediatrics (1993).

An example of whether a community is meeting student's health and education needs would be the correction of visual defects identified through routine school screening. Data from one large urban district in southern California, however, illustrate the difficulties involved in assessing whether follow-up and correction are occurring. Data at the district level, drawn from nurses' monthly reports of screening activities, suggested that only about one-half of students failing vision screening actually received care. However, an in-depth review, including parental phone interviews of two school clusters, found that closer to 85 percent of parents had followed through with the referral but did not inform the school (nor did the providers of care) (Nader, 1995). This situation points out the need for improved communication between parents and/or providers and the school. The targeting of 15 percent of those children still needing referral is a much more feasible task than attempting to define barriers to care for a presumed 50 percent of students found to fail a vision screen.

Other health and educational problems may be much more difficult than visual defects to diagnose, follow up, and treat, particularly problems deriving from mental health conditions and family circumstances. Utilizing the full range of mental health, social work, and family services professionals—both school and community based—is essential in dealing with the most complex problems. It may be that the solution required for certain communities is a full set of comprehensive family and social services made available at the school or accessed through the school. Interestingly, informal feedback from such programs suggests that for families needing mental health and social services, it is often physical health concerns that prompt them initially to seek help and make contact with the program.

In developing its Guidelines for Adolescent Preventive Services (GAPS), the American Medical Association has recognized the broad range of health, mental health, and behavioral concerns that affect students' ability to learn and develop into healthy adults (American Medical Association, 1992). GAPS provides recommendations for the systematic, routine health care of adolescents and calls for annual preventive visits to a primary provider for all adolescents between the ages of 11 and 21. These visits should address not only physical health problems but also psychosocial difficulties such as depression, substance abuse, and risky sexual behavior. The detailed GAPS recommendations are found in Appendix E.

The initial implementation of GAPS recommendations in many communities may be limited by such problems as cost, access, and insufficient numbers of primary providers trained or interested in providing these services. Questions have also been raised about how willing adolescents would be to discuss sensitive issues with a relative stranger—a physician seen only once a year. A more feasible approach, especially in communities with limited resources, might be a strong prevention program for all students, offered in a large group setting in school, with mechanisms for individual peer and professional counseling and referral to specialized providers when warranted. GAPS defines primary care providers not only as physicians but as those who work with physicians in the primary care setting, including nurses, health educators, and other allied health professionals. In many communities, certain GAPS-recommended procedures might be adapted to local needs and carried out more efficiently by appropriately trained school-based personnel—school nurses and nurse practitioners, physicians assistants, school counselors and psychologists—in the school setting. At the time of writing this report, the American School Health Association is working with the American Medical Association to explore ways in which some GAPS recommendations might be performed by the school nurse.

Initial questions that a community should ask to improve identification and resolution of students' problems include the following:

1. How are problems currently identified and tracked?

2. Do community sources of services interact with school services? Do community providers utilize school resources to track students, follow up on identified problems, or give feedback to schools on referrals received from schools? How is confidentiality maintained?

3. What method exists to involve and empower families to work on resolution of identified problems?

4. For students and families requiring an array of services, is there a centralized, user-friendly point of access?

5. Are students, families, primary providers, and the school aware of the GAPS recommendations? What steps have been taken to adapt GAPS to the local community?

Provide Comprehensive and Appropriate Health Education

Health services personnel can be involved in classroom health education, both in developing the instructional program and perhaps in delivering classroom lessons. Health education can also be carried out on an individual or group basis by school health services personnel outside the classroom. In fact, health services personnel often may be more knowledgeable and comfortable with sensitive topics and may be more accessible for confidential discussions with students than are teachers or others working in a classroom situation.

Since utilization of a school health room or clinic is a simulation of a relatively barrier-free health care system, it could become a laboratory where students can learn skills to assess their own needs and become more informed consumers of health care services. Studies have shown that children's use of the school health room mirrors adults' use of community health care services (Nader and Brink, 1981).

Initial questions that should be addressed by a community in beginning to implement a coordinated approach to health education include the following:

1. What are the content and scope of current health education? Have topics been identified through a needs assessment to be the most important issues for the community and particular age groups? What is the acceptance of the program by students?

2. Does health education cut across all aspects of the school—class-

room instruction; health room or clinic; parent involvement; school environment; school nutrition; physical education; and health policies on
smoking, drinking, drugs, or violence?

3. How are health and mental health services personnel involved in
the classroom instructional program and in individual and group health
education?

4. What is the comfort level of school service providers in working
with children and adolescents, particularly in dealing with a complex or
controversial topic? What referral mechanisms are established when problems are identified?

Provide a Healthful and Safe School Environment That Promotes Learning

As discussed in Chapter 2, the school environment is comprised of
the broad areas of the physical, psychosocial, and policy environment. A
range of issues is involved; included are policies regarding the possession
of drugs and alcohol, the existence of a supportive nurturing atmosphere,
and the presence of environmental hazards and pollutants. Staff wellness
is also an important aspect of the environment, as is safety, including
safety in pedestrian, bicycle, and school bus transportation to and from
school.

Initial questions to consider in improving the school environment
include the following:

1. Are policies in place that will lead to an environment that is free of
tobacco, alcohol, drugs, and violence? What disciplinary measures are
taken for violation of these policies? What support groups or services are
available for students who are already participating in these prohibited
behaviors?

2. How might communication and mutual respect and support be
promoted among students, families, and staff?

3. Is the school clean, safe, secure, and free of hazards and sources of
pollution? How can community efforts—for example, community watch
or cleanup programs—promote a clean and safe campus?

4. Are the school lunch and breakfast programs, as well as other foods
available at school, following up-to-date nutrition guidelines and reinforcing classroom health instruction?

5. Are health promotion programs available to school staff?

*Provide a System of Evaluation of the Effectiveness of the School Health
Program*

Improved evaluation of school health programs is critical, both for strengthening programs and for maintaining accountability, and commu- nities must be prepared to allocate sufficient resources to evaluation. Chapter 6 discusses the level of evaluation that might be appropriate for local programs. It may be that individuals and relevant agencies within the community have expertise in evaluation, but many communities are likely to need technical assistance in developing the necessary evaluation methodologies and strategies (American Academy of Pediatrics, 1994).

Suggested initial steps and questions to improve evaluation of local programs include the following:

1. Consider evaluation in the context of improving the health and educational status of children and youth in the community.

2. Establish a district school health coordinating council to oversee the evaluation system, if one does not already exist.

3. What data are available to document students' current health sta- tus and needs? What new data should be collected?

4. What are the goals and specific objectives that the community would like to achieve through the program?

5. Do local agencies have evaluation expertise, or will technical assis- tance be required to help assess needs and develop evaluation strategies and methodologies?

SUMMARY OF FINDINGS AND CONCLUSIONS

Although the scope of school health services varies from one school district to another, many common elements exist throughout the country. Most schools provide screenings, monitor student immunization status, and administer first aid and medication. Schools are also required to pro- vide a wide range of health services for students with disabilities and special health care needs.

There is agreement that a core set of services is needed in schools, but the topic currently generating a great deal of discussion is the role of the school in providing access to extended services that go beyond traditional basic services, such as primary care, social, and family services. The com- mittee believes that extended services should not be the sole—or even the major—responsibility of the schools; instead, the school should be consid- ered by other community agencies and providers as a partner and a po- tentially effective site for provision of needed services—services that will ultimately advance the primary academic mission of the school.

Although the demands and complexity of basic school services have increased, these services are often supervised by education-based admin- istrators who have no clinical preparation in the delivery of health services. Thus, it is important to develop closer links between the school and community health systems and to encourage greater involvement of community health care professionals in the planning and implementation of basic services. School-based health centers and other extended services are a relatively new phenomenon, and research in this area is in the early stages. Studies have shown that SBHCs provide access to care for needy students and increase students' health knowledge significantly. However, it has been difficult to measure the impact of SBHCs on students' health status or high-risk behavior, such as sexual activity or drug use. This is consistent, however, with other interventions to reduce high-risk behavior—increased knowledge has little effect unless the environment and perceived norms are changed. The committee believes that access, utilization, and possibly a reduction in absenteeism may be more appropriate measures of the impact of SBHCs than change in health status or high-risk behavior.

RECOMMENDATIONS

School health services should be formally planned, and the quality of services should be continuously monitored as an integral part of the community public health and primary care systems.

In the planning process, school health services should be considered an integral part of the overall community public health and primary care system. The range of services actually provided at the school site must be determined locally, based on community characteristics and needs. Special concerns should be emphasized about two areas of services that a significant proportion of students need—mental health or psychological counseling and school foodservice. The committee believes that mental health and psychological services are essential in enabling many students to achieve academically; these should be considered mainstream, not optional, services. The committee also believes that the school foodservice should serve as a learning laboratory for developing healthful eating habits and should not be driven by profit-making or forced to compete with other food options in school that may undermine nutrition goals.

Many questions remain unanswered about school services, particularly questions regarding the relative advantages, disadvantages, quality, and effectiveness of providing extended services at the school rather than at other sites in the community. Thus the committee recommends the following:

Research should be conducted on school-based services, particularly on the organization, management, efficacy, and cost-effectiveness of extended services.

In order to facilitate school health research of all kinds, all school health providers should immediately institute uniform data collection protocols and standards.

So that the privacy of families and adolescents be maintained, the committee recommends the following:

Confidentiality of health records should be given high priority by the school. Confidential health records of students should be handled and shared in the school setting in a manner that is consistent with the manner in which health records are handled in nonschool health care settings in the state.

The lack of a consistent and adequate funding base has been a barrier to establishing school health services. Thus, the committee recommends the following:

Established sources of funding for school health services should continue from public health, agriculture, and education funds, and new approaches must be developed.

Strategies that have shown promise and should be further explored include billing Medicaid for services to eligible students, developing school-based insurance groupings, forming alliances with managed care organizations and other providers, instituting special taxes, and placing surcharges or special premiums on existing insurance policies.

REFERENCES

Abt Associates. 1990. Final Report: Study of Income Verification in the National School Lunch Program. Arlington, Va: Abt Associates.

Adelman, H., and Taylor, L. 1991. Mental health facets of the school-based health center movement: Need and opportunity for research and development. *Journal of Mental Health Administration* 18:272–283.

Adelman, H., and Taylor, L. 1997. Addressing barriers to learning: Beyond school-linked services and full-service schools. *American Journal of Orthopsychiatry* 67(3):408–421.

Adelman, H., Barker, L., and Nelson, P. 1993. A study of a school-based clinic: Who uses it and who doesn't? *Journal of Clinical Child Psychology* 22(1):52–59.

Alpha Center. 1995. *State Initiatives in Health Care Reform.* Washington, D.C.: Alpha Center, September/October, No. 14.

American Academy of Pediatrics. 1993. *School Health: Policy and Practice,* 5th ed., P.R. Nader, ed. Elk Grove Village, Ill.: American Academy of Pediatrics.

American Academy of Pediatrics. 1994. *Principles to Link By: Integrating Education Health and Human Services*. The National Consensus Building Conference Final Report, Centers for Disease Control and Prevention. Washington, D.C.: U.S. Department of Health and Human Services.

American Dietetic Association. 1991. Position of the American Dietetic Association: Competitive foods in schools. *Journal of the American Dietetic Association* 93:334–336.

American Dietetic Association, Society for Nutrition Education, and American School Food Service Association. 1995. Joint position of American Dietetic Association, Society for Nutrition Education, and American School Food Service Association: School-based nutrition programs and services. *Journal of American Dietetic Association* 95(3):367–369.

American Medical Association. 1992. *Guidelines for Adolescent Preventive Services*. Chicago: American Medical Association, Department of Adolescent Medicine.

American Medical Association Council on Scientific Affairs. 1990. Providing medical services through school-based health programs. *Journal of School Health* 60(3):87–91.

American School Food Service Association. 1994. *Creating Policy for Nutrition Integrity in Schools*. Alexandria, Va.: American School Food Service Association.

American School Food Service Association. 1995. *Keys to Excellence: Standards of Practice for School Foodservice and Nutrition*. Alexandria, Va.: American School Food Service Association.

Appelboom, T.M. 1985. A history of vision screening. *Journal of School Health* 55(4):138–141.

Bachman, J. 1995. A university's response to a need for school nurse education. *Journal of School Nursing* 11(3):20–22, 24.

Barnett, S.E., Niebuhr, V.H., Baldwin, C., and Levine, H. 1992. Community-oriented primary care: A process for school health intervention. *Journal of School Health* 62(6):246–248.

Barrett, D.C., Radke-Yarrow, M., and Klein, R.E. 1983. Chronic malnutrition and child behavior: Effects of early caloric supplementation on social and emotional function at school age. *Developmental Psychology* 18(4):541–556.

Basco, D. 1963. Evaluation of school nursing activities. *Nursing Research* (Fall):211–212.

Berg, A.O. 1993. Screening for adolescent idiopathic scoliosis: A report from the United States Preventive Services Task Force. *Journal of the American Board of Family Practice* 6(5):497–501.

Brellochs, C. 1995. School health services in the United States: A 100-year tradition and a place for innovation. Paper prepared by School Health Policy Initiative, Montefiore Medical Center, New York, N.Y., May.

Brellochs, C., and Fothergill, K., eds. 1993. *1993 School Health Policy Initiative Special Report: Current Issues of Comprehensive School-Based Health Centers*. New York: Columbia University School of Public Health.

Bricco, E. 1985. Impacted cerumen as a reason for failure in hearing conservation programs. *Journal of School Health* 55(6):240–241.

Brindis, C., Starbuck-Morales, S., Wolfe, A.L., and McCarter, V. 1994. Characteristics associated with contraceptive use among adolescent females in school-based family planning programs. *Family Planning Perspectives* 26:160–164.

Brindis, C., Kapphahnn, C. McCarter, V., and Wolfe, A. 1995. The impact of health insurance status on adolescents' utilization of school-based clinic services: Implications for health reform. *Journal of Adolescent Health Care* 16:18–25.

Brown, J.O., Grubb, S.B., Wicker, T.E. and O'Tuel, F.S. 1985. Health variables and school achievement. *Journal of School Health* 55(1):21–23.

Bryan, D.S. 1970. Skin problems of school age children and youth—A nursing responsibility? *Journal of School Health* 40(October): 437–439.

Burghardt, J.A., and Devaney, B.L. 1993. The School Nutrition Dietary Assessment Study: Summary of Findings. Princeton, N.J.: Mathematica Policy Research.

Burghardt, J.A., and Devaney, B.L., eds. 1995. *American Journal of Clinical Nutrition* 61(1): Suppl.

Cauffman, J.G., Affleck, M., Warburton, E.A. and Schultz, C.S. 1969. Health care of school children: Variations among ethnic groups. *Journal of School Health* 39(5):296–304.

Center for Health Economics Research. 1993. *Access to Health Care: Key Indicators for Policy.* Princeton, N.J.: Robert Wood Johnson Foundation.

Center on Hunger, Poverty, and Nutrition Policy. 1993. Statement on the Link Between Nutrition and Cognitive Development in Children. Medford, Mass.: Tufts University School of Nutrition.

Centers for Disease Control and Prevention. 1996. Guidelines for school health programs to promote healthy eating. *Morbidity and Mortality Weekly Report* 45(RR-9).

Chaskin, R.J., and Richman, H.A. 1992. Concerns about school-linked services: Institution-based versus community-based models. In *The Future of Children: School Linked Services,* R.E. Behrman, ed. Los Altos, Calif.: Center for the Future of Children, David and Lucille Packard Foundation 2(1):107-117, Spring.

Chen, S.C. 1975. Role relationships in a school health interdisciplinary team. *Journal of School Health* 45(3):172–176.

Cities-in-Schools. 1988. *Fact Sheet and Questions About Cities-in-Schools.* Washington D.C.: Cities-in-Schools.

Citizens' Commission on School Nutrition. 1990. *White Paper on School Lunch Nutrition.* Washington, D.C.: Center for Science in the Public Interest.

Clawson, D.K., and Osterweis, M., eds. 1993. *The Roles of Physician Assistants and Nurse Practitioners in Primary Care.* Washington, D.C.: Association of Academic Health Centers.

Committee for Economic Development, Research and Policy Committee, ed. 1994. *Putting Learning First: Governing and Managing the Schools for High Achievement.* Washington, D.C.: Committee for Economic Development.

Cook, B.A., Schaller, K. and Krischer, J.P. 1985. School absence among children with chronic illness. *Journal of School Health* 55(7):265–267.

Crowley, E.A., and Johnson, J.L. 1977. Multiprofessional perceptions of school health: Definition and scope. *Journal of School Health* 47(Sept):398–404.

Davis, M., Fryer, G.E., White, S. and Igoe, J.B. 1995. A Closer Look: A Report of Select Findings from the National School Health Survey 1993–1994. Denver: Office of School Health, University of Colorado Health Sciences Center.

DeAngelis, C. 1981. The Robert Wood Johnson Foundation National School Health Program: A presentation and progress report. *Clinical Pediatrics* 20:344–348.

Dryfoos, J. 1994a. *Full-Service Schools: A Revolution in Health and Social Services for Children, Youth, and Families.* San Francisco: Jossey-Bass.

Dryfoos, J. 1994b. Medical clinics in junior high school: Changing the model to meet demands. *Journal of Adolescent Health* 15(7):549–557.

Dungy, C.I., and Mullins, R.G. 1981. School nurse practitioners: Analysis of questionnaire and time/motion data. *Journal of School Health* 51(Sept):475–478.

Edwards, L.E., Steinman, M.E., Arnold, K.A., and Hakanson, E.Y. 1980. Adolescent pregnancy prevention services in high school clinics. *Family Planning Perspectives* 12(1):7.

Eisner, V. 1970. Health services under the Elementary and Secondary Education Act. *Journal of School Health* 40(Nov.):464–466.

Elias, M.J., Kress, J.S., Gager, P.J., and Hancock, M.E. 1994. Adolescent health promotion and risk reduction: Cementing the social contract between pediatricians and the schools. *Bulletin of the New York Academy of Medicine* 71(1):87–110.

Ellison, C., Capper, A., Goldberg, R., Witschi, J., and Stare, F. 1989. The environmental component: Changing food service to promote cardiovascular health. *Health Education* 16(2):285–297.

Employee Benefit Research Institute. 1993. *Source of Health Insurance and Characteristics of the Uninsured: Analysis of the March 1992 Current Population Survey*. Issue Brief No. 133, January.

English, A., Matthews, M., Extavour, K., Palamountain, C., and Yang, J. 1995. State Minor Consent Statutes: A Summary. Cincinnati, Ohio: Center for Continuing Education in Adolescent Health, Children's Hospital Medical Center.

Food Research and Action Center. 1996. *School Breakfast Score Card: A Status Report on the School Breakfast Program 1995-1996 (Sixth Edition)*. Food Research and Action Center. Washington, D.C. p.2.

Forbes, O. 1965. The role and functions of the school nurse as perceived by 115 public school teachers from three selected counties. *Journal of School Health* 34:101–106.

Frank, G., Vaden, A., and Martin, J. 1987. School health promotion: Child nutrition programs. *Journal of School Health* 57:451–460.

Freedman, S., Klepper, B., Duncan, P., and Bell, S. 1988. Coverage of the uninsured and underinsured: A proposal for school enrollment-based family health insurance. *New England Journal of Medicine* 381(July):843–847.

Frels, L. 1985. Employment trends of school personnel and staff 1980–1990. *Journal of School Health* 55(4):142–144.

Frerichs, A.H. 1969. Relationship of elementary school absence to psychosomatic ailments. *Journal of School Health* 39(2):92–95.

Fryer, G.E., and Igoe, J.B. 1995. Report: A relationship between availability of school nurses and child well–being. *Journal of School Nursing* 11(3):12–16,18.

Fryer, G.E., and Igoe, J.B. 1996. Functions of school nurses and health assistants in U.S. school health programs. *Journal of School Health* 66(2):55–58.

Goldberg, C.J., Dowling, F.E., Fogarty, E.E., and Moore, D.P. 1995. School scoliosis screening and the United States Preventive Services Task Force: An examination of long-term results. *Spine* 20(12):1368–1374.

Goodwin, L.D., and Keefe, M.R. 1984. The views of school principals and teachers on the role of the school nurse with handicapped students. *Journal of School Health* 54(3):105–109.

Gordon, A., and McKinney, P. 1995. Sources of nutrients in students' diets. *American Journal of Clinical Nutrition* 61(S): 232–240.

Greenhill, E.D. 1979. Perceptions of the school nurse's role. *Journal of School Health* 49:368–371.

Hack, M., Breslau, N., Weissman, B., Aram, D., Klein, N., and Borawski, E. 1991. Effect of very low birth weight and subnormal health size on cognitive abilities at school age. *New England Journal of Medicine* 325(4):231–237.

Harrelson, O.A., Ferguson, D.G., Killian, G.P., and Zimmer, I. 1969. Comparison of hearing screening methods. *Journal of School Health* 39(March):161–164.

Hauser-McKinney, D., and Peak, G. 1995. *Update 1994: Advocates for Youth, Support Center for School-Based and School-Linked Health Care*. Washington, D.C.: Advocates for Youth.

Hilmar, N.A., and McAtee, P.A. 1973. The school nurse practitioner and her practice: A study of traditional and expanded health care responsibilities for nurses in elementary schools. *Journal of School Health* 43(7):431–441.

Hobbs, N., Perrin, J.M., and Ireys, H.T. 1983. *Summary of Findings and Recommendations: Public Policies Affecting Chronically Ill Children and Their Families*. Nashville, Tenn.: Vanderbilt University Institute for Public Policy Studies.

Howell, K.A., and Martin, J.E. 1978. An evaluation model for school health services. *Journal of School Health* 48(Sept.):433–441.

Igoe, J.B., and Campos, E.L. 1991. Report of a national survey of school health nurse supervisors. *School Nurse* 6:8–20.

Igoe, J.B., and Giordano, B. 1992. *Expanding School Health Services to Serve Families in the 21st Century.* Washington, D.C.: American Nurses Publishing.

Igoe, J.B., and Stephens, R. 1994. School health activities within educational service agencies. Unpublished final report submitted to the Robert Wood Johnson Foundation.

Innui, T.S. 1992. The social contract and the medical school's responsibilities. In *The Medical School's Mission and Population Health: Medical Education in Canada, the United Kingdom, the United States and Australia,* K. White and J. Connelly, eds. New York: Springer-Verlag.

Institute of Medicine. 1993. *Emergency Medical Services for Children.* Washington, D.C.: National Academy Press.

Institute of Medicine. 1994. *Defining Primary Care: An Interim Report.* Washington, D.C.: National Academy Press.

International Food Information Council. 1995. The healthy attitude of today's kids. *In Food Insight: Current Topics in Food Safety and Nutrition.* Washington, D.C.: International Food Information Council Foundation, May/June.

Jenne, F.H. 1970. Variations in nursing service characteristics and teachers' health observation practices. *Journal of School Health* 40:248–250.

Johnson, J.L., Spellman, C.R., Cress, P.J., Sizemore, A.C. and Shores, R.E. 1983. The school nurse's role in vision screening for the difficult-to-test student. *Journal of School Health* 53(6):345–350.

Kagan, S.L. 1991. *United We Stand: Collaboration for Child Care and Early Education Services.* New York: Teachers College Press.

Kalisch, B.J., Kalisch, P.A., and McHugh, M. 1983. School nursing in the news. *Journal of School Health* 53(9):548–553.

Kaplan, D. 1995. *School HealthCare ONLINE!!!*. Denver: National Center for School-Based Health Information Systems, Children's Hospital, Version 4.1.

Kirby, D. 1994. Findings from other studies of school-based clinics. Presentation given at Meeting on Evaluation sponsored by the Robert Wood Johnson Foundation, Washington, D.C., September 23.

Kirby, D., Resnick., M.D., Downes, B. Kocher, T., Gunderson, P., Potthoff, S., Zelterman, D., and Blum, R.W. 1993. The effects of school-based health clinics in St. Paul on school-wide birth rates. *Family Planning Perspectives* 25:12–16.

Kisker, E.E., Brown, R.S., and Hill, J. 1994a. *Healthy Caring: Outcomes of the Robert Wood Johnson Foundations's School-Based Adolescent Health Care Program.* Princeton N.J.: Mathematica Policy Research.

Kisker, E.E., Marks, E.L., Morrill, W.A., and Brown, R.S. 1994b. *Healthy Caring: An Evaluation Summary of the Robert Wood Johnson Foundation's School-Based Adolescent Health Care Program.* Princeton, N.J.: Mathematica Policy Research.

Klerman, L. 1988. School absence—A health perspective. *Pediatric Clinics of North America* 35:1253–1269.

Kornguth, M.L. 1990. School illnesses: Who's absent and why? *Pediatric Nursing* 16:95–99.

Korup, U.L. 1985. Parent and teacher perception of depression in children. *Journal of School Health* 55(9):367–369.

Knitzer, J. 1989. *Collaborations Between Child Welfare and Mental Health: Emerging Patterns and Challenges.* New York: Bank Street College of Education.

Larson, C.S. 1992. Confidentiality. In *The Future of Children: School Linked Services*, R.E. Behrman, ed. Los Altos, Calif.: Center for the Future of Children, David and Lucille Packard Foundation 2(1):131-134, Spring.

Leonard, W. 1992. Keeping kids in school. *Focus*: June 4–5.

Levine, M.D., Palfrey, J.S., Lamb, G.A., Weisberg, H.I., and Bryk, A.S. 1977. Infants in a public school system: The indicators of early health and education need. *Pediatrics* 60(4 pt 2):579–587.

Lewis, C., and Lewis, M.A. 1990. Consequences of empowering children to care for themselves. *Pediatrician* 17:63–67.

Lewis, C.E., Lorimer, A., Lindeman, C., Palmer, B.B., and Lewis, M.A. 1974. An evaluation of the impact of school nurse practitioners. *Journal of School Health* 44(6):331–335.

Lewit, E.M., Schuurmann-Baker, L., Corman, H., and Shiono, P.H. 1995. The direct cost of low birth weight. In *The Future of Children: Low Birth Weight*, R.E. Behrman, ed. Los Altos, Calif: David and Lucille Packard Foundation 5(1):35-56, Spring.

Lowis, E.M. 1964. An appraisal of the amount of time spent on functions by Los Angeles city school nurses. *Journal of School Health* 34:254–257.

Luepker, R.V., Perry, C.L., McKinlay, S.M., Nader, P.R., Parcel, G.S., Stone, E.J., Webber, L.S., Elder, J.P., Feldman, H.A., Johnson, C.C., Kelder, S.H., and Wu, M. 1996. Outcomes of a field trial to improve children's dietary patterns and physical activity: The Child and Adolescent Trial for Cardiovascular Health (CATCH). *Journal of the American Medical Association* 275(10):768–776.

MacBriar, B.R., Burgess, M. Kottke, S. and Maddox, K. 1995. Development of a health concerns inventory for school-age children. *Journal of School Nursing* 11(3):25–29.

Marcinak, J.F., and Yount, S.C.W. 1995. Evaluation of vision screening practices of Illinois pediatricians. *Clinical Pediatrics* 34:353–357.

Marks, E.L., and Marzke, C.H. 1993. *Healthy Caring: A Process Evaluation of the Robert Wood Johnson Foundation's School-Based Adolescent Health Care Program*. Princeton, N.J.: Mathtech.

McCord, M.D., Klein, J.D., Foy, J.M., and Fothergill, K. 1993. School-based clinic use and school performance. *Journal of Adolescent Health* 14:91–98.

McKaig, C., Hindi-Alexander, M., Myers, T.R. and Castiglia, P. 1984. Implementation of the school nurse practitioner role: Barriers and facilitators. *Journal of School Health* 54(1):21–23.

Meeker, R., DeAngelis, C., Berman, B., Freeman, H.E., and Oda, D. 1986. A comprehensive school health initiative. *Image* 18:86–91.

Meyer, J.S., and Regenstein, M. 1994. *How to Fund Public Health Activities*. Washington, D.C.: Partnership for Prevention.

Meyers, A.F., Sampson, A.D., Weitzman, M., Rogers, B.L., and Kayne, H. 1989. School breakfast program and school performance. *American Journal of Diseases and Children* 143:1234.

Miller, D.F., and Shunk, S. 1972. A survey of elementary school health services with emphasis on preparation for emergency care procedures of sick and injured students. *Journal of School Health* 42(2):114–117.

Missouri School Children's Health Services Committee. 1993. Opening doors to Improved Health for Missouri's School Age Children: Recommendations of the Missouri School Children's Health Services Committee. Jefferson City: Missouri Department of Health.

Murray-Garcia, J. 1995. African-American youth: Essential prevention strategies for every pediatrician. *Pediatrics* 96:132–137.

Nader, P.R. (ed.) 1993. *School Health: Policy and Practice*. Elk Grove Village, Ill.: American Academy of Pediatrics.

Nader, P.R. 1995. San Diego Unified School District, personal communication.

Nader, P.R., and Brink, S.G. 1981. Does visiting the school health room teach appropriate or inappropriate use of health services? *American Journal of Public Health* 71:416–419.

National Adolescent Health Resource Center Evaluative Review. 1993. Findings from a Study of Selected High School Wellness Centers in Delaware. University of Minnesota, Division of General Pediatrics and Adolescent Health.

National Alliance of Pupil Services Organizations. 1992. Mission statement. Washington, D.C. December 9.

National Health Education Consortium. 1992. *Creating Sound Minds: Health and Education Working Together*. Washington, D.C.: National Health Education Consortium.

National Health Education Consortium. 1993. *Eat to Learn, Learn to Eat: The Link Between Nutrition and Learning in Children*. Washington, D.C. National Health Education Consortium.

National Institute of Dental Research. 1995. Personal communication.

National Nursing Coalition for School Health. 1995. School health nursing services: Exploring national issues and priorities. *Journal of School Health* 65(9):370–389.

National Research Council. 1989. *Diet and Health: Implications for Reducing Chronic Disease Risk*. Washington, D.C.: National Academy Press.

Nestle, M. 1992. Societal barriers to improved school lunch programs: Rationale for recent policy recommendations. *School Food Service Research Review* 16(1):5–10.

Newacheck, P.W., Hughes, D.C., English, A., Fox, H.B., Perrin, J., and Halfon, N. 1995. The effect on children of curtailing Medicaid spending. *Journal of the American Medical Association* 274(18):1468–1471.

New York State Department of Health. 1994. Unpublished data from School Health Division. Albany: New York State Department of Health.

Nicklas, T., Forcier, J. Farris R., Hunter, S., Webber L., and Berenson, G. 1989. Heart Smart School Lunch Program: Vehicle for cardiovascular health promotion. *American Journal of Health Promotion* 14(2):91–100.

Oda, D.S., Barysh, N., and Setear, S.J. 1979. Increasing role effectiveness of school nurses. *American Journal of Public Health* 64:591–595.

Oda, D.S., DeAngelis, C., Berman, B., and Meeker, R. 1985. The resolution of health problems in school children. *Journal of School Health* 55(3):96–98.

Office of Technology Assessment, Congress of the United States. 1991. *Adolescent Health*. Washington, D.C.: U.S. Government Printing Office.

O'Neil, S.L., Barysh, N., and Setear, S.J. 1985. Determining school programming needs of special population groups: A study of asthmatic children. *Journal of School Health* 55(6):237–239.

Palfrey, J.S., Haynie, M., Porter, S., Bierle, T., Cooperman, P., and Lowcock, J. 1992. Project school care: Integrating children assisted by medical technology into educational settings. *Journal of School Health* 62(2):50–54.

Palfrey, J.S., Mervis, R.C., and Butler, J.A. 1978. New directions in the evaluation and education of handicapped children. *New England Journal of Medicine* 298(15):819–824.

Pateman, B.C., McKinney, P., Kann, L., Small, M.L., Warren, C.W., and Collins, J.L. 1995. School food services. *Journal of School Health* 65(8):327–332.

Patterson, J. 1967. Effectiveness of follow-up of health referrals for school health services under two different administrative patterns. *Journal of School Health* 37:687–692.

Perino, J.P., and Brindis, C. 1994. Payment for Services Rendered: Expanding the Revenue Base of School-Based Clinics. San Francisco: Center for Reproductive Health Policy Research, Institute for Health Policy Studies, University of California.

Perry, C., Stone, E., Parcel, G., Ellison, R., Nader, P., Webber, L., and Luepker, R. 1990. School-based cardiovascular health promotion: The Child and Adolescent Trial for Cardiovascular Health (CATCH). *Journal of School Health* 60(8):406–413.

Piessens, P., King, M.C., Ryan, J., Millette, B., Sheetz, A., Douglas, J.B., and Rissmiller, P.N. 1995. A statewide institute to delivery professional development programs to school health personnel in Massachusetts. *Journal of School Health* 65(5):176–180.

Poehlman, B., and Manager, A. 1992. Comprehensive School Health Programs Project: Listings of schools provided. Alexandria, Va: National School Boards Association.

Proctor, S.E. 1986. Evaluation of nursing practice in schools. *Journal of School Health* 56(7):272–275.

Proctor, S.T., Lordi, S.L., and Zarger, D.S. 1993. *School Nursing Practice Roles and Standards*. Scarborough, Maine: National Association for School Nurses.

Ratchick, I. 1968. Evaluation of school health services for disadvantaged children under Title I, Elementary and Secondary Education Act. *Journal of School Health* 38:140–146.

Risser, W.L., Hoffman, H.M., Bellah, G.G., and Green, L.W. 1985. A cost–benefit analysis of preparticipation sports examinations of adolescent athletes. *Journal of School Health* 55(7):270–273.

Robert Wood Johnson Foundation. 1988. *Serving Handicapped Children: A Special Report*. Princeton, N.J.: Robert Wood Johnson Foundation.

Roberts, D.E., Basco, D., Slome, C., Glasser, J.H., and Handy, G. 1969. Epidemiologic analysis in school populations as a basis for change in school nursing practice. *American Journal of Public Health* 59(12):2157–2167.

Rosenberg and Associates. 1995. Issues in Financing School-Based Health Centers: A Guide for State Officials. Washington, D.C.: Making the Grade National Program Office, George Washington University.

Rousseau, R. 1995. R and I's school giants: Marketing and motivating are keys to excellence. *Restaurants and Institutions Report* (September):18–30.

Russo, R.M., Harvey, B., Kukafka, R., Supino, P., Freis, P.C., and Hamilton, P. 1982. The use of community health aides in a school health program. *Journal of School Health* 52:425–427.

Rustia, J., Hartley, R., Hansen, G. Schulte, D., and Spielman, L. 1984. Redefinition of school nursing practice: Integrating the developmentally disabled. *Journal of School Health* 54(2):58–62.

Sampson, A., Dixit, S., Meyers, A., and Houser, R. 1995. The nutritional impact of breakfast consumption on the diets of inner city African-American elementary school children. *Journal of the National Medical Association* 87(3):195–202.

Santelli, J., Morreale, M., Wigton, A., and Grason, H. 1995. Improving Access to Primary Care for Adolescents: School Health Centers as a Service Delivery Strategy. MCH Policy Research Brief. Baltimore: Johns Hopkins University School of Hygiene and Public Health.

Santelli, J., Kouzis, A., and Newcomer, S. 1996. School-based health centers and adolescent use of primary care and hospitals. *Journal of Adolescent Health* 19(4):267–275.

Schlitt, J.J., and Rickett, K.D., Montgomery, L.L., and Lear, J.G. 1994. *State Initiatives to Support School-Based Health Centers: A National Survey*. Washington, D.C.: Making the Grade National Program Office.

Shearer, C.A. 1995. *Where the Kids Are: How to Work with Schools to Create Elementary School-Based Health Centers, A Primer for Health Professionals*. Washington, D.C.: National Health and Education Consortium.

Shearer, C.A., and Holschneider, S.O.M. 1995. *Starting Young: School-Based Health Centers at the Elementary Level*. Washington, D.C.: National Health and Education Consortium.

Shenkman, E., Pendergast, J., Reiss, J., Walther, E., and Freedman, S. 1996. The school enrollment-based health insurance program: Socioeconomic factors in enrollees' use of health care. *American Journal of Public Health* 86(12):1791–1793.

Silvetta, M.B., and Swartz, K. 1986. *The Uninsured and Uncompensated Care: A Chart Book.* Washington, D.C.: National Health Policy Forum.

Simons-Morton, B., Parcel, G.S., Baranowski, T., Forthofer, F., and O'Hara, N. 1991. Promoting physical activity and a healthful diet among children: Results of a school-based intervention study. *American Journal of Health Promotion* 81:986–991.

Small, M.L., Majer, L.S., Allensworth, D.D., Farquhar, B.K., Kann, L., and Pateman, B.C. 1995. School health services. *Journal of School Health* 65(8):319–325.

Sneed, J., and White, K. 1993. Continuing education needs of school-level managers in child nutrition programs. *School Food Service Research Review* 17(2):103–108.

Snyder, M., Obarzanek, E., Montgomery, D., Feldman, H., Nicklas, T., Raizman, D., Rupp J., Bibelow, C., and Lakatos, E. 1994. Reducing the fat content of ground beef in a school foodservice setting. *Journal of the American Dietetic Association* 94:1135–1139.

Soler, M.I., Shotton, A.C., and Bell, J.R. 1993. *Glass Walls: Confidentiality Provisions and Interagency Collaborations.* San Francisco: Youth Law Center.

Solloway, M.R., and Budetti, P.P., eds. 1995. *Child Health Supervision: Analytical Studies on the Financing, Delivery, and Cost-Effectiveness of Preventive and Health Promotion Services for Infants, Children, and Adolescents.* Arlington, Va.: National Center for Education in Maternal and Child Health.

Spollen, J.J., and Davidson, D.W. 1978. An analysis of vision defects in high and low income preschool children. *Journal of School Health* 48:177–180.

Starfield, B. 1982. Family income, ill health, and medical care of U.S. children. *Journal of Public Health Policy* 3(September):244–259.

Starfield, B. 1992. Child and adolescent health status measures. *In The Future of Children: U.S. Health Care for Children*, R.E. Behrman, ed. Los Altos, Calif.: Center for the Future of Children, David and Lucille Packard Foundation. 2(2):25-39, Winter.

Starfield, B., and Vivier, P.M. 1995. Population and selective (high-risk) approaches to prevention in well-child care. In *Child Health Supervision: Analytical Studies on the Financing, Delivery, and Cost-Effectiveness of Preventive and Health Promotion Services for Infants, Children, and Adolescents*, M.R. Solloway and P.P. Budetti, eds. Arlington, Va.: National Center for Education in Maternal and Child Health.

Stout, J. 1991. School-Based Health Clinics: Are They Addressing the Needs of the Students? M.P.H. thesis, University of Washington, Seattle.

Strickland, O.L. 1995. Executive Summary: Primary Care in Public Schools. Atlanta: Southern Council on Collegiate Education for Nursing of the Southern Regional Education Board.

Thurber, F., Berry, B. and Cameron, M.E. 1991. The role of school nursing in the United States. *Journal of Pediatric Health Care* 5(3):135–140.

Tuthill, R.W., Williams, C., Long, G., and Whitman, C. 1972. Evaluating a school health program focused on high absence pupils: A research design. *American Journal of Public Health* (January):40–42.

U.S. Department of Agriculture. 1986. Competitive food service. *Federal Register.* FNS, 7CFR. Parts 210.2, 210.12, 220.2, and 220.12. January 1.

U.S. Department of Agriculture. 1994. *Nutrition Objectives for School Meals.* Washington, D.C.: USDA Child Nutrition Programs.

U.S. Department of Health and Human Services. 1988. *The Surgeon General's Report on Nutrition and Health.* Washington, D.C.: U.S. Government Printing Office.

U.S. Department of Health and Human Services. 1991. Healthy People 2000: National Health Promotion and Disease Prevention Objectives. DHHS Publication No. (PHS) 91-50213, Public Health Service. Washington, D.C.: U.S. Government Printing Office.

U.S. Department of Health and Human Services, 1993a. *School-Based Health Centers and Managed Care*. DHEW Publication No. OEI-05-92-00680, Office of the Inspector General. Washington, D.C.: U.S. Government Printing Office.

U.S. Department of Health and Human Services, 1993b. *School-Based Clinics That Work*. Washington D.C.: Public Health Service, Health Resources and Services Administration, Bureau of Primary Health Care, HRSA 93-248P.

U.S. General Accounting Office, 1993a. *School-Linked Human Services: A Comprehensive Strategy for Aiding Students At Risk for School Failure*. GAO/HRD-94-21, Washington, D.C.: U.S. General Accounting Office.

U.S. General Accounting Office. 1993b. *Food Assistance: Schools That Left the National School Lunch Program*. GAO/RCED-94-36BR. Washington, D.C.: U.S. General Accounting Office.

U.S. General Accounting Office. 1994a. *School-Based Health Centers Can Promote Access to Care*. GAO/HEHS-94-166. Washington, D.C.: U.S. General Accounting Office.

U.S. General Accounting Office. 1994b. *School-Based Health Centers Can Expand Access for Children*. GAO/HEHS-95-35. Washington, D.C.: U.S. General Accounting Office.

Wagner, M., Golan, S., Shaver, D., Newman, L., Wechsler, M., and Kelley, F. 1994. A Healthy Start for California's Children and Families: Early Findings from a Statewide Evaluation of School-Linked Services. Menlo Park, Calif.: SRI International.

Walker, D.K. 1992. Children and youth with special health care needs. In *Principles and Practices of Student Health*, Volume One: Foundations, H.M. Wallace, K. Patrick, G.S. Parcel, and J.B. Igoe, eds. Oakland, Calif.: Third Party Publishing.

Wallace, H.M., Patrick, K., Parcel, G.S., and Igoe, J.B., eds. 1992. *Principles and Practices of Student Health*, Volume Two: School Health. Oakland, Calif.: Third Party Publishing.

Whitaker, R., Wright, J., Finch, A., and Psaty, B. 1993. An environmental intervention to reduce dietary fat in school lunches. *Pediatrics* 91(6):1107–1111.

Wolfe, B.L. 1985. The influence of health on school outcomes. *Medical Care* 23(10):1127–1138.

Wolk, L.I., and Kaplan, D.W. 1993. Frequent school-based clinic utilization: A comparative profile of problems and service needs. *Journal of Adolescent Health* 14:458–463.

World Health Organization. 1995. *The European Network of Health Promoting Schools: A Joint WHO-CE-CEC Project*. Denmark: Council of Europe, Commission of the European Communities.

Yankauer, A., and Lawrence, R.A. 1961. A study of case-finding methods in elementary schools: Methodology and initial results. *American Journal of Public Health* 51(Oct.):1532–1540.

Zimmerman, D.J., and Reif, C.J. 1995. School-based health centers and managed care health plans: Partners in primary care. *Journal of Public Health Management Practice* 1(1):33–39.

5
Building the Infrastructure for Comprehensive School Health Programs

The vision of a comprehensive school health program (CSHP) in each of our nation's schools at first may seem daunting and out of reach, but a closer look suggests that this vision is in fact not so far from reality. Many parts of the infrastructure needed to support CSHPs—the basic underlying framework of policies, financial and human resources, organizational structures, and communication channels that will be needed for programs to become established and grow—already exist or are emerging. This chapter examines the resources already available and what needs to be done to build the CSHP infrastructure, from the national level to the local neighborhood school.

The order of the infrastructure discussion reflects the order of potential impact; the national infrastructure establishes various policies, programs, and funding streams that have an effect on and provide the framework for states, which, in turn, coordinate policies, programs, and funding streams that impact on the local level. The committee is certainly aware that in the current policy environment, there is an emphasis on minimizing the federal role and on devolving, or transferring, decisionmaking regarding education and other social programs to the state and local levels. Therefore, it is important to acknowledge that the decisionmaking that directly impacts students occurs at the local level. In reality, the only thing that matters is what happens school by school.

THE NATIONAL INFRASTRUCTURE

Soon after *Goals 2000—Educate America Act*, became law in March 1994, the Secretary of Education, Richard Riley, and the Secretary of Health and Human Services, Donna Shalala, released a joint statement announcing a new level of cooperation between their two departments and affirming the importance of school health programs in accomplishing education goals. Their joint statement (U.S. Departments of Education and Health and Human Services, 1994) made the following points:

- America's children face many compelling educational and health and developmental challenges that affect their lives and their futures.
- To help children meet these challenges, education and health must be linked in partnership.
- School health programs support the education process, integrate services for disadvantaged and disabled children, and improve children's prospects.
- Reforms in health care and in education offer opportunities to forge the partnerships needed for our children in the 1990s.
- Goals 2000 and Healthy People 2000 provide complementary visions that, together, can support our joint efforts in pursuit of a healthier and better-educated nation for the next century.

As part of this new level of cooperation, the secretaries announced the formation of an Interagency Committee on School Health (ICSH) and a National Coordinating Committee on School Health (NCCSH).

Federal Interagency Committee on School Health

The Interagency Committee on School Health consists of representatives from all federal agencies and offices that provide funding and other resources for programs related to school health. The U.S. Department of Agriculture (USDA) has joined the initial efforts of the U.S. Department of Education (DOEd) and the U.S. Department of Health and Human Services (DHHS) in convening the ICSH. The ICSH is concerned with all federal policies and programs related to school health, and its mission is to increase the overall effectiveness of federal agencies in this area. According to its charter (U.S. Department of Education et al., 1994), the ICSH will do the following:

- Improve communication, planning, coordination, and collaboration among federal agencies engaged in ongoing activities of relevance to school health or planning such activities.
- Identify needs and facilitate the planning and updating of strategies to improve federal leadership for school health.
- Identify opportunities for federal policies to facilitate the develop-

ment and implementation of school health programs and identify and address policies and practices which may be acting as barriers to effective school health programs.

• Facilitate the identification, coordination, and dissemination of promising programs, information, or materials relevant to school health generated by federally conducted or supported programs or activities.

• Provide a focal point for identification of, and interaction and coordination with, efforts in the private and voluntary sectors to promote the implementation of school health programs.

• Assist private and voluntary sectors in identifying federal policies, programs, initiatives, and materials that support the implementation of school health programs.

• Prepare reports and make policy recommendations to the relevant officials on special topics identified by the committee.

The ICSH is still in the formative stages, but the committee believes that the ICSH has the potential to serve as an anchor for the national infrastructure and provide increased national leadership and visibility for school health. The committee believes that the capacity of the ICSH should be strengthened by giving it the authority, staff, and funding necessary to carry out its basic functions as listed above. In addition, there is a wide range of additional needs and issues that could benefit from receiving attention from the ICSH.

For example, the ICSH could promote much needed coordination among federal funding streams related to school health and child or family services in order to help states and localities cope with the current broad array of separate programs, each with its own requirements and regulations. The ICSH could be instrumental in catalyzing and supporting state-level infrastructure development and in encouraging dialogue and information-sharing among states. Federal agencies, through the leadership of the ICSH, could help promote awareness and adoption of national standards in health education, physical education, school nutrition, school nursing, and school-based health care.[1] Grantees of federal programs for school health should be expected to give attention to these standards, and funded projects should be aligned with the concept of a comprehensive program.

The position of health education in the K–12 curriculum is ambiguous, because health education is not one of the core subjects specified in the National Education Goals (although it is mentioned in the context of Goal 7 on safe, disciplined, and alcohol- and drug-free schools). Since

---

[1]These standards, as well as standards in other core academic subjects, should be regarded as "national," not "federal" standards, based on a national consensus in each field, to be voluntarily adopted and adapted in each state.

common wisdom holds that schools pay attention to what is tested, the ICSH could elevate the importance of health education by promoting the inclusion of health-related topics in assessments such as the National Assessment for Educational Progress, and by encouraging the use of state assessments that follow the Health Education Standards, such as the State Collaborative on Assessment and Student Standards (SCASS) materials being developed by the Council of Chief State School Officers.

Basic research on school health is also an important area needing attention. Many critical questions remain unanswered,[2] but there is no unified federal program that focuses on supporting basic research in comprehensive school health programming. The ICSH could be instrumental in organizing a coordinated research agenda, facilitating communication among researchers, and interpreting and disseminating research findings to state and local practitioners.

To achieve its basic objectives, as well as the expanded goals mentioned above, the ICSH should be elevated from committee status to a coordinating council with influence and authority. In this reinvigorated role it can serve as a model for collaboration at the state and local levels. The ICSH would also monitor and guide the activities of state-level coordinating bodies.

National Coordinating Committee on School Health

The National Coordinating Committee on School Health brings together federal departments with approximately 40 national nongovernmental organizations to support quality comprehensive school health programs in the nation's schools. The NCCSH is staffed by the same office as ICSH, and the committees work closely with each other. According to its mission statement, the responsibilities of NCCSH include the following:

- Providing national leadership for the promotion of quality comprehensive school health programs.
- Improving communication, collaboration, and sharing of information among national organizations.
- Developing a clear vision of the role of school health programs in improving the health and educational achievement of children.
- Identifying local, state, and federal barriers to the development and implementation of effective school health programs.
- Collecting and disseminating information on effective school health programs.
- Establishing and monitoring national goals for strengthening school health programs.

[2]Some of these questions are outlined in Chapter 6.

The NCCSH consists of organizations that have a local presence, such as the National Parent Teachers Association, National School Boards Association, American Medical Association, American Dental Association, American Academy of Pediatrics, American Nurses Association, National Associations of Elementary and Secondary School Principals, National Association of School Nurses, National Education Association, and the Council of Great City Schools, to name a few. Local communities can thus be connected to the NCCSH—and through the NCCSH to the ICSH—through these organizations. The committee suggests that the NCCSH should be considered the official advisory council to the ICSH and that participating NCCSH organizations should mobilize their memberships to promote the development of the comprehensive school health infrastructure at the state and local levels. The committee feels that the NCCSH currently may be limited in its influence because managed care, indemnity insurance providers, and others key to resolving critical financial issues seem to be missing from its membership; the committee suggests that the NCCSH might be strengthened by actively soliciting the participation of those with financial interests in CSHPs.

States can develop structures similar to the ICSH-NCCSH collaboration by establishing a state interagency coordinating council with regulatory powers. These councils could involve the major agencies that have a mandate for improving the health and education of students, along with an advisory council representing professional and voluntary health organizations, educational organizations, and others dedicated to the health, education, and welfare of children and families.

Federal Programs and Funding Streams for School Health

Many federal agencies have developed programs to improve the health of children and adolescents. These programs can be a source of funding and technical assistance that states and local communities can use to develop their infrastructure and to implement their programs. The following examples demonstrate the range of federal resources for school health. These examples are intended to be brief and illustrative; there are many additional programs. It should be noted that some of the following may be subject to change.

- The U.S. Department of Education programs provide major sources of funding to the local level that can be used for school health programs. Title I of the Elementary and Secondary Education Act (ESEA) gives grants to local education agencies based on the number of disadvantaged students they serve in order to help these students meet high academic standards. Title I funds may be used to provide educationally related support services, such as counseling and health services, for conditions that interfere with learning. Title IV of ESEA, Safe and Drug-Free Schools, provides funds for drug and violence prevention that can be used for school health education. Title XI of ESEA, Coordinated Services Projects, allows local education agencies to use up to 5 percent of their ESEA funding to plan, develop, and implement coordinated health and human services for students and families. The Individuals with Disabilities Education Act (IDEA) provides funding for schools to provide health, counseling, and related services to students with disabilities. DOEd also provides assistance to local curriculum developers by reviewing and disseminating exemplary health education curricula through its National Diffusion Network.

• Since 1992, the Division of Adolescent and School Health (DASH) of the Centers for Disease Control and Prevention (CDC) has funded 12 states and the District of Columbia to develop their own infrastructure to strengthen comprehensive school health programs and student educational achievement.[3] The goal of this initiative is not only to build programs and increase understanding about the process but also to have states serve as models for and provide technical assistance to other states. In each of these states, funding has been provided to hire a senior staff member in the state department of education and department of health and human services in order to ensure program coordination between these agencies and efficient utilization of health and education resources. These comprehensive school health programs are emphasizing the prevention of the priority health-risk behaviors identified by CDC: sexual behaviors that result in HIV infection, other sexually transmitted diseases (STDs), and unintended pregnancy; alcohol and other drug use; behaviors that result in unintentional and intentional injuries; tobacco use; dietary patterns that result in disease; and sedentary lifestyle. In addition to supporting infrastructure development in these states, DASH/CDC also provides funds for HIV/AIDS education in all states and territories.

• CDC/DASH supports the Adolescent and School Health Initiative, a cooperative agreement with the National Association of Community Health Centers. This initiative provides information, training, and technical assistance to help federally qualified health centers and state and regional primary care associations in establishing and strengthening health center partnerships with schools. A database on health center school-based and school-linked programs is being developed, and information about effective programs is being showcased and disseminated.

---

[3]The demonstration states are Arkansas, California, Florida, Michigan, Minnesota, New Mexico, New York, Rhode Island, South Carolina, South Dakota, West Virginia, and Wisconsin, as well as the District of Columbia.

- The Maternal and Child Health Bureau (MCH) of the Department of Health and Human Services administers the MCH Title V state block grants, which can be used to support a state MCH director and the delivery of school-based services. MCH also supports a group of national resource centers that conduct studies, disseminate information, and provide materials, networking, professional development, and technical assistance.[4] MCH has joined with the Bureau of Primary Health Care of DHHS in the "Healthy Schools, Healthy Communities" program, which provides funding to establish school-based health centers to serve high-risk students in disadvantaged communities and to develop health education and promotion programs to complement and support the school-based health centers. The Bureau of Primary Health Care also supports school-based health centers through its Community and Migrant Health Centers initiative.

- The U.S. Department of Agriculture provides financial support for the School Lunch, School Breakfast, Special Milk, and Snack Programs. USDA standards require compliance with the Recommended Daily Allowances of key nutrients and the principles stated in the Dietary Guidelines for Americans, which include limitations on the amount of fat and saturated fat. The Nutrition Education and Training (NET) Program places a NET coordinator in each state and provides limited funding for nutrition education for foodservice directors and classroom health education teachers. Team Nutrition, a program recently announced by the USDA, promotes healthful eating habits in children and young people through media campaigns and school-based promotions, as well as through training of school staff.

- Medicaid, as discussed in Chapter 4, is a potentially significant source of funding for school-based health and rehabilitative services to eligible students. The Medicaid Early and Periodic Screening, Diagnostic, and Treatment Program (EPSDT) can reimburse schools for screenings,

---

[4]These resource centers include the National Center for Education in Maternal and Child Health at Georgetown University, which maintains an extensive database on maternal and child health projects and resources; National Center for Leadership Enhancement of Adolescent Programs at the Colorado Department of Public Health and Environment; National Adolescent Health Information Center at the University of California, San Francisco; Child and Adolescent Health Policy Center at George Washington University; National School-Based Oral Health/Dental Sealant Resource Center at the University of Illinois at Chicago; Child and Adolescent Health Policy Center at Johns Hopkins University; School Health Resource Services at the University of Colorado Health Services Center; National Adolescent Health Resource Center at the University of Minnesota; and the School Mental Health Centers at the University of California at Los Angeles and the University of Maryland at Baltimore.

treatment, case management, and administrative expenses. Many schools are not yet receiving such reimbursement, however, since the process and requirements for qualifying as a Medicaid provider can be complex. Another obstacle is the statutory requirement that Medicaid will not reimburse schools for services that are provided free to other students. Since there is no such limitation on services provided with IDEA or MCH Title V funds, some schools are using these sources to support services for non-Medicaid students, thus removing the free care obstacle (Sullivan, 1995).

• CDC/DASH has recently initiated an effort to identify and disseminate effective curricula that have been shown to reduce health risk behaviors among young people. Curricula that have been credibly evaluated and have demonstrated a positive behavioral impact are further examined, updated, and revised by outside program and evaluation experts. These curricula are then introduced to state and local DASH grantees and to members of an already established network of state level teacher training centers, which in turn introduce the materials to school districts for their consideration. CDC, national organizations, and curriculum developers arrange for the training of "master teachers" and provide technical assistance to state and local education agencies in implementing curricula. The first cycle of curricula examined under the project deals with sexual risk behaviors for HIV, other STDs, and unintended pregnancy.

• In recent years, CDC/DASH has convened an annual National School Health Leadership Conference. Participants include representatives from federal agencies, higher education institutions, state and local education agencies, and nonprofit and professional organizations involved in school health. This conference meets in conjunction with the NCCSH meeting and offers an excellent opportunity for participants to network and gather information to help build local programs.

In addition to the sources mentioned above, other federal agencies have programs and funds for school health. Appendix F contains a budget overview of these programs for fiscal year 1995. At the time of writing this report, it seems possible that some of these programs may undergo change—some may be eliminated or downsized and others reconfigured or transferred to the states as block grants. However, Appendix F gives a sense of the diversity of federal agencies and programs that have connections to school health.

This diversity has its drawbacks at the state and local levels, however. Some federal programs may be categorical, such as Drug-Free Schools, with funds restricted to specifically defined activities. Other programs—such as IDEA, Medicaid, and School Lunch—have particular eligibility requirements for individual student participation. States and localities are often faced with an array of related programs that may be used for school health with different or conflicting criteria, eligibility standards, and application and reporting requirements. Further, many of these funds are stopgap, short-term measures that cannot be relied upon for ongoing support over the long haul. Also, some observers maintain that these funding streams often require substantial resources and know-how to obtain, weave together, and use to produce a coherent, comprehensive program.

Widespread, consistent implementation of CSHPs in the future will require funding and other resources that are adequate, stable, and flexible. Many are calling for a reduction of restrictions on the use of various categorical funds so that funding streams can be coordinated and used for a wider range of needs. A possible downside to this increased flexibility is that specific problems originally targeted by categorical programs might be neglected. A response to this concern is that even if categorical restrictions are eased, the critical needs of a community will still be met if program priorities are determined at the local level through a broad-based needs assessment.

Other National Efforts

Many national organizations are becoming involved in school health. The scope of involvement is illustrated by *Creating An Agenda for School-Based Health Promotion: A Review of Selected Reports*, published by the Harvard School of Public Health (Lavin et al., 1992). This review focused on 25 recent landmark reports published by a variety of national organizations. These reports address the interconnectedness of children's health and education and they incorporate a comprehensive approach to health rather that focusing on a single categorical concern such as AIDS or tobacco use. The reports reflect the following recurring themes: education and health are interrelated; the biggest threats to health are the new "social morbidities;" a more comprehensive, integrated approach is needed; health promotion and education efforts should be centered in and around schools; prevention efforts are cost-effective; and the social and economic costs of inaction are too high and still escalating.

The reports covered in the review, as well as the review itself, provide a wealth of information on comprehensive school health programs. Examples of report publishers include the American Association of School Administrators, American Medical Association, Carnegie Council on Adolescent Development, Children's Defense Fund, Council of Chief State School Officers, National Association of State Boards of Education, National Commission on Children, and the National School Boards Association. Many of these organizations are continuing to undertake initiatives promoting comprehensive school health programs.

Nonprofit and philanthropic organizations have also joined in the national movement to support CSHPs. As examples, the American Cancer Society (ACS) convened a conference in June 1992 (ACS, 1993) to develop a "National Action Plan for Comprehensive School Health Education" and provided support for the production and dissemination of the National Health Education Standards in 1995 (Joint Committee on National Health Education Standards, 1995). The Robert Wood Johnson Foundation has taken the lead in promoting and supporting school-based clinics through its "National School Health Project, School-Based Adolescent Health Care" and "Making the Grade" initiatives.

Comprehensive, integrated school-based services is an area receiving increased attention nationally. Several national conferences have taken place, and reports on comprehensive services been issued in recent years (Melaville and Blank, 1991; Melaville et al., 1993; U.S. DOEd., 1995). As mentioned in Chapter 2, one particularly significant event was a consensus conference held in January 1994, at which representatives of more than 50 national organizations concerned with the well-being of children, youth, and families came together to develop a broad set of principles for community-based, school-linked collaboration (American Academy of Pediatrics, 1994).

THE STATE AND LOCAL INFRASTRUCTURE

At both the state and local levels, the objectives of the school health infrastructure are:

- secure high-level commitment to the program,
- assess state and community needs and capacity for program development,
- define outcome expectations for the program,
- develop policies and regulations needed to ensure quality program implementation,
- ensure coordination, communication, and effective utilization of personnel and resources,
- identify best practices and develop curricula and preservice and inservice programs based on these practices,
- coordinate with other health and education reform efforts,
- establish mechanisms for collecting information about program implementation and outcomes to assure accountability, and
- regularly communicate and disseminate program information to policymakers and the public.

The State Infrastructure

Leadership of the State Infrastructure

The overall task of the state's leadership should be to integrate education, physical and mental health, and other related programs and services for children and families. As mentioned earlier, the committee suggests that an effective approach for anchoring the state infrastructure is to establish an official state interagency coordinating council for school health with designated authority and responsibilities, along with an advisory council of representatives from relevant public and private sector agencies, including representatives from managed care and indemnity insurers. This structure mirrors the ICSH and NCCSH arrangement at the national level. The committee realizes that virtually every new education program requires oversight by some type of collaborative body. Perhaps an existing collaborative body—children's cabinet, state *Goals 2000* committee, or similar group—could assume responsibility for school health. Among its duties, the interagency council should be responsible for developing state plans and policies for school health, promoting collaboration among agencies and programs, coordinating existing funding streams and developing new funding mechanisms, and providing information and technical assistance to local districts.

Currently, collaboration and coordination already exist at the state level, and strengthening collaborative links should not be a prohibitively large step. According to the School Health Policies and Programs Study (SHPPS), in all but two states health education program staff have conducted joint activities or projects with staff from other components of the school health program (Collins et al., 1995). Similar interagency collaborative activities were also conducted by 86 percent of state school health services programs (Small et al., 1995), 92 percent of state foodservice programs (Pateman et al., 1995), and 84 percent of state physical education programs (Pate et al., 1995).

CDC/DASH Models of State Infrastructure Development

The CDC/DASH infrastructure demonstration project, mentioned previously, assists participating states in developing their CSHP infrastructure and documenting the process. Each state is developing its own unique infrastructure, based on its own situation and needs. The goal is to have the states disseminate the lessons learned to other states, including those not participating in the project. A process evaluation manual is being developed to help states understand the essential ingredients of their infrastructure, assess the current status of that infrastructure, and strengthen their system (Academy for Educational Development, 1995). According to this manual, a state-level CSHP infrastructure refers to the basic support system on which the larger, statewide CSHP program depends for continuance and growth. The four primary state CSHP infrastructure ingredients identified in the manual are funding and authorization, personnel and organizational placement, resources, and communication linkages (see Box 5-1).

To provide a sense of the kinds of infrastructure activities under way in states, Appendix G-2 describes some of the experiences and accomplishments in West Virginia—a lead state in the CDC/DASH infrastructure demonstration initiative—as well as Maine's plan (Appendix G-1) for collaboration and integration among education, health, and family services.

Coordination of Funding Streams

A critical function of the state infrastructure is managing the flow of the almost 200 federal funding streams that target children and families, many of which deal with health, education, and social or family services. States, in turn, pass many of these funds on to the local level, perhaps with particular state priorities or stipulations attached. The state and local infrastructures must work together to develop creative approaches for funding local programs from the variety of potential funding sources available.

Examples of federal funding streams arriving at state education agencies and their possible uses for school health include the following:

• Funds for AIDS/HIV prevention education from CDC/DASH can be used to improve health education in the classroom by training teachers and to improve health services by training school nurses to care for students who may be HIV infected. Funds can also be used for improvement of the school environment and for policy development.

• Individuals with Disabilities Education Act funds can be used to support the employment of counselors, school psychologists, and school nurses who work with children with special needs.

• Elementary and Secondary Education Act Title I funds can be used for the delivery of health and counseling services, as well as to increase parent involvement in schools.

• U.S. Department of Agriculture funds for Nutrition Education Training Programs can be used for teacher training related to nutrition education in the classroom and for training foodservice workers. (In a few states, this program is administered by the health or human services department.)

BOX 5-1
Description of a State Comprehensive
School Health Program Infrastructure

1. Funding and Authorization

Funding and authorization establish the purpose, structure, and function of the infrastructure and a commitment to infrastructure development. The subcategories include:

- Directives (laws, statutes, codes, policies, regulations, mandates, operating procedures, and written agreements at multiple levels).
- Financial Resources (federal, state, county/city, local, and private sources).

2. Personnel and Organizational Placement

Personnel and organizational placement provide for access to decision makers at the highest levels, effective management and operation of the infrastructure, accountability for the completion of tasks, authority for making decisions, and commitment to the CSHP. Important subcategories include:

- People (key decision makers, persons with responsibility, individuals with appropriate preparation, experience, and maturity).
- Positions (CDC-funded and non-CDC-funded agency infrastructure positions, responsibilities, parameters, position descriptions, position requirements).
- Hierarchial/Organizational Placement (location in state education agency (SEA), state health agency (SHA), and other agency structures, lines of responsibility, lines of authority and decision making, team membership).
- Physical Placement (office space, proximity to others, meeting space, location and quality of space).

3. Resources

Resources maintain commitment to infrastructure and provide for the development, continued functioning and administration of the CSHP. Important subcategories include:

- Human Resources (support staff, consultants, contractors).
- Technological Resources (hardware, software).
- Data and Data Systems/Sources (health risk data, epidemiological data, epidemiological data systems, libraries, and information centers).
- Inservice Supports (training systems, resource centers, statewide networks).
- External Supports (volunteer/professional/philanthropic agencies, institutions of higher education, parent and community groups).

continued on next page

BOX 5-1 Continued

4. Communications

Communications build capacity, establish or strengthen linkages and collaboration, facilitate advocacy and constituency recruitment efforts, promote broad based decision making, and allow for effective resolution of disagreements. Important subcategories include:

- SHA intra-agency communication (informal networks, formal networks, technical networks, social marketing efforts).
- SEA intra-agency communications (informal networks, formal networks, technical networks, social marketing campaigns).
- SHA/SEA interagency communications (informal networks, formal networks, technical networks, social marketing campaigns).
- External communications (informal networks, formal networks, technical networks, social marketing campaigns).

SOURCE: Reprinted from the Process Evaluation Manual, CSHP Infrastructure Project, Centers for Disease Control and Prevention/Division of Adolescent and School Health.

- Funds from Title IV of ESEA, Safe and Drug-Free Schools, can be used to deliver drug prevention and conflict resolution education within a CSHP. Funds can also be used to train counselors and school nurses to develop policies that improve the school environment and to work with physical educators to develop ways to keep athletes from becoming involved with drugs. Student Assistance Programs, Peer Mediation Training, and other early intervention activities may also be implemented with Safe and Drug-Free Schools funds.

Other federal funding streams arrive at state health agencies. Although these funds may not be specifically targeted to schools, some might logically be used for CSHPs, including the following:

- Chronic Disease and Health Promotion funds from the CDC for tobacco prevention, promotion of physical activity, and diabetes prevention, can be used for training teachers who deliver focused health education dealing with these topics. CDC funding for HIV/AIDS prevention can often be used by schools for classroom programs.
- Maternal and Child Health block grant funds (Title V) are often used to employ school nurses and to develop school-based health centers.
- Specific disease prevention initiatives can be undertaken in schools

with funds received from such sources as the National Cancer Institute ASSIST grant program, in which tobacco prevention is a primary concern. These funds can be used for policy development, public awareness, and development of educational programs.

Certainly, federal funds cannot be expected to serve as the only support for programs, and some states are developing their own strategies to support school health. As examples, Massachusetts uses a tobacco tax and Florida uses proceeds from a tax on health club memberships to help support programs. State lottery revenues also are often available for education and represent a possible source of funds.

Technical Assistance

A critical function of the state infrastructure is to develop mechanisms for providing the local level with information and technical assistance that will help in establishing programs. West Virginia, one of the early participants in the CDC/DASH infrastructure initiative, found that local districts had difficulty getting started when asked to develop implementation plans. Although programs must be designed locally, a certain threshold of basic understanding at the local level is necessary to begin the process. Since the goal is for all districts within a state to develop CSHPs, a great deal of wasted effort and "reinventing the wheel" can be avoided if states provide districts with the necessary assistance and understanding to get started. Priority should be given to those districts with the greatest needs.

The committee suggests that a state technical assistance network—a "school health extension service" modeled after the Agricultural Extension Service—could be an effective mechanism for conveying assistance from the state level through the regional level to the local level.[5] Regional educational service agencies, Boards of Cooperative Educational Services (BOCES), county extension services, area health education centers, and other regional health and/or education service agencies could be linked in a manner similar to that used in the state school health coordinating council; this would provide a regional focal point for school health that

---

[5]USDA's Extension Service—a national cooperative effort by federal, state, and local governments—was established in 1914 to bring new agricultural information and technologies from government and university laboratories to the local farmer. Extension specialists are located at every land grant college of agriculture, and extension agents operate in almost every county in the nation. Since 1988, the Extension Service has expanded its statement of purpose to include activities aimed at the development of communities, families, youth, and leadership (National Research Council, 1995).

would coordinate efforts among districts and provide technical assistance and staff development.

The Local Infrastructure

As emphasized throughout this report, there is no single "best" comprehensive school health program model that will work in every community. Programs must be designed locally, and collaboration among all stakeholders in the community is essential if programs are to be accepted and effective.

District School Health Advisory and Coordinating Councils

The value of collaborative efforts at the local level has been documented by Wang and coworkers (1995), and a number of papers and reports have been published in recent years describing actions on the local level necessary to implement CSHPs (Allensworth, 1987; Kane, 1994; Killip et al., 1987; Penfield and Shannon, 1991). Most of these reports call for establishing a local advisory or coordinating council that involves a variety of health and education professionals, parents, and other community members, in order to mobilize community resources, represent the diverse interests and opinions within the community, and provide advice and guidance to the school board. The premise underlying the establishment of advisory councils is that involving lay representatives enhances the processes of decisionmaking and educational change and that support for change is more forthcoming if the community is involved.

Advisory councils have existed in many districts for decades, and their importance to the implementation of a school health program has long been documented (Dorman and Foulk, 1987; Hackenburg, 1959; Marx, 1968; Spurling, 1948; Valente and Humb, 1981; Zimmerli, 1981). In recent years, however, it has been suggested that a more formalized structure is inherently more effective than an informal advisory group. An official school health coordinating council, with designated authority and responsibilities, can have greater influence, provide continuity, and enable long-range planning (Allensworth, 1987).

According to SHPPS (Collins et al., 1995), only one-third of all districts have a "district-wide school health advisory council that addresses policies and programs related to health education." Further, the roles and extent of influence and responsibilities of these councils are not clear.

The committee believes that the establishment of a district coordinating council for school health is essential; this group should include representatives from all stakeholder groups in the community, including managed care organizations, indemnity insurers, and others who can provide resources to school health programs. In some cases, leadership of the council might best be provided by a neutral party, someone not directly associated with the schools, so that the program is not viewed as "owned" by the schools. The coordinating council should have the authority necessary to carry out such functions as involving the community in assessing needs and resources and in establishing program goals; developing a district school health plan; coordinating school health programs with other community programs and resources; and providing leadership and assistance for local schools.

District School Health Coordinator

Numerous reports have asserted that the coordination and management of the various components of the school health program deserve, even demand, the attention of a central person at the district level who has authority for program administration, implementation, evaluation, and accountability (Education Development Center and the CDC, 1994; Ohio State Board of Education, 1980; Penfield and Shannon, 1991). In its report on comprehensive school health programs, the National School Boards Association highlighted the programs of approximately 25 exemplary districts—all of which had in common the designation of a central person as program coordinator. This coordinator devoted from 10 to 100 percent of his or her time to this task; according to the study, the important factor was not so much the amount of time spent as the interest and organizational abilities of the individual (Penfield and Shannon, 1991).

Some have questioned whether it may be overly ambitious to call for establishing a school health coordinating council and appointing a school health coordinator in each of the nation's approximately 15,000 school districts. The committee's response is that these elements are an integral part of the infrastructure to support CSHPs. Certainly, the size and complexity of the coordinating council and the allotted time for the coordinator should reflect the needs and characteristics of the district; a district with only a few schools might have only a small coordinating council and limited released time for the coordinator. It should also be recognized, however, that the needs of a small district requiring facilitation by a council and coordinator may be large, especially in terms of acquiring technical assistance and seeking interdistrict collaboration.

The Infrastructure at the Individual School Level

A formal organizational arrangement at each individual school is also essential, and the organizational structure in place at the district level may be repeated at the school level. A school health council and an individual assigned to coordinate the program have been proposed as an effective arrangement. Ideally, the school-based program coordinator or member of the health council would serve as a representative to the district coordinating council. In large schools, in addition to the overarching school health council, the work may be divided among subcommittees or work teams, with each responsible for a particular aspect of the program (Gurevitsch, 1991). Ideally, two types of teams might work simultaneously: (1) professional or disciplinary groups focusing on one particular program component, such as health education or food and nutrition services, and (2) cross-disciplinary groups that cut across all program components and major health and educational issues facing students, such as reducing substance abuse or promoting cardiovascular fitness. Cross-disciplinary teams allow for enhanced communication and dissemination of ideas as team members share information and receive advice from other members of their professional team (see Figure 5-1).

It should be emphasized that the school-based infrastructure can be built on existing personnel and programs. A school nurse or a health education teacher might serve as the program coordinator and be given appropriate compensation or "released time" from his or her normal duties. Existing faculty and staff, including those from all disciplines and levels, should serve on school teams.

Extending the Infrastructure through Interdisciplinary and School–Community Collaboration

In the current era of limited resources for both health care and education, it is essential that school health professionals purposefully collaborate with each other and with members of the mainstream health and social services systems in the community. School programs and services that are disconnected from the student's family, primary care provider, social support system, and the larger community merely add a fragmented layer of care that may be either contradictory or redundant.

Existing resources can be maximized by considering schools as an essential, integral part of the overall community health and service system. Although school health programs are often called "comprehensive," it should be emphasized that programs and services actually delivered at the school site may not provide complete coverage by themselves. Instead, on-site school programs and services should work with and complement the efforts of families, primary sources of health care, and other health and social service resources in the community to provide a continuous, complete, and seamless system to promote and protect students' health. In fact, the suggestion has been ventured that the term "coordi-

Participants Matrix	Work Groups/Teams			
	A	B	C	D
Professional Group 1				
Professional Group 2				
Professional Group 3				
Professional Group 4				
Professional Group 5				
Professional Group 6				
Professional Group 7				

- A work group/team has an interdisciplinary membership.
- A professional group consists of participants with the same job function or the same range of work.
- Interdisciplinary team members communicate interventions and new techniques developed by the interdisciplinary work team to professional colleagues in their discipline.

The work groups/teams might focus on the following issues:

Work Group A: Promoting cardiovascular health
Work Group B: Reducing substance abuse
Work Group C: Improving health services
Work Group D: Reducing violence

The Professional groups might have the following composition:

Professional Group 1: School administrators
Professional Group 2: School nurses
Professional Group 3: Health teachers
Professional Group 4: Guidance counselors
Professional Group 5: Physical education teachers
Professional Group 6: Psychologists
Professional Group 7: Science teachers

FIGURE 5-1 Interdisciplinary teams within the school. SOURCE: Healthy Students 2000: An Agenda for Continuous Improvement in America's Schools, 1993. Reprinted with permission. American School Health Association, Kent, OH.

nated school health program" might be more appropriate than "comprehensive school health program" to emphasize this notion.

Often, a variety of professionals must work together within the school to determine appropriate interventions for students with academic or behavioral problems or those who require special education or have special needs. Students receiving special attention at school may also be undergoing assessment and treatment in health and social services systems outside the school; they may be seen and/or treated by psychologists, psychometrists, social workers, counselors, nurse practitioners, physicians, physical therapists, occupational therapists, adaptive physical education specialists, speech pathologists, case managers, and so on. School and community professionals may or may not have similar professional credentials and licensure; assessments may be varied or duplicated; and interventions may occur in both settings or neither setting.

Professional communication across disciplines and settings is therefore critical for the benefit of these students. Ideally, assessment results for common clients are shared, needs are determined jointly, and intervention plans are made with active involvement of the student and his or her family, along with appropriate staff from the school and the individuals or agency staff providing health and social services in the community. This level of integration would result in a truly "seamless" delivery system for children and their families, reduce fragmentation or duplication of care, and maximize existing resources.

Two major barriers have been identified regarding interagency collaboration: the confidentiality of medical records and the varied qualifications of staff among agencies doing the same tasks for shared clients. However, as pointed out in Chapter 4, confidentiality is a barrier only if the clients or the parents or guardians of clients who are minors refuse to consent to the sharing of medical information. The issue of staff qualifications among agencies can be addressed with protocols to ensure standardization of care and administrative support from the agencies involved. For example, assessments done by nurse practitioners, registered nurses, and certified assistive personnel (such as psychometrists and physician assistants) may not be as consistently accepted as those done by physicians. Interagency protocols and agreements can address those inconsistencies so that clients do not have repetitious assessments and duplicated medical, laboratory, or psychological tests from a variety of agencies.

Personnel Training Needs

Appropriately prepared professionals and paraprofessionals—teachers, administrators, counselors, psychologists, social workers, school nurses, foodservice personnel, and other team members from the school and community—will be crucial for the implementation of effective CSHPs, and collaboration among these professionals will be essential to produce a strong CSHP infrastructure within a district or school. However, some observers suggest that many professionals do not understand disciplines beyond their own and that discipline-based views and terminology inhibit the fullest exchange of ideas. Thus, there is a critical need to take an interdisciplinary approach to preservice and inservice training, not just for personnel assigned directly to school health but for educators in all fields and for administrators as well. Interdisciplinary interaction should be an integral part of preservice preparation at the university level, and preservice programs should be aligned with the concepts embodied by CSHPs. University faculty providing preservice preparation in school health and related fields should create models of collaboration with colleagues in other relevant departments, and students should be exposed to interdisciplinary experiences in field placements and internships (Gingiss, 1995; Lawson and Hooper-Briar, 1994). Consideration should also be given to creating a new category of personnel—comprehensive school health coordinators—who can work with both the school and the community and who have the management skills to oversee complex partnership programs.

School administrators, both at the district level and in individual schools, can be pivotal in developing and supporting the CSHP infrastructure. Thus, the preparation of administrators should include providing them with an understanding of all facets of a CSHP—what programs are about and what they can do; the mobilization of support among staff and community members; sources of financing; organization of the school day, facilities, and existing resources to support the program; and the responsibilities that departments and individuals must assume.

Overcoming Controversy

The ultimate authority for all local school policies and programs belongs to the local board of education, which operates within the federal, state, and local legislative framework. Whether appointed or elected directly, these boards are political bodies. As in other arenas, with politics come controversies. Indeed, many of the most visible and controversial issues that school boards encounter—sexuality and family life education, mental health counseling, reproductive health counseling and services— are associated with school health programs (Marks and Marzke, 1993; Rienzo and Button, 1993).

Thus, supporters of comprehensive school health programs must become activists at school board meetings and in the media—although they must take special care not to ride roughshod over general community and parental concerns. Where criticism is ill-informed or unwarranted, supporters must operate with a clear understanding of the health status, behaviors, and needs of children and young people in the community. Supporters can also be armed with facts such as the results of the national Gallup and Harris surveys, discussed in Chapter 3, which show overwhelming support for school health education from parents and students. They can cite studies of parents' perceptions of school-based health centers, such as the one carried out in the vicinity of Portland, Oregon, which found that parents overwhelmingly favored the provision of all general health, counseling, parent education, and reproductive health services in the school (Glick et al., 1995).[6]

Healthy Caring, the process evaluation of the Robert Wood Johnson School-Based Adolescent Health Care Program, found that controversy surrounded the start-up of school-based health centers at almost all program sites (Marks and Marzke, 1993). Objections were reported to have come from limited but vocal segments of the community, often from individuals or representatives of organizations who themselves did not have children attending the schools. One effective strategy for deflecting controversy was to involve the parents of school students in program planning and advocacy. Another successful approach was to establish an advisory committee for the school-based health center that included respected leaders in the medical and health professions, educators, parents, and other community leaders.

Supporters of school health programs must respect the concern that some—perhaps many—parents have about the possible loss of control over what is taught in the health education classroom or over services that their children might receive in school. Proposed health education curricula and materials should be reviewed and accepted by a majority of parents and community leaders, including religious leaders, and they should be available to all parents for examination. *Healthy Caring* reported that planners of school-based health centers eased parents' concerns by allowing parents to choose services they wished to exclude for their children. The committee emphasizes the importance of compromising on small issues for the sake of advancing the larger program. For example,

---

[6]Parents in the region recognized the need for a range of reproductive health services at school-based health centers. They showed strong support for abstinence counseling, treatment of sexually transmitted diseases, counseling for birth control, provision of birth control, and services for pregnant teens. According to the authors of the study, perhaps the most intriguing finding was that school-based health centers were overwhelmingly supported by the parents of students who used the centers as well as by the parents of students who did not use them.

Healthy Caring noted that several sites dropped plans for making contraceptives available to students at the school site when it became apparent that this single issue could seriously impede, if not completely derail, attempts to establish a school-based health center.

Overcoming Other Barriers

Inertia and resistance to change are often obstacles that local communities must be prepared to confront in establishing a CSHP infrastructure. Time will also be an issue—especially finding time for teachers and other professionals on school teams to meet and plan. Resource constraints will likely exist. Turf battles may arise over who has authority. Unconvinced or uncommitted administrators may not understand the importance of programs or may refuse to assume leadership for promoting collaboration. Professional training differences could lead to misunderstandings and communication gaps. Some staff may feel overly burdened or threatened as traditional roles give way to new responsibilities.

Several recent articles provide advice on overcoming barriers to collaboration, but they also concede that progress may often be difficult (Allensworth, 1994; Lawson and Hooper-Briar, 1994; Melaville and Blank, 1991; Melaville et al., 1993; Russell, 1994). Districts and schools should expect occasional problems, but they should maintain the leadership and commitment to persevere. The committee believes that communities faced with seemingly insurmountable barriers would benefit from technical assistance provided by a school health extension service and from communication with other communities that have overcome similar problems.

Mobilizing Community Support

Economics may provide the ultimate argument in persuading unconvinced community members of the importance of a CSHP. Today's world of work requires employees to think critically and make decisions, to solve problems individually or as part of a team, to analyze and interpret new information, to develop convincing arguments, and to apply knowledge and skills. Moreover, employers value "healthy" employees—those who practice good nutrition and keep fit, avoid risky behavior, do not smoke or abuse alcohol or drugs, are well adjusted socially and emotionally, and have less health-related absenteeism. The school's mission is to ensure that its graduates have the skills and qualities that are needed to succeed in the world of work, and a comprehensive school health program can play a central role in meeting this goal. Therefore, an important task of the community coordinating council is to help the community come to see the school health program as a critical and primary component in achieving the mission of preparing students for the future—not to see the program as a separate, unconnected, or secondary "add-on."

Peer, family, and community influences are as integral to the adoption of health-promoting behaviors as is the acquisition of knowledge. The discussion of health education in Chapters 3 and 6 points out that perceived norms are a critical factor that influences behavior. No matter how high the quality of the school program, its effects will likely be diminished if the community environment does not support and reinforce the program. A strong community coordinating council can work to ensure that all health messages received in the school are reinforced in the community. The council can also marshal forces to develop desirable health-related policies, to provide opportunities to practice health-promoting behaviors, and to foster role modeling by community members. For example, when schools educate students about the laws and hazards regarding the use of illegal substances such as tobacco and alcohol, and prohibit the use of these substances in school, the community should also establish policies and expectations that will help establish a perceived community norm that "alcohol and tobacco are not acceptable substances to use, they are not available to students, and other alternatives are available for students to explore their emerging independence." Students must also see that adults in the community practice responsible behavior with regard to the use of alcohol and tobacco. Another example of community reinforcement of school health messages is that when health classes are discussing access to health care and emphasizing the importance of periodic health assessment, the message will be strengthened if students see that these needed services are accessible to all students.

Principles for Collaboration

A number of articles on collaboration have appeared in the literature in recent years. A review of this literature found that some elements were consistently mentioned as essential for successful collaboration and integration of education and health-related services (Thomas et al., 1993). These elements include

  • family-centered service delivery that responds to the diversity of youth and families,
    • coordinated and comprehensive services,
    • local community and empowerment focus,
    • evaluation of processes and cost,
    • joint data collection,
    • strategies to ensure that youth and families have easy access to

services and that they actually receive the services they need (e.g., colloca-tion, one-stop shopping, case management), and

- restructuring of funding streams to achieve integrated budgets.

A set of principles for integrating local education, health, and human services for children, youth, and families was affirmed by the more than 50 national organizations that met at the consensus conference in January 1994 (American Academy of Pediatrics, 1994). The conference report, *Principles to Link By*, outlines eight principles for building stronger structures for coordination in the development of the CSHP infrastructure:

1. Coordinating structures should be collaborative.
2. Coordinating structures should be community-based and reflect the diversity and uniqueness of the community.
3. Coordinating structures should be empowered to guide systems change and assure collaboration.
4. Coordinating structures should have flexibility in defining geo-graphic boundaries and institutional relationships.
5. Coordinating structures should establish and maintain a results-based accountability system.
6. Coordinating structures should be encouraged without prescrib-ing a specific structure or authority.
7. Federal and state levels should model collaboration that supports community efforts.
8. Federal and state policies should provide incentives that encour-age collaboration among public, private, and community agencies.

SUMMARY OF FINDINGS AND CONCLUSIONS

Many parts of the infrastructure—the basic framework of policies, resources, organizational structures, and communication channels—needed to support CSHPs already exist or are emerging. However, these parts are often fragmented and uncoordinated, and resources are typi-cally transient or limited to specific categorical activities. Leadership and coordination at all levels—national, state, local—will be crucial for pro-grams to become established and grow.

RECOMMENDATIONS

The committee believes that a strong interconnected infrastructure will be essential if CSHPs are to become established and flourish. What happens school by school is ultimately the important outcome. The na-tional infrastructure establishes certain policies and programs that serve as a foundation for the state infrastructure; in turn, the state infrastructure develops and coordinates policies and programs that further add to the foundation for the infrastructure at the district and local school levels. Below is a summary of the committee's recommendations for the infrastructure at each level.

National Level

At the national level, the federal Interagency Committee on School Health (ICSH) was established in 1994 to improve coordination among federal agencies, identify national needs and strategies, and serve as a national focal point for school health. The National Coordinating Committee on School Health (NCCSH), which works closely with the ICSH, brings together federal departments with approximately 40 national nongovernmental organizations to provide national leadership in school health.

The committee recommends that the mission of the federal Interagency Committee on School Health be revitalized so that the ICSH fulfills its potential to provide national leadership and to carry out critical new national initiatives in school health. In addition, the committee recommends that the National Coordinating Committee on School Health serve as an official advisory body to the ICSH and that individual NCCSH organizations mobilize their memberships to promote the development of a CSHP infrastructure at the state and local levels. The committee also recommends that the membership of the NCCSH be expanded to include representatives from managed care organizations, indemnity insurers, and others who will be key to resolving financial issues of CSHPs.

The ICSH and the NCCSH are poised to provide national leadership, and expanding the missions of these organizations may help them to fulfill the leadership role. Specifically, the ICSH and the NCCSH should develop a national action plan for school health and, in so doing, promote the adoption of the national standards in health education, physical education, school nutrition, school nursing, and school-based health care.

To provide leadership in research, the ICSH and NCCSH could establish a grants program for basic research and outcome evaluation in school health programming; ensure that national data about student health behaviors and health status as well as school health programs and practices are collected, monitored, and tracked; encourage the inclusion of health topics in national and state assessment programs, develop national and state "school health report cards," and establish a national clearinghouse, accessible through the Internet, that analyzes and disseminates in useful form, research findings and effective practices in school health for state and local practitioners.

Other leadership roles could include providing funding and technical assistance to help states establish a state-level coordinating council on school health; assisting states in establishing a school health extension service by uniting regional educational service units, agricultural extension services, and area health education coordinators; providing mechanisms for communication between the local and national level to share information, such as an Internet discussion group, annual conferences, and newsletters; identifying and publicizing information about federal funding streams and various strategies for financing school health programs at the state and local levels; promoting the flexible use of federal funds for school health programming; and coordinating relevant federal programs so that states and local communities are not faced with an array of related programs with different or conflicting requirements regarding eligibility, application and reporting processes, personnel, funding, and so forth.

To finance these initiatives without an increase in overall spending, each ICSH agency could receive from a common pool of each of the participating agencies an appropriate fraction of its budget for school health programming.

State Level

At the state level, the infrastructure can be anchored by a structure similar to the ICSH-NCCSH arrangement at the national level.

The committee recommends that an official state interagency coordinating council for school health be established in each state to integrate health education, physical education, health services, physical and social environment policies and practices, mental health, and other related efforts for children and families. Further, an advisory committee of representatives from relevant public and private sector agencies, including representatives from managed care organizations and indemnity insurers, should be added.

This state coordinating council should develop a state plan for school health and institute appropriate policies and legislation; serve as a link for communication about funding and local concerns between the federal and local or regional levels; increase cross-agency integration of programs, funding streams, and research; coordinate federal funding streams by developing mechanisms to allow categorical funds to be used for CSHPs; find new sources of funding for school health, such as lottery revenues or taxes on items such as tobacco, alcoholic beverages, health club memberships, or Medicaid and private insurers; coordinate state programs and funding streams; provide technical assistance to establish district school health coordinating councils and demonstration models, training, curriculum development, program evaluation, and so forth (especially targeting districts that have the greatest number of students at risk); and sponsor research and evaluation studies on multicomponent-multistrategy programs. Establishing a regional school health extension service, modeled after the Agricultural Extension Service and educational service agencies offers a particularly promising approach for providing technical assistance.

Community or District Level[7]

To anchor the infrastructure at the community or district level, the committee recommends the following:

A formal organization with broad representation—a coordinating council for school health—should be established in every school district.

Among its duties, the district coordinating council should appoint a district school health coordinator to oversee the program; involve the community in conducting a needs and resource assessment; develop plans and policies for delivery and ongoing assessment of quality programs (with special attention to students at greater risk); provide information to individual schools about standards, practice, and technological developments; coordinate programs and resources; increase cross-agency integration of funding streams and research; assist each individual school in designating a school health coordinator and a school health committee; coordinate school health and social service programs with other community programs and resources, including the private health care sector; ensure that all students have a medical home—a stable, accessible source of primary care; collaborate with nearby districts, regional, or state providers of technical assistance, information, and inservice programs; support the employment, involvement, and continuing professional development of appropriately prepared professional school health staff; and

---

[7]A "community" may consist of a single school district or be divided into two or more districts. See Figure 5-2 for a distinction between community and district responsibilities.

provide a monitoring and tracking program for feedback to the community, and to the state coordinating council. Communities must be prepared to confront barriers in building their CSHP infrastructures, including time and resource constraints, turf battles, indifference, or controversy over sensitive aspects of programs. An effective method for mobilizing support has been to enlist parents, students, and other community leaders as program advocates. Compromise on small issues may be essential for the sake of advancing the larger program.

School Level

The committee recommends that at the school level, individual schools should establish a school health committee and appoint a school health coordinator to oversee the school health program.

Under this leadership, schools should address the major health issues facing students and/or the continuous improvement of the various components of the CSHP; develop policies and plans for periodic reports of all aspects of the CSHP (current activities, student outcomes, and plans for improvement); appoint representatives to the district school health coordinating council; coordinate activities and resources with the district coordinating council for assessment of students' needs and behaviors; coordinate funding, time, space, personnel, and other resources to implement comprehensive school health education and provide needed health services for students at the school or at school-linked sites; coordinate case management of services for students at risk; support the employment, involvement, and continuing professional development of appropriately prepared professional school health staff; and seek the active involvement of students and families in designing and implementing programs.

The comprehensive school health infrastructure—the basic interconnected framework on which programs can be built—is summarized in Figure 5-2.

In order to implement quality comprehensive school health programs, the training and utilization of competent, properly prepared personnel should be expanded.

In general, the committee believes that an interdisciplinary approach is needed in the preservice and inservice preparation of CSHP professionals to enable them to communicate and collaborate with each other. In addition, the committee believes that educators in all disciplines—particularly administrators—need preparation in order to understand the phi-

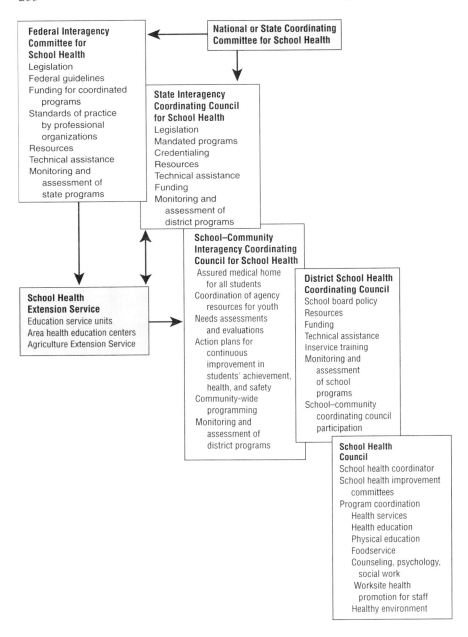

FIGURE 5-2 Comprehensive school health infrastructure. SOURCE: Healthy Students 2000: An Agenda for Continuous Improvement in America's Schools, 1993. Reprinted with permission. American School Health Association, Kent, OH.

losophy and potential of CSHPs. Important personnel needs include the following:

- employment of more certified health education specialists at the middle and secondary school levels,
- enhanced preparation of elementary teachers to deliver quality health instruction and deal with student health problems,
- increased utilization of certified physical education specialists to provide instruction at the elementary level,
- enhanced preparation of school administrators in order that they more thoroughly understand school health programs and fully utilize school health personnel,
- employment of more certified school nurses, nurse practitioners, and other midlevel providers,
- retraining and shifting existing service providers (especially nurse practitioners and other midlevel providers) from one setting to another in order to respond to changing health delivery demands,
- designation of a school health coordinator at each school site, with appropriate released time or compensation,
- employment of professionally prepared foodservice or nutrition directors and managers,
- increased emphasis on interdisciplinary health-related experiences in the preservice preparation of all educators and school personnel,
- additional and ongoing training of school health professionals, especially in the ability to translate and adapt research findings to field practice,
- increased health-related knowledge of individuals in disciplines outside health education so that they are better able to see the relationships between their own disciplines and health promotion,
- increased emphasis on school health in pediatric and family practice training for physicians, including the roles of physicians in primary and specialty care, as well as roles for physicians from academic health centers and hospitals, in these programs,
- possible creation of a new category of personnel—comprehensive school health coordinators—who can work with both the school and the community and who have the management skills to operate complex partnership programs.

The call for proper professional preparation is not intended to be self-serving or to promote narrow professional interests; instead, the committee believes that CSHPs and the health of our children are important enough to merit a requirement for well-prepared, qualified professionals. Ideally, all personnel involved in school health programs should have the appropriate academic credentials and certification before initial employment, and this should be the goal for the future with all new hires. The committee recognizes, however, that there are currently many personnel serving in school health programs without the necessary paper credentials who have received their training on the job. It would not be practical to attempt to replace these individuals, because many are performing well; furthermore, there would be a shortage of credentialed personnel to fill these positions. However, it is important that all school health personnel—whether initially credentialed or trained on the job—be evaluated regularly by knowledgeable supervisors, participate in ongoing inservice training, and maintain active connections with the professional organizations in their respective fields.

REFERENCES

Academy for Educational Development. 1995. *Comprehensive School Health Program Infrastructure Development: Process Evaluation Manual* (Draft III). Washington, D.C.: Academy for Educational Development.

Allensworth, D.D. 1987. Building community support for quality school health programs. *Health Education* (Oct./Nov.):7.

Allensworth, D.D. 1994. *Building Effective Coalitions to Prevent the Spread of HIV/AIDS.* Kent, Ohio: American School Health Association.

American Academy of Pediatrics. 1994. *Principles to Link By: Integrating Education Health, and Human Services for Children, Youth, and Families.* Report of the Consensus Conference. Washington, D.C.

American Cancer Society. 1993. National action plan for comprehensive school health education. *Journal of School Health* 63(1):46–66.

Collins, J.L., Small, M.L., Kann, L., Pateman, B.C., Gold, R.S., and Kolbe, L.J. 1995. School health education. *Journal of School Health* 65(8):302–311.

Dorman, S.M., and Foulk, D.F. 1987. Characteristics of school health education advisory councils. *Journal of School Health* 57(8):337–339.

Education Development Center and the Centers for Disease Control and Prevention. 1994. *Educating for Health: A Guide to Implementing a Comprehensive Approach to School Health Education.* Newton, Mass.: Education Development Center.

Gingiss, P.L. 1995. Education and Training for Interprofessional Collaboration. Presentation to the Institute of Medicine Committee on Comprehensive School Health Programs in Grades K–12, Washington, D.C., June 28.

Glick, B., Doyle, L., Ni, H., Gao, D., and Pham, C. 1995. School-Based Health Center Program Evaluation: Perceptions, Knowledge, and Attitudes of Parents/Guardians of Eleventh Graders. A limited dataset presented to the Multnomah County (Oregon) Commissioners, March 21.

Gurevitsch, G. 1991. The Nordberg Project: A model for the development of a health-promoting school in Denmark. In *Youth Health Promotion: From Theory to Practice in School and Community*, D. Nutbeam, B. Hagland, P. Farley, and P. Tillgren, eds. London: Forbes Publication.

Hackenburg, H. 1959. School health by citizen's council. *Journal of School Health* 29(9):330–332.

Joint Committee on National Health Education Standards. 1995. *National Health Education Standards: Achieving Health Literacy.* Atlanta: American Cancer Society.

Kane, W.M. 1994. Planning for a comprehensive school health program. In *The Comprehensive School Health Challenge*, P. Cortese and K. Middleton, eds. Santa Cruz, Calif.: Education, Training, and Research, Associates.

Killip, D.C., Lovick, S.R., Goldman, L., and Allensworth, D.D. 1987. Integrated school and community programs. *Journal of School Health* 57(10):437–444.

Lavin, A.T., Shapiro, G.R., and Weill, K.S. eds. 1992. *Creating an Agenda for School-Based Health Promotion: A Review of Selected Reports.* Boston: Harvard School of Public Health.

Lawson, H.S., and Hooper-Briar, K. 1994. *Expanding Partnerships: Involving Colleges and Universities in Interprofessional Collaboration and Service Integration.* Oxford, Ohio: Danforth Foundation and the Institute for Educational Renewal at Miami University.

Marks, E.L., and Marzke, C.H. 1993. Healthy Caring: *A Process Evaluation of the Robert Wood Johnson Foundation's School-Based Adolescent Health Care Program.* Princeton, N.J.: Mathtech.

Marx, S.H. 1968. How a health council developed a narcotics education program. *Journal of School Health* 38(4):243–246.

Melaville, A.I., and Blank, M.J. 1991. *What it Takes: Structuring Interagency Partnerships to Connect Children and Families with Comprehensive Services.* Washington, D.C.: Education and Human Services Consortium.

Melaville, A.I., Blank, M.J., and Asayesh, G. 1993. *Together We Can: A Guide for Crafting A Profamily System of Education and Human Services.* Washington, D.C.: Superintendent of Documents.

National Research Council. 1995. *Colleges of Agriculture at the Land Grant Universities.* Washington, D.C.: National Academy Press.

Ohio State Board of Education. 1980. *Guidelines for Improving School Health Education K–12.* Columbus, Ohio: State Board of Education.

Pate, R.R., Small, M.L., Ross., J.G., Young, J.C., Flint, K.H., and Warren, C.W. 1995. School physical education. *Journal of School Health* 65(8):312–318.

Pateman, B.C., McKinney, P., Kann, L., Small, M.L., Warren, C.W., and Collins, J.L. 1995. School food service. *Journal of School Health* 65(8):327–332.

Penfield, A.R., and Shannon, T.A. 1991. *School Health: Helping Children Learn.* Alexandria, Va.: National School Boards Association.

Rienzo, B.A., and Button, J.W. 1993. The politics of school-based clinics: A community-level analysis. *Journal of School Health* 63(6):266–272.

Russell, W.R. 1994. *Preparing Collaborative Leaders: A Facilitator's Guide.* Washington, D.C.: Institute for Educational Leadership.

Small, M.L., Majer, L.S., Allensworth, D.D., Farquhar, B.K., Kann, L., and Pateman, B.C. 1995. School health services. *Journal of School Health* 65(8):319–326.

Spurling, D. 1948. A school health council in action. *Journal of School Health* 18(2):50–54.

Sullivan, C.J. 1995. *School Health Programs: A Time for Action.* Washington, D.C.: National School Health Education Coalition.

Thomas, C.F., English, J.L., and Bickel, A.S. 1993. *Moving Toward Integrated Services: A Literature Review for Prevention Specialists.* Portland, Ore.: Northwest Regional Educational Laboratory.

U.S. Department of Education. 1995. *School-Linked Comprehensive Services for Children and Families: What We Know and What We Need to Know.* Washington, D.C.: SAI 9503025, U.S. Department of Education.

U.S. Department of Education and U.S. Department of Health and Human Services. 1994. Joint Statement on School Health by the Secretaries of Education and Health and Human Services.

U.S. Department of Education, U.S. Department of Health and Human Services, and U.S. Department of Agriculture. 1994. *Interagency Committee on School Health Charter.* Washington, D.C: U.S. Department of Health and Human Services, Public Health Service.

Valente, C.W., and Humb, K.J. 1981. Organization and function of a school health council. *Journal of School Health* 51(7):446–468.

Wang, M.C., Haertel, G.D., and Walberg, H.J. 1995. Effective features of collaborative school-linked services for children in elementary schools: What do we know from research and practice? Paper commissioned for the Invitational Conference of the U.S. Department of Education and the American Educational Research Association: School-Linked Comprehensive Services for Children and Families, Leesburg, Va., September 28 to October 2, 1994.

Zimmerli, W.H. 1981. Organizing for school health education at the local level. *Health Education Quarterly* 8:39–42.

RECOMMENDED READING

Allensworth, D.D. 1994. The Comprehensive School Health Program: Essential Elements. Paper commissioned by the World Health Organization.

American Academy of Pediatrics. 1994. Task force on integrated school health services: Integrated school health services. *Pediatrics* 4(3):400–402.

Children's Defense Fund. 1989. *Vision for America's Future: An Agenda for the 90's.* Washington D.C.: Children's Defense Fund.

Davies, D. 1981. Citizen participation in decision making in the school. In *Communities and Their Schools*, D. Davies, ed. New York: McGraw Hill.

Davies, D., Burch, P., and Palanki, A. 1993. *Fitting Policy to Family Needs: Delivering Comprehensive Services Through Collaboration and Family Empowerment.* Boston: Center on Families, Communities, Schools and Children's Learning.

Dryfoos, J. 1991. *Adolescents at Risk: Prevalence and Prevention.* New York: Oxford University Press.

Gingiss, P.L. 1992. Enhancing program implementation and maintenance through a multiphase approach to peer-based staff development. *Journal of School Health* 62(5):161–166.

Gingiss, P.L. 1993. Peer coaching: Building collegial support for using innovative health programs. *Journal of School Health.* 63(2):79–85.

Green, W., and Krueter, M.W. 1991. *Health Promotion Planning: An Educational and Environmental Approach.* Toronto: Mayfield Publishing.

Jehl, J., and Kirst, M. 1992. Spinning a family support web. *The School Administrator* (September):8–15.

Jivanjee, P., Moore, K., Friesen, B.J., and Schultze, K.H. 1995. Education for Interprofessional Collaboration: A Status Report. Portland, Ore.: Regional Research Institute for Human Services, Portland State University.

Liontos, L.B. 1991. Why is collaboration mandatory? Eric Digest: Collaboration Between Schools and Social Services. Eugene, Oreg.

Palanki, A., Burch, P., and Davies, D. 1992. Mapping the Policy Landscape: *What Federal and State Governments Are Doing to Promote Family-School-Community Partnerships.* Boston: Center on Families, Communities, Schools and Children's Learning.

Resnicow, K. 1995. Conducting a Comprehensive School Health Program. Unpublished paper.

Saxl, E.R., Miles, M.B., and Lieberman, A. 1990. *Assisting Change in Education: Trainer's Manual.* Alexandria, Va.: Association for Supervision and Curriculum Development.

Sujansky, J.G. 1991. *The Power of Partnerships.* San Diego: Pfeiffer.

Thompson, R. 1988. *Primary School Drug Education Evaluation: A School Team Approach.* Canberra, Australia: CPO/Communications.

6

Challenges in School Health Research and Evaluation

OVERVIEW OF RESEARCH AND EVALUATION

One of the primary arguments for establishing comprehensive school health programs (CSHPs) has been that they will improve students' academic performance and therefore improve the employability and productivity of our future adult citizens. Another argument relates to public health impact—since one-third of the *Healthy People 2000* objectives can be directly attained or significantly influenced through the schools, CSHPs are seen as a means to reduce not only morbidity and mortality but also health care expenditures. It is likely that the future of CSHPs will be determined by the degree to which they are able to demonstrate a significant impact on educational and/or health outcomes.

Evaluation of any health promotion program poses numerous challenges such as measurement validity, respondent bias, attrition, and statistical power. The situation is even more challenging for CSHPs, for several reasons. First, these programs comprise multiple, interactive components, such as classroom, family, and community interventions, each employing multiple intervention strategies. Therefore, it is often difficult to determine which intervention components and specific messages, activities, and services are responsible for observed treatment effects. Second, given the broad scope of CSHPs, it is difficult to determine what the realistic outcomes should be, and measuring these outcomes in school-age children (be it the actual behavior or precursors such as communication skills) is often problematic, especially when outcomes have to do with such sensitive matters as drug use or sexual behavior. Finally, though some aspects of a CSHP (e.g., classroom curricula) can be replicated, many aspects of the CSHP (e.g., staffing patterns, local norms, and community resources) differ across schools, cities, states, and regions. Consequently, the results of even the most rigorous evaluations may not be generalizable to other settings.

This chapter examines these and other issues related to the evaluation of CSHPs. First, general principles of research and evaluation, as applied to school health programs, are reviewed. Then the challenges and difficulties associated with research and evaluation of comprehensive, multi-component programs are examined. Finally, the difficulties and uncertainties related to research and evaluation of even a single, relatively well-defined component of comprehensive programs—the health education component—are be considered. The committee felt that it was appropriate to focus on health education in this chapter, because of the relative maturity of research in this area. Specific aspects of health education research have been chosen that highlight challenges in evaluating school-based interventions, as well as in interpreting ambiguous, if not conflicting, results relevant to other components of the comprehensive program. Discussion of the research and evaluation of other components of CSHPs—health services, nutrition or foodservices, physical education, and so forth—is found in the general discussion of these components in earlier chapters.

Types of School Health Research

Research and evaluation of comprehensive school health programs can be divided into three categories: basic research, outcome evaluation, and process evaluation.

Basic Research

An ultimate goal of CSHPs is to influence behavior. Basic research in CSHPs involves inquiry into the fundamental determinants of behavior as well as mechanisms of behavior change. Basic research includes examination of factors thought to influence health behavior—such as peer norms, self-efficacy, legal factors, health knowledge, and parental attitudes—as well as specific behavior change strategies. Basic research often employs epidemiologic strategies, such as cross-sectional or longitudinal analyses, as well as pilot intervention studies designed to isolate specific behavior change strategies, although often on a smaller scale than full outcome trials. A primary function of basic behavioral research is to inform the development of interventions, whose effects can then be tested in outcome evaluation trials.

Outcome Evaluation

Outcome evaluation includes empirical examination of the impact of interventions on targeted outcomes. Possible outcomes (or dependent variables) include health knowledge, attitudes, skills, behaviors, biologic measures, morbidity, mortality, and cost-effectiveness. Interventions (or independent variables) include specific health education curricula, teaching strategies, organizational change, environmental change, or health service delivery models. This type of evaluation in its most basic form resembles the randomized clinical trial with experimental and control groups, along with the requisite null hypothesis assumptions and concern for internal and external validity. Outcome evaluation can further be divided into three stages: efficacy, effectiveness, and implementation effectiveness trials (Flay, 1986).

Efficacy. Efficacy testing involves the evaluation of an intervention under ideal, controlled implementation conditions. During this stage, for example, teachers may be paid to ensure that they implement a health curriculum, or other motivational strategies may be used to ensure fidelity. The goal of efficacy testing is to determine the potential effect of an intervention, with less concern for feasibility or replicability. In drug study parlance, during this stage of research efforts are made to ensure that the "drug" is taken so that biologic effects, or lack thereof, can be attributed to the drug rather than to degree of compliance.

Effectiveness. In effectiveness trials, interventions are implemented under real-world circumstances with the associated variations in implementation and participant exposure. Effectiveness trials help determine if interventions can reliably be used under real-world conditions and the extent to which effects observed under efficacy conditions are reproduced in natural settings. Some programs, despite being efficacious, may not be effective if they are difficult to implement or are not accepted by staff or students. Effectiveness research is of particular concern because the results of efficacy testing and, to a lesser extent, of effectiveness trials may not always be generalizable to the real world.

Implementation Effectiveness. In implementation effectiveness trials, variations in implementation methods are manipulated experimentally and outcomes are measured (Flay, 1986). For example, the outcomes can be compared when a CSHP is implemented with or without a school coordinator or when a health education program is implemented by peers rather than adults.

Process Evaluation

Once an intervention has demonstrated adequate evidence for efficacy and effectiveness, it can be assumed that replications of the intervention will yield effects similar to those observed in prior outcomes research trials. The validity of this assumption is enhanced when multiple effectiveness trials have been successfully conducted under varying conditions and the intervention is delivered with fidelity in a setting and with a target population similar to those used in the initial testing.

It is at this point that process evaluation becomes the desired level of assessment. The goal of process evaluation is not to determine the basic impact of an intervention but rather to determine whether a proven intervention was properly implemented, and what factors may have contributed to the intervention's success or failure at the particular site. Implementation and/or participant exposure can be used as proxies for formal outcome evaluation. Key process evaluation strategies include implementation monitoring (e.g., teacher observation), quality assurance, and assessing consumer reactions (e.g., student, teacher, and parent response to the program).

Evaluation at this level may include some elements of outcome evaluation. Desired outcomes are often stated as objectives to be achieved by the program, which can be evaluated pre- and post-intervention, and may include a comparison group or references to normative data. Random selection and assignment of participants are typically not employed, however, and the level of rigor used to collect and analyze data is often less stringent than in formal outcome evaluation. This type of evaluation is sometimes referred to as program evaluation.

Although program evaluation can include rigorous design and analyses, in many real world program evaluations the assessment is often secondary to the intervention. Such interventions often do not bother with randomized design, control groups, or complex statistics. The evaluation is adapted to the intervention, rather than the inverse. For example, pragmatic issues, more than experimental design, often determine sample size and which sites are assigned to treatment or comparison conditions. In basic research and outcome evaluation on the other hand, evaluation is the principal reason that the intervention is being conducted; pragmatic issues often yield to methodologic concerns, and evaluation procedures largely are determined prior to initiating intervention activities.

Linking Outcome and Process Evaluations

Although outcome and process evaluation are described above as being sequential, the two often are conducted concurrently by linking process data to outcome data in order to determine causal pathways. One application of linking process and outcome data is the dose–response analysis—measuring the relationship between intervention dose and level of outcomes. For example, student behavioral outcomes can be examined relative to levels of teachers' curriculum implementation in a health education study or to students' level of clinic usage in a health services study. A positive dose–response relationship is seen as evidence for construct validity—that is, observed outcomes are attributed to the intervention rather than to other influences. Numerous health education studies have established a dose–response relationship between curriculum exposure and student outcomes (Connell et al., 1985; Parcel et al., 1991; Resnicow et al., 1992; Rohrbach et al., 1993; Taggart et al., 1990). Less is known about dose–response in other components of CSHPs.

Who Conducts the Research?

The various types of school health research are conducted by a diverse group of professionals. Basic research and outcome evaluation are typically conducted by doctoral-level professionals from university and freestanding research centers, often with funding from the federal government (though such studies also are supported by private foundations or corporations). Evaluating CSHPs at the level of basic research or outcome evaluation is largely beyond the fiscal and professional capacity of most local and even state education agencies. Process evaluation, on the other hand, can be conducted by local education agencies, perhaps in partnership with local public health agencies. Many models of CSHPs include an evaluation component, and it is important to delineate what type of evaluation schools and education agencies should reasonably be expected to conduct on the local level.

Although carried out by research professionals, basic research and outcome evaluation should not be abstract academic pursuits that are an end in themselves. Greater interaction is needed between researchers and those who actually implement programs. It would be desirable to stimulate and support research and evaluation alliances among colleges of education, schools of public health, and colleges of medicine. Bringing together the expertise from all three sectors in school health research and evaluation centers may enhance the understanding and interaction between these sectors and produce research and evaluation methods that can address cross-sector issues more accurately. This also will lead to developing programs that can be disseminated more easily and to reducing the number of researchers working in isolation.

Uses for Research and Evaluation

Basic research, outcome evaluation, and process evaluation are also conducted for different audiences and intentions. The first two are largely intended to build scientific knowledge and are generally published in the peer-reviewed literature. The latter generally is used to demonstrate feasibility of an intervention, as well as to document the facts that program implementation objectives were met and funds were properly spent. Such reports are typically requested by or intended for state education agencies, local education agencies, or funding sources that may have sponsored the local project. Local program evaluations of pilot programs also are used to justify expanding dissemination efforts.

All three types of evaluation can contribute to the development and dissemination of comprehensive school health programs, although it is important that they be applied in their proper sequence. Process evaluation studies are inappropriate for demonstrating intervention efficacy or measuring cost-effectiveness, just as basic research approaches may go beyond what is necessary for local program evaluation. To merit dissemination, programs should first undergo formal experimental efficacy and effectiveness testing; lower standards may result in adoption of suboptimal programs and ultimately impair the credibility of school health programs among their educational and public health constituencies (Ennett et al., 1994).

METHODOLOGICAL CHALLENGES

Although traditional experimental studies using control or comparison groups are appropriate for testing individual program components and specific intervention strategies, this may not be the case for the overall CSHP, which is a complex entity and varies from site to site. In a recent discussion of methods to evaluate such complex systems as CSHPs, Shaw (1995) proposed that the use of the classic experimental design to conduct outcome evaluations may be outmoded and inadequate for several reasons. First, the randomized clinical trial, with its tightly controlled and defined independent and dependent variables, cannot measure and capture large-scale, rapidly changing systems. Traditional experimental design ignores the need for timely formative descriptive data, maintains the artificial roles of the researcher as external expert and the subject as passive recipient of a defined treatment, and fails to recognize the complex nature of multifaceted programs that vary according to community needs.

Furthermore, there may be ethical dilemmas in randomly assigning students to treatment versus control groups when children's health and well-being are at stake.

It will be difficult—and possibly not feasible—to conduct traditional randomized trials on entire comprehensive programs. However, interventions associated with individual program components should be developed and tested by using rigorous methods that involve experimental and control groups, with the requisite concern for internal and external validity. In this section, some of the methodological challenges of demonstrating program impacts are examined.

Challenges in Assessing Validity

A goal of studying CSHPs at the level of efficacy testing is to measure the extent to which programs produce the desired outcomes (internal validity)—that is, to determine whether there is a causal relationship between the independent variable (CSHP) and defined outcomes such as knowledge, health practices, or health status.

Defining the Independent Variable

The first measurement challenge is the difficulty in defining the independent variable (the CSHP) or "treatment." Knapp (1995) has described this dilemma: "The 'independent variable' is elusive. It can be many different kinds of things, even within the same intervention; far from being a fixed treatment, as assessed by many research designs, the target of study is more often a menu of possibilities."

Ironically, the most successful programs—which are, in fact, comprehensive, multifaceted, interdisciplinary and well integrated into the community—may be the most difficult to define and segregate into components readily identifiable as the independent variable. It may be impossible, for example, to separate effects of the school from those of the community (Perry et al., 1992). This poses an important assessment dilemma. While it is vital that comprehensive programs be evaluated as a whole (Lopez and Weiss, 1994), it is unlikely that any individual program could be replicated in its entirety in a different community with its varying infrastructure, needs, and values. Thus, internal validity—the extent to which the effectiveness of the entire program is being accurately measured—may be high, but external validity—the extent to which the findings can be generalized and replicated beyond a single setting—is sacrificed.

Because of limited resources, one might wish to prioritize individual program components based on their relative efficacy. However, the overall effect of comprehensive programs may well be more than or different from the sum of its parts. Using a factorial design to examine the effects of individual components or combinations of components would require an unwieldy number of experimental conditions and large sample size. Thus, the independent variables in a CSHP not only may be difficult to define and measure, but it is unlikely that a consensus of what should comprise the intervention can or even should be reached.

Defining the Dependent Variable

In similar ways, defining the appropriate, feasible, and measurable outcomes (dependent variables) of a CSHP is equally challenging. Is it necessary to use change in health-related behaviors, such as smoking or drug use, to measure effectiveness of health education programs, or is the acquisition of knowledge and skills sufficient? If behavior change outside the school is required to declare effectiveness, this would seem to represent an educational double standard. For example, the quality and effectiveness of mathematics education are measured by determining mathematics knowledge and skills, using some sort of school-based assessment, not by determining whether the student actually balances a checkbook or accurately fills out an income tax form as an adult. Likewise, the quality of instruction in literature or political science is measured by the acquisition of knowledge, not by whether the student writes novels, reads poetry, votes, or becomes a contributing citizen.

Similarly, should appropriate outcomes for school health services be improved health status, behaviors, and long-term health outcomes, or is simply access to and utilization of services a sufficient end point? Is a reduction in absenteeism a proxy for improved health status and a reasonable indicator of health outcomes? Dependent variables used to measure effectiveness of school-linked health services have included linking students with no prior care to health services, decreased use of the emergency room for primary care, identification of previously unidentified health problems, access to and utilization of services by students and families, perceptions and health knowledge of students and their parents, decreasing involvement in risk behaviors, and health status indicators (Glick et al., 1995; Kisker et al., 1994; Lewin-VHI and Institute of Health Policy Studies, 1995). Some of these measures simply determine whether school services provide access and utilization, whereas other measures look for a change in health status and behavior. However, if improved health status and behaviors are declared to be the expectation for school health services, does this hold the school to higher standards than those of other health care providers?

The committee points out that, although influencing health behavior and health status are ultimate goals of CSHPs, such end points involve personal decisionmaking beyond the control of the school. Other factors—family, peers, community, and the media—exert tremendous influence on students, and schools should not bear total responsibility for students' health behavior and health status. Schools should be held accountable for conveying health knowledge, providing a health-promoting environment, and ensuring access to high-quality services; these are the reasonable outcomes for judging the merit of a CSHP.[1] Other outcomes—improved attendance, better cardiovascular fitness, less drug abuse, or fewer teen pregnancies, for example—may also be considered, but the committee believes that such measures must be interpreted with caution, since they are influenced by personal decisionmaking and factors beyond the control of the school. In particular, null or negative outcomes for these measures should not necessarily lead to declaring the CSHP a failure; rather, they may imply that other sources of influence on children and young people oppose and outweigh the influence of the CSHP.

Other Issues

In addition to the above difficulties, all of the potential biases and challenges inherent in any research also apply. Serious threats to validity in measuring effects of CSHP include:

- the Hawthorne effect—positive outcomes simply due to being part of an investigation, regardless of the nature of the intervention;
- self-reporting biases—responding with answers that are thought to be "correct" and socially desirable;
- Type III error—incorrectly concluding that an intervention is not effective, when in fact ineffectiveness is due to the incorrect implementation of the intervention.
  - ensuring even and consistent distribution of the intervention;
  - sorting out effects of confounding and extraneous variables;
  - isolating effective ingredients of multifaceted programs;
  - control groups that are not comparable;
  - differential and selective attrition in longitudinal studies;
  - inadequate reliability and validity of measurement tools; and
  - vague or inadequate conceptualization of study variables.

---

[1]This view is consistent with earlier discussion in this chapter that for the local school, the desired level of evaluation is process evaluation. If the school is providing health curricula and health services that have been shown through basic research and outcome evaluation to produce positive health outcomes, the committee suggests that the crucial question at the school level should be whether the interventions are implemented properly.

Another problem in drawing conclusions from reported research is "reporting bias"—the fact that only positive findings tend to be reported in the literature while studies with negative or inconclusive results are not often published. It is also important to remember that results that are statistically significant may not always have educational and public health significance.

Challenges Related to Feasibility

The kinds of large-scale research studies necessary to assess long-term outcomes of CSHPs are extremely costly and require extensive coordination. Since such programs are usually implemented for entire schools, communities, regions, or states, a majority of the children who participate are at relatively low risk for a number of outcomes of potential relevance. In addition, often only small to moderate outcome effects are sought. Hence, sample size needs are large, particularly when the unit of measurement is the school or the community rather than the individual.

Once efficacy and effectiveness have been demonstrated, the problem of developing a feasible program evaluation plan is compounded by the lack of evaluation expertise at the local or regional level and the inadequate or incompatible information systems for collecting, analyzing, and disseminating information. Local planners often need assistance in selecting and implementing evaluation strategies and in identifying means to make existing data more useful. For school health education, there are numerous guidelines and evaluation manuals from the Centers for Disease Control and Prevention (CDC), the Department of Health and Human Service's Center for Substance Abuse Prevention at the Substance Abuse and Mental Health Services Administration, and the Educational Development Center, to help states develop an evaluation plan. The national evaluation plan for the Healthy Schools, Healthy Communities Program provides helpful information for the evaluation of school health services (Lewin-VHI and Institute of Health Policy Studies, 1995). This plan is facilitated by a standardized data collection system and marks the first time that health education and health services will be systematically analyzed with a management information system that records different types of health education interventions, utilization of health services, and outcomes.

CHALLENGES AND FUTURE DIRECTIONS FOR SCHOOL HEALTH EDUCATION RESEARCH

Health education is one of the essential components of CSHPs. As described in earlier chapters, health instruction has taken place in schools for many years, and the field is reasonably well defined and developed compared to some of the other aspects of a CSHP. Health education research has been an active field, but considerable knowledge gaps exist and research findings are often ambiguous, unexpected, or sometimes seemingly contradictory. This section focuses on some of the challenges and unresolved questions in classroom health education and suggests issues that merit further study.

Effects of Comprehensive Health Education

The preponderance of school health education research has consisted of outcome evaluations focusing on categorical risk behavior, such as smoking, drug use, sexual behavior, and nutrition. A few notable studies have examined several risk behaviors simultaneously—such as nutrition, physical activity, and smoking—as risk reduction interventions for cardiovascular disease or cancer (Luepker et al., 1996; Resnicow et al., 1991) or have looked at efforts to prevent drug, alcohol, and tobacco abuse (Pentz, 1989a), but there have been very few studies that evaluate comprehensive, multitopic health education programs (Connell et al., 1985; Errecart et al., 1991). The lack of evaluation studies of comprehensive health education is to a large extent the result of how school health research has been funded at the federal level. Generally, health concerns are divided into categorical areas for research and demonstration funding; the result is that funding agencies are interested in funding only research and development projects that address their particular disease area of responsibility. There is a scarcity of hard data about the potential impact of overall comprehensive classroom health education programs. Only a few commercially available multitopic school health curricula have been evaluated to test their effectiveness (e.g., the Know Your Body program). Some of these either are old and or have not made use of the methods demonstrated to be effective in categorical research and demonstration projects, which means that schools are faced with adopting programs that have not been evaluated or attempting to piece together evaluated programs.

How Much Health Education Is Enough?

There is consensus that health education programming should span kindergarten through grade 12 (Lohrman et al., 1987). However, the precise number and sequence of lessons required to achieve significant enduring effects have not been clearly defined. As mentioned previously, such determinations are complicated by uncertainties in what end points are desirable or feasible—behavior change versus change in knowledge and attitudes. If the desired end point is change in behavior, a greater dose will likely be required. ("Dose" involves two dimensions: intensity, or amount of programming per year, and duration, the number of years of programming.) Moreover, if the end point is long-term behavior change or reductions in adult morbidity and mortality, an even greater dose may be necessary that provides more intensive programming for a longer time.

The ideal means to determine adequate dose would be to deliver the same curriculum using various levels of intensity and duration and then examine differences in student outcomes by differences in curriculum exposure. However, few studies have been designed a priori to test varying format and amount of programming. Instead, most of the evidence derives from post hoc analyses examining dose–response effects between health education programming and student outcomes—that is, the relationship between level of student outcomes and how much intervention students actually received. Despite the methodologic limitations, establishing a dose–response relationship from post hoc analysis is helpful for two reasons. First, a positive dose–response relationship provides evidence for construct validity—observed changes can be attributed to the health education program rather than to other variables. Second, results of these analyses have implications regarding the proper amount and sequence of health education programming.

One of the first major studies to demonstrate a dose–response effect was the School Health Education Evaluation project (Connell et al., 1985). Students from classrooms in which health programs were implemented more fully demonstrated significantly greater improvements in attitude and behaviors, compared to the entire intervention cohort. In addition, students exposed to two years versus one year of programming showed considerably greater changes in attitudes and practices. With regard to specific dose, there was evidence that between 15 and 20 hours of classroom instruction was required to produce meaningful student effects.

Dose–response effects were also evident in the Teenage Health Teaching Modules evaluation. This study found that changes in health knowledge as well as some priority health behaviors were related to teacher proficiency and to how well teachers adhered to the program materials, although these effects were somewhat equivocal (Parcel et al., 1991). In a third study, a three-year evaluation of the Know Your Body program, Resnicow et al. (1992) found significantly larger intervention effects for blood lipids, systolic blood pressure, health knowledge, self-efficacy, and dietary behavior among students exposed to "high-implementation" teachers relative to moderate- and low-implementation teachers, as well as to comparison youth receiving no programming.

There is additional evidence regarding dose–response from a survey conducted for the Metropolitan Life Insurance Company in 1988. This survey of 4,738 students in grades 3 through 12 in 199 public schools revealed that as the years of health instruction increased, students' health-related knowledge and healthy habits increased. With one year of health instruction, 43 percent of the students drank alcohol "sometimes or more often," a level that decreased to 33 percent for students who had received three years of health instruction. With only one year of health instruction, 13 percent of the students had taken drugs, compared with only 6 percent who had received three years of health instruction. In regard to exercising outside of the school, 80 percent of the students who had three years of health instruction did so, but only 72 percent of those who had one year of instruction exercised outside of school (Harris, 1988).

Duration, Sequence, and Timing of Health Education

Two other aspects of dose include intensity of programming (i.e., concentrated versus dispersed) and booster treatments. With regard to the former, Botvin and colleagues (1983) found that students who received a substance use education program several times a week for 4 to 6 weeks (a "concentrated" format) showed stronger treatment effects than youth receiving the program once a week for 12 weeks (a "dispersed" format). Additionally, in two separate studies, students receiving booster sessions following a year of primary intervention showed larger and more sustained behavior effects than youth receiving only the initial intervention (Botvin et al., 1983; Botvin et al., 1995). Taken together, these findings suggest that the greater the intensity and duration of health education programming, the greater is the effect. It is important to note that "increased dose" can include two elements. The first relates to the number of lessons contained in a curriculum; the second is a function of implementation fidelity on the part of classroom teachers. Thus, a complex, non-user-friendly health education program containing many lessons may, due to low teacher implementation, result in a lower dose than will a more user-friendly program containing fewer lessons.

With regard to specific policy recommendations, there are insufficient data to delineate a requisite number of lessons across content areas and grades. There is, however, some evidence to suggest that at least 10 to 15 initial lessons, plus 8 to 15 booster sessions in subsequent years, are required to produce lasting behavioral effects (Botvin et al., 1983, 1995; Connell et al., 1985). These data, however, are derived primarily from substance use prevention studies of middle school youth. Little is known about the requisite intensity and duration of programming for other content areas or other age groups. It is also unclear to what extent general life skills training, which targets substance use or sexual risk behaviors, may positively influence other behavioral domains. If spillover, synergistic effects from skills training or other common elements of health education programs (e.g., modifying normative expectations and increasing self-efficacy) occur when categorical programs are delivered within a comprehensive framework, the total number of lessons ultimately required for comprehensive curricula may be fewer than the sum of lessons from isolated categorical programs.

Additionally, whether these findings, which are based on a categorical topic, can be applied to a comprehensive curriculum merits discussion. It may be necessary to stagger content across K–12 and to target programming by developmental needs. For example, programming could be concentrated more heavily on substance use prevention at the middle school level, while in primary grades, nutrition and safety education could comprise the areas of focus. This developmental needs approach is a deviation from currently proposed curriculum frameworks, which suggest that health education address 8 to 12 content areas at each grade level. In view of the research that suggests a minimal number of lessons per grade for each content area, more serious attention should be given to setting priority areas for each stage of student development.

Lasting Effects of School Health Education

In several long-term follow-up studies of substance prevention programs delivered in grades 5 through 8 (Bell et al., 1993; Flay et al., 1989; Murray et al., 1989), positive program effects observed one to four years following the intervention had decayed by grade 12, or shortly after graduation from high school. Decay of program effects has also been observed for curricula addressing other content areas (Bush et al., 1989). There are studies, however, in which behavioral effects decayed but significant effects for knowledge and attitude were maintained (Bell et al., 1993; Flay et al., 1995).

Recently, however, Botvin and colleagues (1995) reported positive long-term results in a study involving more than 3,500 students in grade 12 who were randomly assigned to receive either the Life Skills Training substance use prevention program in grades 7 through 9 or "treatment as usual." Significant reductions in tobacco, alcohol, and marijuana use were evident at the follow-up in grade 12, and effects were greater among students whose teachers taught the program with higher fidelity (i.e., high implementors).

How can the positive effects reported by Botvin et al. be reconciled with the null results reported in prior studies? One explanation is dose. The previous interventions comprised only six to eight lessons in the first year and, in the Ellickson and Bell (1990) and Flay et al. (1989) studies, three to five booster sessions in subsequent years. Botvin's intervention contained 15 lessons in the first year and 15 additional lessons over the next two years. Other explanations include superiority of the Life Skills Training curriculum, including its content, format, and teacher training procedures, as well as higher levels of teacher implementation. Although the results of Botvin's study of substance use prevention are encouraging, research regarding the optimal dose and timing of curricula addressing other health behaviors is still needed. Given that achieving change in language arts and mathematics skills requires daily instruction for 12 academic years, it is reasonable to conclude that changes in health knowledge and in health behaviors also will require more instruction than one semester, the standard middle and secondary school requirement.

Active Ingredients of Health Education

Many successful health education programs employ several conceptually diverse intervention strategies such as didactic, affective, and behavioral activities directed at students, as well as environmental and policy change. Although there is considerable evidence that such programs as a whole can work, the construct validity of specific subcomponents—that is, "why" programs achieve or fail to achieve their desired effects—remains unclear (McCaul and Glasgow, 1985). Consider, for example, skills training. During the 1980s, numerous skills-based interventions aimed at increasing general and behavior-specific skills were developed and evaluated (Botvin et al., 1984; Donaldson et al., 1995; Flay, 1985; Kirby, 1992; McCaul and Glasgow, 1985). While initial results were encouraging and skills training has become an integral component of many school health education programs (Botvin et al., 1980; CDC, 1988, 1994; Flay, 1985; Glynn, 1989; Kirby, 1992; Pentz et al., 1989b; Schinke et al., 1985; Walter et al., 1988), many "skills-based" programs include other intervention strategies, such as modifying personal and group norms and outcome expectations, which also may have contributed to the reported intervention effects (Botvin et al., 1984; Ellickson and Bell, 1990; Murray et al., 1989; Pentz et al., 1989a; Walter et al., 1987). Several studies specifically designed to test the independent effects of skills training have found this approach to be largely ineffective (Elder et al., 1993; Hansen and Graham, 1991; Sussman et al., 1993). Instead, these studies indicate that modifying normative beliefs—students' assumptions regarding the prevalence and acceptability of substance use—appears to be the "active ingredient" of many of the skills training programs. Despite the questionable effectiveness of skills training in substance use prevention, skills may be important in other behavioral domains such as sexuality, nutrition, and exercise (Baranowksi, 1989; Perry et al., 1990; Sikkema et al., 1995; St. Lawrence et al., 1995; Warzak et al., 1995).

Similarly, although there is acceptance on the part of many health educators that peers are effective "messengers," the evidence for the effectiveness of peer-based health education is also somewhat equivocal (Bangert-Drowns, 1988; Clarke et al., 1986; Ellickson et al., 1993; Johnson et al., 1986; McCaul and Glasgow, 1985; Murray et al., 1988; Perry et al., 1989; Telch et al., 1990). The effectiveness of peer-based programs is likely to depend more on how peers are included in the program than on simply having peer-led activities.

In a review of programs to reduce sexual risk behavior, Kirby and coworkers found several differences between programs that had an impact on behavior and those that did not (Kirby et al., 1994). Although the authors warn that generalizations must be made cautiously, ineffective curricula tended to be broader and less focused. Effective curricula clearly focused on the specific values, norms, and skills necessary to avoid sex or unprotected sex, whereas ineffective curricula covered a broad range of topics and discussed many values and skills. Interestingly, the length of the program or the amount of skills practice did not appear to predict the success of programs. The authors suggest, however, that skills practice may be effective only when clear values or norms are emphasized or when skills focus specifically on avoiding undesirable sexual behavior rather than on developing more general communication skills.

Given the limited funding and classroom time available for health education, it is important that school health education programs include primarily those approaches known to influence health behavior. Providing health information is a necessary but certainly not sufficient condition for affecting behavior. Identifying "active ingredients" can be achieved through factorial designs as well as post hoc statistical techniques such as structural models, and discriminant analysis can be used to elucidate mediating variables and specific intervention components that may account for program effects (Botvin and Dusenbury, 1992; Dielman et al., 1989; MacKinnon et al., 1991).

Risk-Factor-Specific Versus Problem Behavior Intervention Models

Numerous studies have found that "problem" behaviors—such as the use of alcohol, marijuana, and tobacco; precocious sexual involvement; and delinquent activity—are positively correlated and occur in clusters. Problem Behavior Theory proposes an underlying psychologic phenomenon of "unconventionality" as the unifying etiologic explanation (see Basen-Engquist et al., 1996; Donovan and Jessor, 1985; Donovan et al., 1988; Resnicow et al., 1995). This conceptualization of health behavior has significant implications for CSHPs. As opposed to commonly used risk-factor-specific interventions that deal with each behavior separately, Problem Behavior Theory suggests that high-risk and problem behaviors can be prevented by an intervention that addresses common predisposing causes. Such interventions may be not only more effective but also more efficient, since fewer total lessons may be required to alter the common "core" causes. In addition to generic interventions, it may also be necessary to apply general strategies to selected high-risk behaviors. However, most school systems do not conceptualize health education from this perspective. Instead, health instruction is broken down into discrete content areas, more akin to the risk-factor-specific approach. Additional research, particularly studies examining the effects of interventions addressing traits that may underlie clusters of risk behaviors, is needed before health education is restructured toward a more targeted model of health behavior change.

Realistic Outcomes for School Health Education

It can be argued that previous studies reporting weak or null behavioral outcomes employed health education interventions of insufficient dose and breadth. Many of the interventions had no more than 10 lessons, delivered over the course of one year, and few or no subsequent booster lessons. As noted earlier, the positive long-term behavioral effects reported by Botvin and colleagues (1995) may be attributed largely to the increased dose. Additionally, had the categorical programs for which no long-term behavioral effects were observed been delivered within the context of a comprehensive school health program, positive effects may have been observed. It is important to set realistic expectations for school health education, particularly since many of the programs used in our schools provide a dose of insufficient intensity and duration, whose effects are further attenuated by inadequate levels of teacher implementation. As stated earlier, although influencing behavior is an ultimate goal of school health education, schools should not bear the total responsibility for student behavior, given all the other influences on students—family, peers, the media, community norms, and expectations—that are beyond the control of the school. Schools should be held accountable for providing a high-quality, up-to-date health education program that is delivered by qualified teachers using curricula that are based on research and have been validated through outcome evaluation. Schools should be held responsible for arming students with the knowledge, attitudes, and skills to adopt health-enhancing behavior and to avoid health-compromising behavior. If these conditions are met but behavioral outcomes are still less than desired, then other sources of influence on students must be examined for alignment with school health education messages. In addition, there may be delayed effects on behavior in later life, even if no immediate behavioral impacts are observed.

There is encouraging evidence that when school-based interventions are delivered along with complementary community-wide or media campaigns, significant long-term behavioral effects can be achieved (Flynn et al., 1994; Kelder et al., 1993; Perry et al., 1992; see Flay et al., 1995, for an exception). Therefore, although health education delivered in isolation may not be able to produce lasting behavioral effects, when combined with other activities or implemented within a comprehensive school health program, significant enduring changes in behavior as well as physical risk factors can be achieved.

There is considerable evidence that comprehensive curricula can produce significant short-term effects on multiple health behaviors, including substance use, diet, and exercise (Bush et al., 1989; Connell et al., 1985; Errecart et al., 1991; Resnicow et al., 1992; Walter et al., 1988, 1989). However, many of the assumptions regarding the effectiveness of classroom health education derive from studies of categorical programs, and it is unclear to what degree the effects observed for categorical programs are diminished or magnified when taught within a comprehensive framework. Although it can be argued that incorporating categorical programs within a comprehensive framework would attenuate effects because the focus on any one behavior or health issue would be diminished, it could also be argued that program effects would be enhanced because comprehensive programs provide extended if not synergistic application and reinforcement of essential skills across a wide range of topics. This is another area that calls for further research.

SUMMARY OF FINDINGS AND CONCLUSIONS

Research and evaluation of CSHPs can be divided into three categories: basic research, outcome evaluation, and process evaluation. Basic research involves inquiry into the fundamental determinants of behavior as well as mechanisms of behavior change. A primary function of basic research is to inform the development of interventions that can then be tested in outcome evaluation trials. Outcome evaluation involves the empirical examination of interventions on targeted outcomes, based on the randomized clinical trial approach with experimental and control groups. Process evaluation determines whether a proven intervention was properly implemented and examines factors that may have contributed to the intervention's success or failure. Basic research and outcome evaluation are typically conducted by professionals from university or other research centers and are largely beyond the capacity of local education agencies.

The committee believes that process evaluation is the appropriate level of evaluation in local programs.

Research and evaluation are particularly challenging for CSHPs. Since these programs comprise multiple interactive components, it is often difficult to attribute observed effects to specific components or to separate program effects from those of the family or community. Determining what outcomes are realistic and measuring outcomes in students are often problematic, especially when outcomes involve sensitive matters such as drug use or sexual behavior. Furthermore, since CSHPs are unique to a particular setting, the results of even the most rigorous evaluations may not be generalizable to other situations.

Interventions associated with the separate, individual components of CSHPs—health education, health services, nutrition services, and so forth—should be developed and tested using rigorous methods involving experimental and control groups. However, such an approach is likely to be difficult—and possibly not feasible—for studying entire comprehensive programs or determining the differential effects of individual components and combinations of components.

A fundamental issue involves determining what outcomes are appropriate and reasonable to expect from CSHPs. The committee recognizes that although influencing health behavior and health status is an ultimate goal of a CSHP, such end points involve factors beyond the control of the school. The committee believes that the reasonable outcomes on which a CSHP should be judged are equipping students with the knowledge, attitudes, and skills necessary for healthful behavior; providing a health-promoting environment; and ensuring access to high-quality services. Other outcomes—improved cardiovascular fitness or a reduction in absenteeism, drug abuse, or teen pregnancies, for example—may also be considered, but the committee believes that such measures must be interpreted with caution, since they are influenced by factors beyond the control of the school. In particular, null or negative measures for these outcomes should not necessarily lead to declaring the CSHP a failure; rather, they may imply that other sources of influence oppose and outweigh that of the CSHP or that the financial investment in the CSHP is so limited that returns are minimal.

RECOMMENDATIONS

In order for CSHPs to accomplish the desired goal of influencing behavior, the committee recommends the following:

An active research agenda on comprehensive school health programs should be pursued in order to fill critical knowledge

gaps; increased emphasis should be placed on basic research and outcome evaluation and on the dissemination of these research and outcome findings.

Research is needed about the effectiveness of specific intervention strategies such as skills training, normative education, or peer education; the effectiveness of specific intervention messages such as abstinence versus harm reduction; and the required intensity and duration of health education programming. Evidence suggests that common underlying factors may be responsible for the clustering of health-compromising behaviors and that interventions may be more effective if they address these underlying factors in addition to intervening to change risk behaviors. Additional research is needed to understand the etiology of problem behavior clusters and to develop optimal problem behavior interventions. And finally, since the acquisition of health-related social skills—such as negotiation, decisionmaking, and refusal skills—is a desired end point of CSHPs, basic research is needed to develop valid measures of social skills that can then be used as proxy measures of program effectiveness. Diffusion-related research is critical to ensure that efforts of research and development lead to improved practice and a greater utilization of effective methods and programs. Therefore, high priority should be given to studying how programs are adopted, implemented, and institutionalized. The feasibility and effectiveness of techniques of integrating concepts of health into science and other school subjects should also be examined.

Since the overall effects of comprehensive school health programs are not yet known and outcome evaluation of such complex systems poses significant challenges, the committee recommends the following:

A major research effort should be launched to establish model comprehensive programs and develop approaches for their study.

Specific outcomes of overall programs should be examined, including education (improved achievement, attendance, and graduation rates), personal health (resistance to "new social morbidities," improved biologic measures), mental health (less depression, stress, and violence), improved functionality, health systems (more students with a "medical home," reduction in use of emergency rooms or hospitals), self-sufficiency (pursuit of higher education or job), and future health literacy and health status. Studies could look at differential impacts of programs produced by such factors as program structure, characteristics of students, and type of school and community.

A thorough understanding of the feasible and effective (including cost-effective) interventions in each separate area of a CSHP will be necessary to provide the basis for combining components to produce a comprehensive program.

The committee recommends that further study of each of the individual components of a CSHP—for example, health education, health services, counseling, nutrition, school environment—is needed.

Additional studies are needed in a number of other areas. First, more data are needed about the advantages (cost and effectiveness) and disadvantages of providing health and social services in schools compared to other community sites—or compared to not providing services anywhere—as a function of community and student characteristics. This information will require overall consensus about the criteria to use for determining the quality of school health programs. It is also important to know how best to influence change in the climate and organizational structure of school districts and individual schools in order to bring about the adoption and implementation of CSHPs. Finally, there is a need for an analysis of the optimal structure, operation, and personnel needs of CSHPs.

REFERENCES

Bangert-Drowns, R.L. 1988. The effects of school-based substance abuse education: A meta-analysis. *Journal of Drug Education* 18:243–264.

Baranowski, T. 1989. Reciprocal determinism at the stages of behavior change: An integration of community, personal and behavioral perspectives. *International Quarterly of Community Health Education* 10(4):297–327.

Basen-Engquist, K., Edmundson, E., and Parcel, G.S. 1996. Structure of health risk behavior among high school students. *Journal of Consulting and Clinical Psychology* 64(4):764–775.

Bell, R.M., Ellickson, P.L., and Harrison, E.R. 1993. Do drug prevention effects persist into high school? How Project Alert did with ninth graders. *Preventive Medicine* 22:463–483.

Botvin, G.J., and Dusenbury, L. 1992. Smoking prevention among urban minority youth: Assessing effects on outcome and mediating variables. *Health Psychology* 11:290–299.

Botvin, G.J., Eng, A., and Williams, C.L. 1980. Preventing the onset of cigarette smoking through life skills training. *Preventive Medicine* 9:135–143.

Botvin, G.J., Renick, N.L., and Baker, E. 1983. The effects of scheduling format and booster sessions on a broad-spectrum psychosocial approach to smoking prevention. *Journal of Behavioral Medicine* 6(4):359–379.

Botvin, G.J., Baker, E., Renick, N.L., Filazzola, A.D., and Botvin, E.M. 1984. A cognitive-behavioral approach to substance abuse prevention. *Addictive Behaviors* 9:137–147.

Botvin, G.J., Baker, E., Dusenbury, L., and Botvin, E.M. 1995. Long-term follow-up results of a randomized drug abuse prevention trial in a white middle class population. *Journal of Behavioral Medicine* 273(14):1106–1112.

Bush, P.J., Zuckerman, A.E., Taggart, V.S., Theiss, P.K., Peleg, E.O., and Smith, S.A. 1989. Cardiovascular risk factor prevention in black school children: The "Know Your Body" evaluation project. *Health Education Quarterly* 16(2):215–227.

Centers for Disease Control and Prevention. 1988. Guidelines for effective school health education to prevent the spread of AIDS. *Morbidity and Mortality Weekly Report* 37(Suppl.)2:1–14.

Centers for Disease Control and Prevention. 1994. Guidelines for school health programs to prevent tobacco use and addiction. *Journal of School Health* 64(9):353–360.

Clarke, J.H., MacPherson, B., Holmes, D.R., and Jones, R. 1986. Reducing adolescent smoking: A comparison of peer-led, teacher-led, and expert interventions. *Journal of School Health* 56(3):102–106.

Connell, D.B., Turner, R.R., and Mason, E.F. 1985. Summary of findings of the school health education evaluation: Health promotion effectiveness, implementation, and costs. *Journal of School Health* 55(8):316–321.

Dielman, T.E., Shope, J.T., Butchart, A.T., Campaneilli, P.C., and Caspar, R.A. 1989. A covariance structure model test of antecedents of adolescent alcohol misuse and a prevention effort. *Journal of Drug Education* 19(4):337–361.

Donaldson, S.I., Graham, J.W., Piccinin, A.M., and Hansen, W.B. 1995. Resistance-skills training and onset of alcohol use: Evidence for beneficial and potentially harmful effects in public schools and in private Catholic schools. *Health Psychology* 14(4):291–300.

Donovan, J.E., and Jessor, R. 1985. Structure of problem behavior in adolescence and young adulthood. *Journal of Consulting and Clinical Psychology* 53:890–904.

Donovan, J.E., Jessor, R., and Costa, F.M. 1988. Syndrome of problem behavior in adolescence: A replication. *Journal of Consulting and Clinical Psychology* 56:762–765.

Elder, J.P., Sallis, J.F., Woodruff, S.I., and Wildey, M.B. 1993. Tobacco-refusal skills and tobacco use among high risk adolescents. *Journal of Behavioral Medicine* 16:629–642.

Ellickson, P.L., and Bell, R.M. 1990. Drug prevention in junior high: A multi-site longitudinal test. *Science* 247:1299–1305.

Ellickson, P.L., Bell, R.M., and Harrison, E.R. 1993. Changing adolescent propensities to use drugs: Results from Project ALERT. *Health Education Quarterly* 20(2):227–242.

Ennett, S.T., Tobler, N.S., Ringwalt, C.L., and Flewelling, R.L. 1994. How effective is drug abuse resistance education? A meta-analysis of Project DARE outcome evaluations. *American Journal of Public Health* 84(9):1394–1401.

Errecart, M.T., Walberg, H.J., Ross, J.G., Gold, R.S., Fielder, J.L., and Kolbe, L.J. 1991. Effectiveness of Teenage Health Teaching Modules. *Journal of School Health* 61(1):26–30.

Flay, B.R. 1985. Psychosocial approaches to smoking prevention: A review of findings. *Health Psychology* 4(5):449–488.

Flay, B.R. 1986. Efficacy and effectiveness trials in the development of health promotion programs. *Preventive Medicine* 15:451–474.

Flay, B.R., Phil, D., Koepke, D., Thomson, S.J., Santi, S., Best, A., and Brown, K.S. 1989. Six-year follow-up of the first Waterloo school smoking prevention trial. *American Journal of Public Health* 79:1371–1376.

Flay, B.R., Miller, T.Q., Hedeker, D., Siddiqui, O., Britton, C.F., Brannon, B.R., Johnson, C.A., Hansen, W.B., Sussman, S., and Dent, C. 1995. The television, school, and family smoking prevention and cessation project. *Preventive Medicine* 24:29–40.

Flynn, B.S., Worden, J.K., Secker-Walker, R.H., Pirie, P.L., Badger, G.J., Carpenter, J.H., and Geller, B.M. 1994. Mass media and school interventions for cigarette smoking prevention: Effects two years after completion. *American Journal of Public Health* 84(7):1148–1150.

Glick, B., Doyle, L., Ni, H., Gao, D., and Pham, C. 1995. School-based health center program evaluation: Perceptions, knowledge, and attitudes of parents/guardians of eleventh graders. A limited dataset presented to the Multnomah County (Oregon) Commissioners, March 21.

Glynn, T.J. 1989. Essential elements of school-based smoking prevention programs. *Journal of School Health* 59(5):181–188.

Hansen, W.B., and Graham, J.W. 1991. Preventing alcohol, marijuana, and cigarette use among adolescents: Peer pressure resistance training versus establishing conservative norms. *Preventive Medicine* 20:414–430.

Harris, L. 1988. Health: *You've Got to be Taught: An Evaluation of Comprehensive Health Education in American Public Schools*. New York: Metropolitan Life Foundation.

Johnson, C.A., Hansen, W.B., Collins, L.M., and Graham, J.W. 1986. High-school smoking prevention: Results of a three-year longitudinal study. *Journal of Behavioral Medicine* 9(5):439–452.

Kelder, S.J., Perry, C.L., and Klepp, K.I. 1993. Community-wide youth exercise promotion: Long-term outcomes of the Minnesota Heart Health Program and the Class of 1989 Study. *Journal of School Health* 53(5):218–223.

Kirby, D. 1992. School-based programs to reduce sexual risk-taking behaviors. *Journal of School Health* 62(7):280–287.

Kirby, D., Short, L., Collins, J., Rugg, D., Kolbe, L., Howard, M., Miller, B., Sonenstein, F., and Zabin, L.S. 1994. School-based programs to reduce sexual risk behaviors: A review of effectiveness. *Public Health Reports* 109(3):339–359.

Kisker, E.E., Marks, E.L., Morrill, W.A., and Brown, R.S. 1994. *Healthy Caring: An Evaluation Summary of the Robert Wood Johnson Foundation's School-Based Adolescent Health Care Program*. Princeton, N.J.: Mathtech.

Knapp, M.S. 1995. How shall we study comprehensive, collaborative services for children and families? *Educational Research* 24(4):5–16.

Lewin-VHI and Institute of Health Policy Studies. 1995. Healthy schools, healthy communities program: National evaluation. Submitted to Bureau of Primary Health Care, Health Resources and Services Administration, U.S. Department of Health and Human Services by Lewin-VHI, Inc., and Institute for Health Policy Studies, University of California at San Francisco, February, 1995.

Lohrman, D.K., Gold, R.S., and Jubb, W.H. 1987. School health education: A foundation for school health programs. *Journal of School Health* 57(10):420–425.

Lopez, M.E., and Weiss, H.B. 1994. Can we get here from there? Examining and expanding the research base for comprehensive, school-linked early childhood services. Paper commissioned for the Invitational Conference of the U.S. Department of Education and the American Educational Research Association: School-Linked Comprehensive Services for Children and Families, Leesburg, Va., September 28–October 2.

Luepker, R.V., Perry, C.L., McKinlay, S.M., Nader, P.R., Parcel, G.S., Stone, E.J., Webber, L.S., Elder, J.P., Feldman, H.A., Johnson, C.C., Kelder, S.H., and Wu, M. 1996. Outcomes of a field trial to improve children's dietary patterns and physical activity: The Child and Adolescent Trial for Cardiovascular Health (CATCH). *Journal of the American Medical Association* 275(10):768–776.

MacKinnon, D.P., Johnson, C.A., Pentz, M.A., Dwyer, J.H., Hansen, W.B., Flay, B.R., and Wang, E.Y. 1991. Mediating mechanisms in a school-based drug prevention program: First-year effects of the Midwestern Prevention Project. *Health Psychology* 10(3):164–172.

McCaul, K.D., and Glasgow, R.E. 1985. Preventing adolescent smoking: What have we learned about treatment construct validity? *Health Psychology* 4:361–387.

Murray, D.M., Davis-Hearn, M., Goldman, A., Pirie, P., and Luepker, R.V. 1988. Four- and five-year follow-up results from four seventh grade smoking prevention strategies. *Journal of Behavioral Medicine* 11(4):395–405.

Murray, D.M., Pirie, P., Luepker, R.V., and Pallonen, U. 1989. Five- and six-year follow-up results from four seventh-grade smoking prevention strategies. *Journal of Behavioral Medicine* 12:207–218.

Parcel, G.S., Ross, J.G., Lavin, A.T., Portnoy, B., Nelson, G.D., and Winters, F. 1991. Enhancing implementation of the Teenage Health Teaching Modules. *Journal of School Health* 61(1):35–38.

Pentz, M.A., Dwyer, J.H., MacKinnon, D.P., Flay, B.R., Hansen, W.B., Wang, E.Y., and Johnson, C.A. 1989a. A multicommunity trial for primary prevention of adolescent drug abuse: Effects on drug use prevalence. *Journal of American Medical Association* 261:3259–3266.

Pentz, M.A., MacKinnon, D.P., and Flay, B.R., Hansen, W.B., Johnson, C.A., and Dwyer, J.H. 1989b. Primary prevention of chronic diseases in adolescence: Effects of the Midwestern Prevention Project on tobacco use. *American Journal of Epidemiology* 130(4):713–724.

Perry, C.L., Grant, M., Ernberg, G., Florenzano, R.U., Langdon, M.C., Myeni, A.D., Waahlberg, R., Berg, S., Andersson, K., and Fisher, K.J. 1989. WHO collaborative study on alcohol education and young people: Outcomes of four-country pilot study. *International Journal of the Addictions* 24(12):1145–1171.

Perry, C.L., Baranowski, T., and Parcel, G. 1990. How individuals, environments and health behavior interact: Social learning theory. In *Health Behavior and Health Education Theory, Research, and Practice*, K. Glanz, F.M. Lewis, and B. Rimer, eds. New York: Jossey-Bass.

Perry, C.L., Kelder, S.H., Murray, D.M., and Klepp, K. 1992. Community-wide smoking prevention: Long-term outcomes of the Minnesota Heart Health Program and the Class of 1989 study. *American Journal of Public Health* 82(9):1210–1216.

Resnicow, K., Cross, D., and Wynder, E. 1991. The role of comprehensive school-based interventions: The results of four "Know Your Body" studies. *Annals of the New York Academy of Sciences* 623:285–297.

Resnicow, K., Cohn, L., Reinhardt, J., Cross, D., Futterman, R., Kirschner, E., Wynder, E.L., and Allegrante, J. 1992. A three-year evaluation of the "Know Your Body" program in minority school children. *Health Education Quarterly* 19(4):463–480.

Resnicow, K., Ross, D., and Vaughan, R. 1995. The structure of problem and conventional behaviors in African-American youth. *Journal of Clinical and Consulting Psychology* 63(4):594–603.

Rohrbach, L.A., Graham, J.W., and Hansen, W.B. 1993. Diffusion of a school-based substance abuse prevention program: Predictors of program implementation. *Preventive Medicine* 22(2):237–260.

Schinke, S.P., Gilchrist, L., and Snow, W.H. 1985. Skills intervention to prevent cigarette smoking among adolescents. *American Journal of Public Health* 75:665–667.

Shaw, K.M. 1995. Challenges in evaluating systems reform. *The Evaluation Exchange: Emerging Strategies in Evaluating Child and Family Services* 1(1):2–3.

Sikkema, K.J., Winett, R.A., and Lombard, D.N. 1995. Development and evaluation of an HIV-risk reduction program for female college students. *AIDS Education and Prevention* 7(2):145–159.

St. Lawrence, J.S., Jefferson, K.W., Alleyne, E., and Brasfield, T.L. 1995. Comparison of education versus behavioral skills training interventions in lowering sexual HIV-risk behavior of substance-dependent adolescents. *Journal of Consulting and Clinical Psychology* 63(1):154–157.

Sussman, S., Dent, C.W., Stacy, A.W., Sun, P., Craig, S., Simon, T.R., Burton D., and Flay, B.R. 1993. Project towards no tobacco use, one-year behavior outcomes. *American Journal of Public Health* 83(9):1245–1250.

Taggart, V.S., Bush, P.J., Zuckerman, A.E., and Theiss, P.K. 1990. A process of evaluation of the District of Columbia "Know Your Body" project. *Journal of School Health* 60(2):60–66.

Telch, M.J., Miller, L.M., Killen, J.D., Cooke, S., and Maccoby, N. 1990. Social influences approach to smoking prevention: The effects of videotape delivery with and without same-age peer leader participation. *Addictive Behaviors* 15(1):21–28.

Walter, H.J., Hofman, A., and Barrett, L.T., Connelly, P.A., Kost, K.L., Walk, E.H., and Patterson, R. 1987. Primary prevention of cardiovascular disease among children: Three-year results of a randomized intervention trial. In *Cardiovascular Risk Factors in Childhood: Epidemiology and Prevention*, B. Hetzel and G.S. Berenson, eds. Netherlands: Elsevier.

Walter, H.J., Hofman, A., Vaughan, R., and Wynder, E.L. 1988. Modification of risk factors for coronary heart disease. *New England Journal of Medicine* 318:1093–1100.

Walter, H.J., Vaughan, R.D., and Wynder, E.L. 1989. Primary prevention of cancer among children: Changes in cigarette smoking and diet after six years of intervention. *Journal of the National Cancer Institute* 81:995–999.

Warzak, W.J., Grow, C.R., Poler, M.M., and Walburn, J.N. 1995. Enhancing refusal skills: Identifying contexts that place adolescents at risk for unwanted sexual activity. *Journal of Developmental and Behavioral Pediatrics* 16(2):98–100.

7

The Path to the Future

Previous chapters of this report have described the concept of a comprehensive school health program (CSHP), examined some of its essential components, and proposed steps that might be taken to build an infrastructure to support and promote CSHPs. Some of the knowledge gaps about these programs and challenges to filling these gaps have also been discussed. Throughout the report, the analysis and rationale for many important recommendations are presented. This final chapter highlights several remaining overarching issues.

THE UNIQUE POSITION OF THE SCHOOL

Many factors—the family, friends or peers, school, and community—exert tremendous influence on children and youth. Each of these systems may have assets or deficits, and each must share responsibility for children's health and well-being.

The basic question might be raised: Why focus on schools? The answer has to do with the unique position of the school. Of the four major "systems of influence" cited—family, friends or peers, school, and community—the *school* is the only one that is an *organized public institution*, amenable to being restructured and mobilized to promote societal goals. Schooling is the only universal entitlement for children in this country, and schools are the only institution that allows access on a daily basis to almost all children between the ages of 5 and 17 in the nation. Schools not only provide academic preparation but are one of the principal formal community institutions responsible for transmitting culture and bringing about the socialization of children and youth.

Realistically, the potential impact of comprehensive school health programs is greatly diminished if deficits in other systems are large. Schools cannot be expected to overcome difficult family situations, pressure from antisocial and rebellious peers, or problems of impoverished and dysfunctional communities. On the other hand, schools are strategically positioned to serve as a linchpin or rallying point, capable of bringing together and aligning the other "systems of influence" to promote the health and well-being of students.

MOVING SCHOOL HEALTH PROGRAMS INTO THE FUTURE

As stated above, schooling is the only universal entitlement for children in this country, and schools are the only institution that allows access on a daily basis to children between the ages of 5 and 17. The committee believes that as a part of this educational entitlement, students should receive the health-related programs and services necessary for them to derive maximum benefit from their education and enable them to become healthy and productive adults. This view appears to be broadly accepted since the committee has found that many of the components of a CSHP already exist in many schools across the country—health education, physical education, nutrition and foodservice programs, basic school services, and policies addressing the school environment (Collins et al., 1995; Davis et al., 1995; Pate et al., 1995; Pateman et al., 1995; Ross et al., 1995; Small et al., 1995). The question then arises: What would it take to transform existing programs in typical communities into a comprehensive school health program?

First, although the many components of a CSHP exist widely, the implementation and quality of many of these components require attention, as earlier chapters have noted. New standards and recommendations have been released in many of these fields that have yet to reach the local level. Further, since the Centers for Disease Control and Prevention's School Health Policies and Programs Study (SHPPS) did not address counseling and psychological services, less is known about their extent and quality, but anecdotal evidence reviewed in Chapter 4 indicates that this is an area of significant need. Another serious deficiency of current programs is the apparent lack of involvement of critical community stakeholders in designing and supporting programs. SHPPS found that only one-third of districts had some sort of district-wide school health advisory council; only about half of these councils had representation from the medical community, and only 14 percent had representation from the mental health community (Collins et al., 1995). In addition, although

SHPPS found that collaboration among the separate disciplines and components of a CSHP exists, by no means was collaboration universal. Interdisciplinary collaboration and communication are likely to be areas requiring constant emphasis and attention.

Perhaps the most difficult issue to resolve before existing programs can be considered "comprehensive" involves the role of the school in providing access to services typically considered the responsibility of the private sector, such as certain preventive and primary health care services. "Providing access" does not necessarily mean that services will be delivered at the school site; rather, it implies ensuring that all students are able to obtain and make use of needed services. Depending on the community, many students may already be receiving such services and be covered through private insurance or Medicaid. However, as mentioned in earlier chapters, increasing numbers of students are uninsured or lack coverage for even the most basic preventive services. Each community must devise appropriate strategies to ensure that all of its students have access to these basic preventive and primary care services.

Even if many students in a community already have access to private care, certain preventive and primary care services might be more efficiently and effectively delivered at the school site, either by school personnel (school nurses, nurse practitioners, psychologists, counselors, or social workers) or community providers, rather than at scattered locations throughout the community. Studies have found that school-based health centers increase access to health care and provide some services more easily and appropriately than other kinds of providers, particularly for adolescents (U.S. Department of Health and Human Services, 1993; U.S. General Accounting Office, 1994b). As discussed in Chapter 4, some of the American Medical Association's Guidelines for Adolescent Preventive Services (GAPS) recommendations might be efficiently and appropriately carried out in schools by school personnel.

Lack of stable and adequate funding appears to be a major obstacle to the development of school-based services, as noted in Chapter 4. Although barriers to cooperation between school health providers and private sector providers are large (Davis et al., 1995; U.S. Department of Health and Human Services, 1993; U.S. General Accounting Office, 1994a, 1994b), some progress is beginning to occur. Examples include the Health Start program in St. Paul, Minnesota (Zimmerman and Reif, 1995), and the program conducted by the Baltimore City Health Department, both of which have negotiated with managed care plans to support the delivery of school-based services. As described in Chapter 4, the Florida legislature has added provisions to the insurance code allowing school districts to become large grouping mechanisms for the purchase of health coverage for students and their families. The state has established a quasi-public, nonprofit corporation (Healthy Kids Corporation) that subsidizes the payment of premiums where necessary and acts as an intermediary between school districts and the insurance community. The Florida program has been effective in negotiating managed care coverage for tens of thousands of children in rural and urban areas. Although such examples of progress exist, school or private sector collaboration and third-party reimbursement for school-based services are still critical issues requiring further study and analysis.

The committee believes that although dedication and cooperation will be required, the goal of a comprehensive school health program is attainable, and the situation is not so complicated that, even today, local communities could not begin working toward this vision. The process itself—mobilizing the various stakeholders in a community to give greater attention to the needs of its children and families—may have significant benefits that extend beyond the school health program.

AN INVESTMENT IN THE FUTURE

Recently, a group of more than 100 distinguished professionals, representing a wide range of child health and related perspectives, came together over a four-year period to develop scientifically based child health supervision guidelines to meet the health promotion and disease prevention needs of children and families into the twenty-first century. The resulting document, *Bright Futures: Guidelines for Health Supervision of Infants, Children, and Adolescents* (Green, 1994), has been widely accepted and endorsed by a broad range of individuals and national organizations concerned with the health and welfare of children and youth.

Bright Futures emphasizes that the "linear model of prevention"— which worked well in the past, as in the case of developing and distributing vaccines that provide immunity—is no longer adequate. Health, educational, and social issues are strongly interrelated and cannot be addressed in isolation from each other. Child health supervision in the future will require a partnership between health professionals and families, attention to the social and cultural context in which children live, and the support of a range of community institutions.

As a basis for preparing the *Bright Futures* guidelines, the study participants adopted the following Children's Health Charter shown in Box 7-1.

The committee believes that this document represents a consensus view of what we owe to our children and young people; the committee also suggests that a comprehensive school health program can make a critical contribution to achieving each of the charter's goals. A CSHP can help all students reach their full potential, assist them in becoming eco-

BOX 7-1
Bright Futures Children's Health Charter

Throughout this century, principles developed by advocates for children have been the foundation for initiatives to improve children's lives. Bright Futures participants have adopted these principles in order to guide their work and meet the unique needs of children and families into the 21st century.

- Every child deserves to be born well, to be physically fit, and to achieve self-responsibility for good health habits.
- Every child and adolescent deserves ready access to coordinated and comprehensive preventive, health-promoting, therapeutic, and rehabilitative medical, mental health, and dental care. Such care is best provided through a continuing relationship with a primary health professional or team, and ready access to secondary and tertiary levels of care.
- Every child and adolescent deserves a nurturing family and supportive relationships with other significant persons who provide security, positive role models, warmth, love, and unconditional acceptance. A child's health begins with the health of his parents.
- Every child and adolescent deserves to grow and develop in a physically and psychologically safe home and school environment free of undue risk of injury, abuse, violence, or exposure to environmental toxins.
- Every child and adolescent deserves satisfactory housing, good nutrition, a quality education, and adequate family income, a supportive social network, and access to community resources.
- Every child deserves quality child care when her parents are working outside the home.
- Every child and adolescent deserves the opportunity to develop ways to cope with stressful life experiences.
- Every child and adolescent deserves the opportunity to be prepared for parenthood.
- Every child and adolescent deserves the opportunity to develop positive values and become a responsible citizen in his community.
- Every child and adolescent deserves to experience joy, have high self-esteem, have friends, acquire a sense of efficacy, and believe that she can succeed in life. She should help the next generation develop the motivation and habits necessary for similar achievement.

SOURCE: Green, 1994.

nomically productive citizens, allow them take personal charge of their own health, and enable them to become informed participants in the health system in the future. A CSHP also represents an investment in the future because, as today's children mature and have their own children, future generations will be affected.

CONCLUDING REMARKS

The committee's one overwhelming finding is that most people think school health programs are an important and a good thing. School health is the focus of many governmental and nongovernmental initiatives and the subject of numerous reports and policy statements, some of which have proposed ambitious recommendations and standards. Yet the committee has found a wide gap between rhetoric and action, between theory and practice. For programs to reach their potential and promise, concerted action and departure from "business as usual" will be needed to coordinate scattered activities, improve the quality and consistency of implementation, engage the participation of crucial stakeholders, and provide adequate and stable funding.

Perhaps the term "comprehensive school health program" does not do justice to these programs, and a different name might better convey their true nature and importance to the general public. Comprehensive school health programs may not be "comprehensive" in and of themselves, but they serve as a critical link to ensure that the broader community health and social services system is comprehensive. The word "school" belies the fact that programs are not the sole responsibility of the school, and the school alone can do very little without the support of families and the community. The term "health" is often regarded in its narrowest sense as the absence of disease, whereas its meaning here involves complete physical, emotional, and social well-being and fulfillment of one's maximum potential. Some observers have suggested that the term "coordinated school health program" might give a better sense of the interdisciplinary and interagency collaboration required. Although the term comprehensive school health program seems firmly entrenched in the vocabulary of those close to these programs, the question remains of whether a different name would give a better sense of the true nature of these programs and more readily capture the attention from the general public that these programs deserve.

Whatever the name given to these programs, this report has underscored their importance for all students, affluent or poor, high achievers or those at risk of dropping out. The committee is not calling for schools to do more on their own; instead, it is asking communities to recognize and take advantage of the key role that schools can play in promoting and protecting the health and well-being of our nation's children and youth. An investment in the health and education of today's children and young people is the ultimate investment for the future.

LIVERPOOL JOHN MOORES UNIVERSITY
LEARNING SERVICES

REFERENCES

Collins, J.L., Small, M.L., Kann, L., Pateman, B.C., Gold, R.S., and Kolbe, L.J. 1995. School health education. *Journal of School Health* 65(8):302–311.

Davis, M., Fryer, G.E., White, S., and Igoe, J.B. 1995. *A Closer Look: A Report of Select Findings from the National School Health Survey 1993–1994.* Denver: Office of School Health, University of Colorado Health Sciences Center.

Green, M., ed. 1994. *Bright Futures: Guidelines for Health Supervision of Infants, Children, and Adolescents.* Arlington, Va.: National Center for Education in Maternal and Child Health.

Pate, R.R., Small, M.L., Ross., J.G., Young, J.C., Flint, K.H., and Warren, C.W. 1995. School physical education. *Journal of School Health* 65(8): 312–318.

Pateman, B.C., McKinney, P., Kann, L., Small, M.L., Warren, C.W., and Collins, J.L. 1995. School food service. *Journal of School Health* 65(8):327–332.

Ross, J.G., Einhaus, K.E., Hohenemser, L.K., Greene, B.Z., Kann, L., and Gold R.S. 1995. School health policies prohibiting tobacco use, alcohol and other drug use, and violence. *Journal of School Health* 65(8):333–338.

Small, M.L., Majer, L.S., Allensworth, D.D., Farquhar, B.K., Kann, L., and Pateman, B.C. 1995. School health services. *Journal of School Health* 65(8):319–326.

U.S. Department of Health and Human Services. 1993. *School-Based Health Centers and Managed Care.* Washington, D.C.: U.S. Department of Health and Human Services, Office of the Inspector General.

U.S. General Accounting Office. 1994a. *School-Based Health Centers Can Promote Access to Care.* Pub. No. GAO/HEHS-94-166. Washington, D.C.: U.S. General Accounting Office, May.

U.S. General Accounting Office. 1994b. *School-Based Health Centers Can Expand Access for Children.* Pub. No. GAO/HEHS-95-35. Washington, D.C.: U.S. General Accounting Office, December.

Zimmerman, D.J., and Reif, C.J. 1995. School-based health centers and managed care health plans: Partners in primary care. *Journal of Public Health Management Practice* 1(1):33–39.

Appendixes

A
The School–Community Interface in Comprehensive School Health Education

Mary Ann Pentz, Ph.D.

The major causes of mortality among youth who attend primary and secondary schools continue to include accidents, homicide, and suicide; major morbidities include drug abuse, violence, nonfatal accidents and lack of safety precautions (e.g., failure to use safety belts or helmets), sexually transmitted diseases and unintended pregnancy, and mental health problems (depression, anxiety, somatic complaints) (1–3). However, for the first time in the history of the United States, morbidity rates for youth—particularly adolescents—have increased and general health has decreased in the past decade (4–6). This alarming trend would appear to fly in the face of the 1977 U.S. Surgeon General's mandate and subsequent national attempts to improve the health of youth, first by the year 1990 and then by 2000 (see 2, 7). The apparent downward trend in health suggests that current efforts to promote health and prevent disease in our youth are failing. While health care reform advocates consider such options as universal health care to offset this trend (8), another option that is complementary to universal health care and that seeks to target youth directly is comprehensive school health education (9, 10). Developing health education efforts that are centered around and reach out from the school is a logical goal for national health, given that upwards of one-third of the 1990 health objectives can be potentially attained through the school (7, 11). These include objectives related to prevention of drug abuse (tobacco, alcohol, other drugs), heart disease (exercise, nutrition), sexually transmitted diseases and unwanted pregnancy, mental distress

(stress), accidents (violence, safety), and infectious diseases in general (immunization) (7).

Several educators and researchers have proposed that for comprehensive school health education programs to be most effective in improving youth health, the programs' comprehensive health education should be integrated with various community efforts. The remainder of this paper selectively reviews the research literature to consider whether current school health education is likely to be more efficacious with the inclusion of community efforts.

CRITERIA FOR LITERATURE REVIEW

The search databases included Medline, Psych Abstracts, and ERIC. Key words were crossed, including community, health promotion, school and health education, and adolescents. Additional sets of key words were crossed to yield information about specific sub areas of prevention. For example, since most prevention programs evaluated have been in the areas of smoking, alcohol, and drug abuse prevention, these were included as key terms. Other key terms included student assistance programs (SAPs), school health centers, and school clinics. With some exceptions, the initial criteria for selection were publication in a nationally disseminated peer-reviewed professional journal, studies or reviews since 1990, U.S. populations, a primary focus on late childhood or adolescence, and report of behavioral outcomes. The exceptions included papers representing models of health education rather than studies (see below), non-peer reviews where peer-reviewed publications were relatively lacking, and a few studies published before 1990 if they were particularly illustrative of a type of program or approach or other studies were lacking. The initial search resulted in 73 community health education citations, plus 37 keyed specifically for drug abuse prevention; 55 keyed for SAPs, school clinics, and health centers; and 15 non-peer review technical reports or monographs on studies from ERIC. The ERIC reports were eliminated. Elimination of redundant studies and studies in which behavioral outcomes were not clear resulted in 16 papers discussing models of health education programs that involved both schools and communities (school and community programs), 22 papers and reviews of school prevention studies, 5 of community prevention, and 25 of school and community prevention studies. The resulting review is intended to provide a selective but representative sample of studies and models, since an in-depth review of separate aspects of health education by health area (e.g., sex education) or type of service (e.g., SAPs) would be beyond the scope of this paper.

MODELS OF INTEGRATED SCHOOL AND COMMUNITY HEALTH EDUCATION

Numerous models of comprehensive school health education have been proposed, most since 1990, and many of them have been published in one or more special issues of the *Journal of School Health*. As part of the literature review for this paper (see criteria below), 16 models with varying degrees of specificity were identified (1, 7, 8, 12–24). Two of the models were general (12, 13). One conceptualizes comprehensive school health education as an educational package within larger population-based health promotion efforts that include community education, worksite wellness programs, and legislative efforts (12). The other conceptualizes health education as part of a "Healthy Children Ready to Learn" initiative that is targeted to the family, rather than the school, and integrates health education with referrals to social services (13). All of the models directly include or assume the following criteria for achievement of comprehensive school health education:

- interaction of personal (educational skills), social or situational (provision of support services, communication, referral), and environmental levels (changing or monitoring school environment, surrounding physical environment) of health promotional activity (see 17, 24);
- integration of school and community efforts;
- extensive, regular school health education programs from kindergarten through grade 12; and
- coordination of school and other health efforts through a coordinating council or team.

However, the models differ on or do not specify several points:

- What constitutes "community efforts" is not well defined, with various models interpreting community as the presence of coalitions or local and state partnerships (e.g., 8), clusters of partnerships such as agencies and universities (e.g., 20, 21), community health councils involving the school and/or teams directly developed within or through the school (e.g., 23), and/or extra-school educational programming (e.g., 24).
- Assumption of the need for integrated school and community efforts is based on practical considerations rather than on theory or empirical evidence.
- With one exception (23), no models articulated specific mechanisms or functions that community efforts could provide in comprehensive health education; none related mechanisms to theoretical principles of health behavior change.

• Although most of the models directly addressed or alluded to school health services as part of comprehensive school health education (e.g., in the form of school health clinics or student assistance programs), none attempted to represent the continuum of school services from primary prevention through early intervention.

• What constitutes community programs is not well defined. Some models assume that community programming is restricted to community health education in the form of courses or materials, whereas others include mass media, parental involvement, community organization, or policy efforts. In addition, some models address the need for health education that is culturally sensitive and that integrates school and community efforts through systems intervention, but neither of these concepts is well defined (e.g., 15).

The remainder of this paper focuses on the first four points. It attempts to differentiate practical from theoretical arguments for integrated school and community programming and articulate specific mechanisms for behavior change according to theory; to delineate several levels of prevention activity in schools and use of mechanisms by each level; and to provide a selective overview of studies that represent school, school and community, or community interventions for health behavior.

RATIONALE FOR INTEGRATING SCHOOL AND COMMUNITY EFFORTS

Practical Considerations

In today's society, it has become too often the case that neither the family nor the community assumes responsibility for caring for youth. Alternatively, schools "house" and care for youth six to seven hours a day, potentially serving as a mini-community for youth. However, common wisdom states that these hours are not sufficient to deliver health education messages that will result in long-term behavior change, and that school programming augmented by complementary community programs and messages is necessary to "boost" the effects of school program to the point of changing youth health behavior. In addition, there is some evidence to suggest that although adults (including parents, community leaders, and representatives of the mass media) do not respond well to direct efforts to change their own health behavior, they do respond somewhat positively to efforts channeled through the school, typically in the form of appeals made by youth as part of a school education activity (25, 26). The integration of school and community efforts can potentially reduce costs and competition related to overlap of services. Community support of school health education can improve teacher and administrator empowerment to deliver health education, particularly in such sensitive areas of health as AIDS (acquired immunodeficiency syndrome) prevention (27–29). Community support in the form of financial, technical (material), or personnel resources can maintain or increase the quality of school health education during periods of shrinking school budgets.

Several of these practical considerations offset barriers in current school-based health education that decrease the possibility of achieving long-term health behavior change in youth. The barriers include insufficient dose and implementation, inappropriate expectations for health, curriculum limitations, attrition of high-risk students, and inappropriate or conflicting health messages (30–32). The problem of insufficient dose of education could be offset by the booster effect of additional community programs and complementary health messages in the media. Insufficient implementation could be offset by teacher empowerment gained from community support and recognition for teaching. Inappropriate expectations for behavior change could be corrected by comparisons with community treatment costs for unhealthy behavior. Curriculum limitations could be expanded by community education, trainers, and health behavior practice opportunities. Attrition could be offset by alternative community education activities and programs that reach high-risk youth in other settings. Inappropriate messages could be offset by coordinating programs, activities, and services in the community that complement school program messages.

In addition to offsetting barriers to effectiveness, the inclusion of community efforts in school health education would likely offset barriers to the initiation of new health education programs and the institutionalization of current programs (33). Community support in the form of positive mass media coverage or financial support could increase the probability that a school health referendum would pass or that a controversial program, such as AIDS prevention, would be adopted by parents. Community support in the form of local policy change, such as increased taxes, could provide long-term funding for smoking prevention.

Theoretical Considerations

One of the models reviewed proposes that schools and communities can integrate their health education efforts as a series of one-way, two-way, and multiple exchanges (23). For example, voluntary community health agencies can distribute health information materials that complement the messages delivered in school (a one-way exchange). Several potential avenues or functions in which school/community exchanges can occur are elaborated, including sharing and extending information, health services, training, and advocacy or policy change. Although both the functions and the exchanges are feasible given that they currently exist and are funded with varying degrees of integration, none of these is related to theories of health behavior change. Consideration of theory is necessary if one intends to design an integrated school/community program that has treatment construct validity and thus is likely to be testable for efficacy and replicable in multiple communities.

Several theories figure prominently in school and school/community programs that have shown significant effects on youth health behavior. These include, but are not limited to, the following. Social learning theory explains how models, practice opportunities, and reinforcement affect behavior; this theory translates to the development and testing of school educational programs that focus on teaching skills and the use of community leaders as models for behavior (34). Reasoned action and expectancy value theories explain how actual and perceived social norms affect behavior; these theories translate to promoting mass media coverage of health behavior and advocacy and formal policy change initiatives for health behavior (35). Social support theories explain the types of support that a community can provide a school and supportive health communications that parents and other adults can provide to youth; these theories translate to parent skills and communications programs; interactive parent/child homework activities; and community coalition, council, or partnership action planning (36). Peer cluster theory explains how and why youth will gravitate toward certain peer groups that represent specific norms for health and serve as models for behavior; this theory translates to group settings for health education (37). Diffusion of innovation theories (and, to a lesser extent, persuasion theories such as spiral-of-silence theory) explain how a small critical mass of community leaders or innovators may influence youth and adults to adopt health programs; these theories translate to lobbying for education referenda and local policy change, as well as the use of mass media to complement school health education programs (38, 39).

Potential mechanisms for integrating community efforts with school health education, according to theory, are summarized in Table A-1. Potentially, each could be evaluated for its contribution to school health education, based on its relevant theoretical principle for behavior change. All of the school + community studies reviewed included distribution of materials to schools and complementary community education or activities; studies varied on the use of other mechanisms. With the exception of parent trainers or participants and mass media coverage, none of the other mechanisms was evaluated for its independent effects.

TABLE A-1 Potential Mechanisms for Interfacing Community Efforts with School Health Education, According to Theory

Mechanism	Operating Principle	Relevant Theory
Community trainer or participant	Modeling behavior	Social learning or training (34)
Parent trainer participant	Modeling, social support	Social learning or training, social support (34, 36)
External peer leader Trainer or discussant	Modeling, changing perceived social norms, peer selections	Social learning or training, reasoned action, peer cluster (34, 35, 37)
Distribution or posting of materials	Cuing	Social learning or training, diffusion (37, 38)
Community review or release of materials to schools	Message consistency	Social learning or training, reasoned action (34, 38)
Complementary community education or activities	Message consistency, changing norms, support, booster	Social learning or training, reasoned action, social support (34, 35, 36)
Lobbying for policy change	Changing norms	Reasoned action, diffusion, persuasion (35, 38, 39)
Mass media coverage	Reinforcement, changing norms	Social learning or training, reasoned action (34, 36)
Collateral referral or health services	Message consistency, booster, support	Social learning or training, social support (34, 36)
Raising external funding	Credibility, support	Social learning or training, social support (34, 36)

THE CONCEPT OF STRATEGIC PREVENTION

Comprehensive school health education can be conceptualized in terms of level of prevention services provided to youth. Four levels are shown in Table A-2. Ideally, these levels of services are reciprocal and synergistic in terms of their effectiveness; thus, inclusion of all four levels in a comprehensive school health education plan would be considered a strategic use of prevention services (40). Level 1 is primary prevention or universal health education involving whole populations of youth in school settings. Because schools are the single most available normative setting

TABLE A-2 Levels of Strategic Prevention

Level	Number of Studies/ Reviews	Primary Mechanisms	Primary Health Area
1. Primary prevention (universal education)	34	Teacher, parent or peer leader trainer, materials distribution	Smoking, drugs, nutrition
2. Self-selective prevention (special topic activities)	7	Complementary community education, mass media coverage	Drugs
3. Secondary prevention (student assistance programs)	4	Complementary community education, peer leaders	Drugs
4. Early intervention (clinics, health centers, referrals)	7	Collateral health services or referral	Reproductive health

for youth, primary prevention programs would be expected to be a major focus of school health education. Some qualitative results of process evaluations suggest that primary prevention programs promote increases in student requests or self-referrals for other levels of programming (40). Level 2 consists of special topic activities and prevention and group counseling programs oriented toward high-risk youth (e.g., children of alcoholics) and underserved youth. These programs are typically voluntary, are scheduled to complement primary prevention programs, and can provide a forum for more detailed discussion and assistance with such health problems as drug abuse (41). Level 3 involves student assistance programs or related core team efforts in schools. This level is aimed at youth who are already experiencing academic difficulties and who probably are experiencing difficulties in health behavior, particularly drug abuse and mental distress. Health problems identified in SAPs may lead to referral to school clinics or health centers for screening or early intervention (42, 43). Level 4 represents the prevention/ treatment linkage within school services (from education to school clinic or health center) as well as outside the school (from education or school clinic to community health clinics, agencies, and hospitals). Innovative use of existing school counselors, nurses, and other personnel in school clinics in Level 4 can link back to services at other levels of prevention (44). Routine referring and mainstreaming of youth across different levels of prevention where appropriate should result in more comprehensive school education service delivery than is available through single-level service (45). Table A-2 illustrates the studies and reviews of studies that focused on each level of prevention, the primary mechanisms for interfacing school and community efforts that were employed, and the primary areas of health addressed by each level. The majority of studies and reviews of studies have been concentrated at Level 1. Mechanisms for school/community interface at this level—when they are used at all—typically include the use of school, community, or peer leader trainers for education and the distribution of materials. The fewest published studies were in Level 3, or SAPs, which used complementary community education or activities to interface with the community. Smoking and drug abuse prevention predominated as the major health areas addressed at all four levels.

THE ARGUMENT FOR SCHOOL + COMMUNITY PROGRAMS

The major question under consideration in this paper is whether school + community programming is more efficacious than school programming alone. Addressing this question requires comparison of school, community, and school + community prevention studies. The working definition of "community" was any health promotion or disease prevention intervention conducted outside of the school and representing potentially significant channels of influence and programming for youth. The community channels included parent programs; mass media programming, campaigns, and materials; community organization and training, including the use of councils, coalitions, and partnerships or the use of extra-school settings for education, such as Boys and Girls Clubs or health agencies; and policy change initiatives, including school and community (46–49). Two types of behavioral outcomes were considered: those representing participation or implementation in prevention and those representing change in health behaviors, such as smoking or nutrition. Several factors were examined, based on assumptions made in the general model and discussion papers described earlier, including evidence of collaboration or integration across community program components, levels of prevention involved, and mechanisms employed for achieving health-behavior outcomes and, where relevant, school/community interface. Results are summarized in Table A-3.

School Programs

Twenty-eight literature studies and reviews, representing more than 246 separate studies, are summarized. A standard for comparison might be the School Health Education Evaluation (SHEE) studies, which showed a 1.5 percent difference in student self-reported health practices after 40 to

TABLE A-3 Effectiveness of School, Community, and School +
Community Programs

Number of Studies	Prevention Level	Program Components or Mechanisms	
		School	Parent
SCHOOL			
5 drug prevention reviews (>175 studies; 30, 51–54)	1	Education	
1 health promotion review (25 studies; 55)	1	Education	
2 reviews of stress prevention for at-risk populations (42, 56)	2, 3	Education + counseling	
1 sex education review (23 studies), 1 study (57, 58)	1, 2	Education	
4 long-term drug prevention studies (59–62)	1	Education	
2 tobacco, HIV prevention studies (63, 64)	1	Training	

Media	Community Organization	Outcomes		
		Policy	Participation	Health Behavior
			Standardized training, increased implementation	2–15% net decreases or 20–67% net change in monthly smoking, smaller effects on monthly alcohol and marijuana use; 6-mo. to 3-yr. effects; no long-term effects (30)
			Some effects on program use rates	Modest effects on knowledge, attitudes
			NS	Varied effects on behavior
			Effectiveness related to support, implementation, participation	Variable effects on condom use, intercourse, no. of partners
			NS	With exception (61), no effects by 5-yr. follow-up; 20% average change in monthly cigarette use, drunkenness, polydrug use
			Receptivity or likely use related to teaching support	

continued on next page

TABLE A-3 Continued

Number of Studies	Prevention Level	Program Components or Mechanisms	
		School	Parent
SCHOOL continued			
2 health promotion studies (66, 67)	3, 4	SAP clinics	
1 pregnancy prevention study (68)	2, 4	Counseling, clinics	
2 heart health studies (69, 70)	1, 4	Education, screening	
1 heart health review (71)	1	Education	
4 health promotion studies (72–75), 2 reviews studies (76, 77)	1	Education, screening	
COMMUNITY			
2 drug prevention studies (83, 84)	2		
1 health services review (85)	4		

| | | | Outcomes | |
Media	Community Organization	Policy	Participation	Health Behavior
			Increase in health services delivery	Increase in communications, intentions to smoke
				Modest effects on sexual risk behaviors
			Effects on dissemination	Not yet available
				Modest effects on nutrition, smoking
			Effects on implementation, organizational change	Modest effects on drug use (77), 40% or greatest reduction in cholesterol levels (72–74, 76), moderate and increase in physical activity (73, 74)
	Community leader and peer training, education, complementary club activities		Increased parent participation in activities	Decrease in cigarette, alcohol, marijuana use
	Collateral health services, fund-raising		Increased health services utilization, funding	NR

continued on next page

TABLE A-3 Continued

		Program Components or Mechanisms	
Number of Studies	Prevention Level	School	Parent

COMMUNITY continued

| 1 pregnancy or child health study (86) | 4 | | |
| 1 smoking prevention review (50 coalitions; 87) | 1, 2 | | |

SCHOOL + COMMUNITY

2 smoking prevention studies (92, 93)	1	Education	
1 smoking prevention study (94), 1 review (4 studies; 25)	1	Education	Homework, education
1 smoking prevention study (95)	1	Education	Homework, education
1 reproductive health review (96)	1	Education	

| | | Outcomes | | |
Media	Community Organization	Policy	Participation	Health Behavior
	Community training, education, collateral clinic services		Increased self- and daily health services utilization	NR
	Coalitions for training, distribution, release of materials, mass media coverage, lobbying for policy change, fund-raising		Effects on purchase decisions, media coverage; fund-raising and training teachers not effective	NR
Education coverage			School + parent	Smoking decreased in duration of intervention
Education			Effects on media use increased with student + parent implementation varied	Effects on smoking increased with school + parent participation
Campaigns			School program implementation questionable	No effects
	Education distribution in clinics of universities			Condom use varied by setting

continued on next page

TABLE A-3 Continued

Number of Studies	Prevention Level	Program Components or Mechanisms	
		School	Parent

SCHOOL + COMMUNITY continued

Number of Studies	Prevention Level	School	Parent
1 physical fitness study (97)	2, 4	Fitness activity	
4 drug prevention studies (98–101)	1, 3	Education, SAPs	
5 cardiovascular health studies (26, 102 and 103 counted as 1, 104–107)	1	Education	Homework
1 accident prevention study (108)	1	Helmet distribution	
1 smokeless tobacco prevention study (109)	1	Education	Education
1 drug prevention study (110)	2	SAPs, core team	
1 health promotion study (111)	1	Involvement in community development process	

Media	Community Organization	Outcomes		
		Policy	Participation	Health Behavior
	Fitness activity in community			Fitness increased, drug use decreased, in all settings
	Police as trainers, task force		High student, parent participation rates	Delayed onset in 1 study; no overall effects
Coverage, campaigns	Task force, distribution of materials, community education	Product availability	High dissemination	11% decrease in cholesterol, increase in nutrition and exercise; 8% difference in weekly smoking at 5-yr. follow-up; 2 studies with no behavior outcomes reported
Campaign				50% more used helmets after program
	Task force			No effects
	Involvement in core team		Increase in teacher drug education implementation, referrals	NR
	Community organization		Possible increased participation, support	NR

continued on next page

TABLE A-3 Continued

		Program Components or Mechanisms	
Number of Studies	Prevention Level	School	Parent
SCHOOL + COMMUNITY continued			
1 alcohol prevention study (112)	1	Peer-led education	Homework, education
1 pregnancy prevention study (113)	2	Education	
2 drug, suicide prevention studies (114, 115)	3	Education, counseling	Parent reinforcement, education
1 drug prevention study (116 and 117 counted as 1)	1	Education and lobbying	Education

NOTE: NR = not reported; NS = not specific; blank spaces = no information or not evaluated.

50 hours of teacher-taught school health education in the 1980s (50). The majority of the studies shown in Table A-3 focused on smoking and drug abuse prevention at Level 1 and used teachers or peer leader trainers as mechanisms for achieving health behavior change. Although some individual studies included participation variables as behavioral outcomes, fewer than 10 percent of studies in review articles did so. Overall, the pattern of school-based studies suggests strong short-term effects on experimental use rates of smoking, drug use, and sexual risk behaviors; few effects on regular use rates; and no effects at five-year follow-up, with one exception, which required 30 sessions of instruction (62). Effects on nutrition and exercise appeared to be smaller overall than effects on smoking or drug use. The magnitude of effects overall appears to be larger than

Media	Community Organization	Outcomes		
		Policy	Participation	Health Behavior
	Task force, education	Policy change	Not yet available	Not yet available
	Clinic education, material distribution, health services			Reduced pregnancy rates
	Peer support		High parent participation	Decreased drug use, depression reported in 1 study
Program, coverage	Task force, training	Policy change		20–40% reduction in monthly and daily tobacco, alcohol, marijuana use through 5-yr. follow-up; effects on parent alcohol, marijuana use and health community + 3-yr. follow-up

those achieved from the SHEE studies averaging 7 percent (122), perhaps attributable to the shift from didactic to interactive education (e.g., 52). None of the studies reviewed emphasized mechanisms to link or interface with the community (78). None reported using a systems or restructuring intervention as suggested in some comprehensive school health education models and none reported placing a special emphasis on cultural sensitivity (15, 79).

Community Programs

Five studies and reviews were found, including one review of 50 community coalitions. Experiences from the community-based adult heart health trials conducted in the United States have shown that a community-based program—exclusive of the school—should include training, education, screening, and policy change efforts to maximize intervention effectiveness (80). A standard of comparison might be the recent results of the COMMIT trial on adults, which resulted in 3 percent difference in the rate at which light-to-moderate smokers quit smoking prevention programs, events, and policy changes for youth. These options were not a main focus of the trial, and results of any effects on youth have not been published; thus, COMMIT is not included in the table (82). The level of prevention targeted varied across studies, as did the mechanisms used to achieve change. All studies reported participation outcomes; only two reported health behavior outcomes. Of the two studies involving educational programs and activities conducted by Boys and Girls Clubs, both showed significant short-term decreases in cigarette, alcohol, and marijuana use comparable to short-term decreases reported for school-based programs; effects of the other studies on health behavior were either smoking but no other effects (81). Although the communities participating in COMMIT had the option to includenot reported or not clear. All studies but one reported beneficial changes in health care utilization. The study of coalitions showed that community training of teachers was ineffective. The effectiveness of fund-raising varied.

School + Community Programs

State-of-the-art school health education should include one or more of the mechanisms shown in Table A-1 to promote cross-referrals, cross-communication, and resource sharing with community agencies for general health, as well as specific prevention services (compare 88). The mechanisms should also include community leaders and parents as participant or discussants in the health education process, particularly for such sensitive health areas as AIDS education (89). Using these mechanisms to integrate school programs with parents, mass media, community organizations, and health policy change efforts may be increasingly necessary to offset the new "social morbidity" posed by youth, families, and schools that are failing in health achievement (90).

A total of 25 studies, including two reviews, was found, representing more than 30 studies. Based on youth-related experiences of the heart health trials, multicomponent community-based programs should include substantial school programming to initiate behavior change, in conjunction with a community organization structure and process that promotes mass media programming and coverage, parent and adult education, and informal or formal policy change (91). A standard for comparison might be the 3 percent decrease in adult smoking found in the COMMIT trial and the 2–15 percent short-term decreases found in school-based studies of smoking.

Overall, school programs that included one or more community program components showed short-term effects on monthly smoking and drug use similar to comprehensive school programs that included a large number of sessions and boosters; however, school + community programs appeared to have a greater range of effects and larger long-term effects on heavier use rates, averaging 8 percent net reductions (122). School + community programs were the only programs to show any effects on parent participation and parent health behavior or any effects on program or materials dissemination and health service delivery in the community. Effects of school + community programs on nutrition and exercise appear to be somewhat larger than effects of school programs; differential effects on sexual risk behaviors are not clear.

Prevention levels varied among the studies, but emphasized Level 1. Most studies used a variety of mechanisms to link the community with the school. The most common were the inclusion of parents, peers, and community leaders in a community task force or council and, to a lesser extent, as leaders or participants in education. About half of the studies reported information on participation or dissemination rates as well as health behavior outcomes.

Twelve studies included parent involvement or programming with a school program. Eight of these suggested that parent involvement increased effects on youth health behavior; two studies suggested that parent involvement increased effects on parent health behavior; all but one study showed increased parent participation in school or other program activities as a result of a parent involvement component.

Twelve studies included a mass media component. Because most of these included mass media as part of additional program components, the independent effects of media are not altogether clear. However, three studies suggest that media involvement increased parent participation and changed parent health behavior.

Nineteen of the studies included the integrating of some type of community organization or education with a school program. Since most integrated community organization with other components, the independent effects of community are not clear. Across studies, however, those with community organization appeared to have greater dissemination and parent and community participation rates, more referrals for health services, and possibly greater rates of implementation of other components.

Only seven studies included some informal or formal policy change component. Policy change mostly involved reducing youth access to substances and controlling product availability. The independent effects of this component are not clear.

Only six studies (two of them reviews) directly compared a school program component with other community program components. Three studies and a review of four other studies compared the effectiveness of school programming with parent and/or mass media involvement versus school programming alone for changing tobacco use. Overall, these studies showed greater effects on youth smoking when school programs included parent and/or mass media programs and showed small effects on parent smoking with inclusion of a parent program. Two studies showed no effects and attributed the findings to poor implementation and/or a resistant cultural norm for tobacco use. Two other studies, one on physical fitness and one a review of reproductive health, compared school programs or activities with programs or activities in alternative community settings (99, 100); the physical fitness study reported no differences among settings, whereas the other study showed variability in condom use among settings.

REMAINING QUESTIONS

What is the community? Most of the studies reviewed here involved efforts by small- to moderate-size communities to integrate efforts with school programs. Involvement of large cities showed a greater range of health services and resources, but also more competition. Communities that consisted of large, sparsely populated rural areas relied on the local school as a community for program dissemination and training. Thus, meaning of and affiliation with community may vary at least by size.

Should the school reach out to the community or should the community "reach in" to the school? Results of studies suggest that school outreach may be both a more feasible and a more acceptable strategy for linking the community with the school for health education. Several studies suggested that attempts by a community organization to reach in to the school to provide training failed.

Can the effects of community be disentangled from those of the school? Because the largest community effects appear with a synergistic relationship to the school, the question should be reconceptualized as, Is school + community better than school or community alone? The present review suggests that, overall, the answer is yes.

Are school + community programs replicable, and can technology be transferred from schools across communities? Given the consistency of positive findings of school + community programs on participation, dissemination, and youth and parent health behavior variables, the general answer would appear to be yes. However, communities show great variability in the structure and action plans of the coalition, council, core team, or task force component used to integrate health education with the school. This type of component may not be replicable in a standardized fashion, and communities report the need for flexibility to develop such a component to reflect their own individual needs.

Is school + community research feasible? Several methodological papers have addressed this question indirectly (e.g., 118–121). The demographics and past health behavior involvement of communities is difficult to match, suggesting that a large number of communities would be necessary for randomizing to experimental conditions, with the community as unit. Such a study would be expensive. Most of the studies reviewed school plus multiple community components versus a control or delayed intervention group. The ability to evaluate the effects of separate components in a school + community intervention would require the use of a factorial design, in which the effect size associated with each component intervention or sets of components compared to each single-component intervention would be assumed to be significantly different. Only a few studies have included enough schools to be able to detect differences between interventions or components of interventions (e.g., 93, 94).

Are school + community programs cost-effective? A recent analysis of prototype integrated school health education programs included projected costs and reported outcomes from seven comprehensive school-based programs and two school + community-based programs (122). Results indicated that annual costs per student for program delivery ranged from $10 to $35, depending on whether the primary focus of the program was on sexual behavior, substance use, or smoking. Effects, measured as percentage net reduction between program and control groups, ranged from 6 to 9 percent. The benefit-to-cost ratio ranged from 5 for sexual behavior to 19 for smoking, for an average of 14. Sensitivity analyses suggested that benefit–cost ratios for comprehensive school health education programs were lower for smoking, higher for drug abuse, and higher for sexual behavior. This suggests that, compared to single health focus, overall a comprehensive multicomponent, multihealth focus school health education program is apt to be more beneficial. A recent analysis of a school + community program for drug abuse prevention supports this finding (123).

Who would coordinate integrated school and community health education programs, and who would fund these programs? To address the first part of the question: the programs examined in the studies and reviews varied in terms of who was responsible for coordinating programming; those responsible needed research staff, health educators, school personnel, and paid and volunteer community leaders. However, none of the studies systematically compared the effectiveness of types of coordinators. In an integrated program, it is more likely that coordination will be the task of a group rather than an individual. A major question, then, is whether school health advisory councils that draw from community leaders but are organized by the school or school district generate more credibility and cooperation than do coalitions that draw from community leaders and are organized by the community (see 18). The studies show that school + community programs are effective, but the studies made no comparisons with community-only programs. The second part of the question is related to the first. If coalitions are used to coordinate school health education, then community agencies and federal and state funds that are allocated to community agencies for health services might be used to augment existing school health education budgets. However, if school-based health advisory councils are used, then accessing community health care funds may be difficult and resented. A long-term alternative would be qualifying school health clinics as managed health care service delivery organizations, which would be reimbursable by insurance and federal funds. In this case, managed care funds could be combined with existing school health education funds to create a unified funding package for school health education. As long as health care reimbursements were forthcoming, this alternative should be more stable than relying on the graces of volunteered community agency funds.

Can integrated school + community programs affect educational outcomes as well as health outcomes? Comprehensive school programs that included more than seven sessions, booster sessions, standardized training, and monitoring of implementation had substantial effects on knowledge change, as did school + community programs. To the extent that knowledge is measured as an educational outcome in health education classes, comprehensive school programs and integrated school + community programs could be considered effective in improving educational achievement. However, no studies reported significant effects of a health program on grade point average, absenteeism, or drop out rates, which are considered overarching indices of educational achievement.

CONCLUSIONS AND FUTURE DIRECTIONS

Review of multiple studies suggests that in a school + community interface, "community" can include the use of mass media, parent programs, community education and organization, and local policy change. Results suggest that community + school health education may yield higher participation, implementation, and dissemination rates of health education; greater effects on the more serious levels of health risk (e.g., on daily smoking compared to monthly smoking), greater effects on parents as well as youth, and perhaps longer effects than are currently obtainable from most school programs alone. Overall, the magnitude of effects on such health behaviors as smoking, substance use, and sexual behavior appears slightly greater for school + community versus school programs alone (6 versus 8 percent net reductions). Benefit-to-cost ratios appear overall higher for comprehensive school health education programs than for single-component (e.g., smoking) programs.

Several caveats apply to these summary conclusions. First, the school + community studies reviewed here were based on a model of intensive community involvement that probably exceeds the realistic capacity, resources, and time of most schools and school systems. The integrated school + community health education program mentioned in general models at the beginning of this paper (e.g., 18) represents much less intensive community involvement than the studies reviewed here, for example, following the Child and Adolescent Trial for Cardiovascular Health (CATCH) model of fliers to parents, invitational health nights held at school, and changes in cafeteria menu choices versus the organized community council activities of the Minnesota Heart Health Project (cf. 70 vs. 102). Less intensive community involvement could also take the form of simple community leader advisement on health education materials or protocols to adopt in schools, facilitation of health service referrals from school to community, and/or assistance in administering or managing health care funds in school health clinics. However, none of these lesser involvement roles has been adequately evaluated in research. Third, for simplicity's sake, studies were not separated for their effects by level of prevention. For example, school health education programs at Level 1 were not separated from school health services at Level 3 or 4. Because of the use of different research designs and outcomes, stratification and comparisons on these levels are not yet feasible.

The review of studies points to several gaps in the literature that should serve as directions for future research. These include:

- more systematic evaluation of cost–benefit and cost-effectiveness of school and school + community programs that rely on true costs;
- evaluation of the efficacy of extensive school programming alone (e.g., 30 sessions or more with boosters delivered over several years) versus the same school programming with additional community components, with school district or community as the unit of assignment and analysis if possible; and
- comparison of school + community programs that vary in intensity or type of community involvement.

REFERENCES

1. Kirby, D. 1990. Comprehensive school health and the larger community: Issues and a possible scenario. *Journal of School Health* 60(4):170–177.

2. McGinnis, J.M. 1993. The year 2000 initiative: Implications for comprehensive school health. *Preventive Medicine* 22(4):493–498.

3. Blum, R. 1987. Contemporary threats to adolescent health in the United States. *Journal of the American Medical Association* 257:3390–3395.

4. United States Congress, Office of Technology Assessment. 1991. *Adolescent Health — Volume I: Summary and Policy Options*, OTA–H–468.Washington, D.C.: U.S. Government Printing Office.

5. Hechinger, FM. 1992. *Fateful Choices: Healthy Youth for the 21st Century*. New York: Carnegie Council on Adolescent Development, Carnegie Corporation.

6. National Commission on the Role of the School and the Community in Improving Adolescent Health. 1989. *Code Blue — Uniting for Healthier Youth 1989*. Washington, D.C. National Association of State Boards of Education and American Medical Association.

7. Allensworth, D.D., and Wolford, C.A. 1988. School as agents for achieving the 1990 health objectives for the nation. *Health Education Quarterly* 15(1):3–15.

8. Schauffler, H.H. 1994. Analysis of prevention benefits in comprehensive health care reform legislation in the 102nd Congress. *American Journal of Preventive Medicine* 10(1):45–51.

9. American Association of School Administrators. 1984. Comprehensive school health education. *Journal of School Health* 53(8):312.

10. Brindis, C. 1993. Health policy reform and comprehensive school health education: the need for an effective partnership. *Journal of School Health* 63(1):33–37.

11. Kolbe, L.J., and Iverson, D.C. 1983. Integrating school and community efforts to promote health: strategies, policies, and methods. *HYGIE* 2(3):40–47.

12. Wynder, E.L. 1995. Editorial: Interdisciplinary centers for tobacco-related cancer research—A health policy issue. *American Journal of Public Health* 85(1):14–16.

13. Norello, A.C., DeGraw, C., and Kleinman, D.V. 1992. Healthy-children ready to learn—An essential collaboration between health and education. *Public Health Reports* 107(1):3–15.

14. Walker, S.M. 1993. Applying community organization to developing health promotion programs in the school community. *Journal of School Health* 63(2):109–111.

15. DeGraw, C. 1994. A community-based school health system: Parameters for developing a comprehensive student health promotion program. *Journal of School Health* 64(5):192–195.

16. DeFriese, G.H., Crossland, C.L., MacPhail-Wilcox, B., and Sowers, J.G. 1990. Implementing comprehensive school health programs: prospects for change in American schools. *Journal of School Health* 60(4):182–187.

17. Perry, C.L., and Kelder, S.H. 1992. Models for effective prevention. *Journal of Adolescent Health* 13(5):355–363.

18. Allensworth, D.D., and Kolbe, L. J. 1987. The comprehensive school health program: Exploring an expanded concept. *Journal of School Health* 57(10):409–411.

19. Brink, S.G., Simons-Morton, D.G., Harvey, C.M., Parcel, G.S., and Tiernan, K.M. 1988. Developing comprehensive smoking control programs in schools. *Journal of School Health* 58(5):177–80.

20. Fox, C.K., S.E. Forbing, and Anderson, P.S., 1988. A comprehensive approach to drug-free schools and communities. *Journal of School Health* 58(9):365–369.

21. Mason, J.O. 1989. Forging working partnerships for school health education. *Journal of School Health* 59(1):18–21.

22. Becker, S.L., Burke, J.A., Arbogast, R.A., Naughton, M.J., Bachman, I., and Spohn, E. 1989. Community programs to enhance in-school anti-tobacco efforts. *Preventive Medicine* 18(2)221–228.

23. Killip, D.C., Lovick, S. R., Goldman, L., and Allensworth, D.D. 1987. Integrated school and community programs. *Journal of School Health* 57(10):437–444.

24. Pentz, M.A. 1986. Community organization and school liaisons: How to get programs started. *Journal of School Health* 56(9):382–388.

25. Flay, B.R., Pentz, M.A., Johnson, C.A., Sussman, S., Mestell, J., Scheier, L., Collins, L.M., and Hansen, W.B. 1985. Reaching children with mass media health promotion programs: The relative effectiveness of an advertising campaign, a community-based program, and a school-based program. In *Health Education and the Media* 2, ed. D.S. Lethare. Oxford: Pergamon Press, Ltd.

26. Kelder, S.H., Perry, C.L., and Klepp, K.I. 1993. Community-wide youth exercise promotion: Long-term outcomes of the Minnesota Heart Health Program and the Class of 1989 study. *Journal of School Health* 63(5):218–223.

27. Slovacek, S.P., et al. 1993. Project Support Evaluation, Los Angeles Unified School District. Report No. 1.

28. Smith, D.W., McCormick, L.K., Steckler, A.B., and McLeroy, K.R. 1993. Teachers' use of heath curricula: Implementation of growing healthy, Project SMART, and the teenage health teaching modules. *Journal of School Health* 63(8):349–354.

29. Swisher, J.D., and Ashby, J.S. 1993. Review of process and outcome evaluations of team training. *Journal of Alcohol and Drug Education* 39(1):66–77.

30. Resnicow, K., and Botvin, G. 1993. School-based substance use prevention programs: why do effects decay? *Preventive Medicine* 22:484–490.

31. Resnicow, K., Cherry, J., and Cross, D. 1993. Ten unanswered questions regarding comprehensive school health promotion. *Journal of School Health* 63(4):171–175.

32. Bartlett, E.E. 1981. The contribution of school health education to community health promotion: What can we reasonably expect? *American Journal of Public Health* 71(12):1384–1391.

33. Oetting, E.R., and Beauvais, F., 1991. Critical incidents: Failure in prevention. *International Journal of the Addictions* 26(7):797–820.

34. Bandura, A. 1977. *Social Learning Theory*. Englewood Cliffs, N.J.: Prentice-Hall.

35. Fishbein, M., and Ajzen, I. 1975. *Belief, Attitude, Intention, and Behavior: An Introduction to Theory and Research*. Reading, Mass.: Addison-Wesley.

36. Barrera, M., Jr. 1986. Distinctions between social support concepts, social support inventory: Measure and models. *American Journal of Community Psychology* 14(4):413–445.

37. Oetting, E.R., and Beauvais, F. 1986. Peer cluster theory: Drugs and the adolescent. *Journal of Counseling and Development* 65:17–22.

38. Rogers, E.M. 1987. The diffusion of innovations perspective. In *Taking Care: Understanding and Encouraging Self-Protective Behavior*, ed. N.D. Weinstein, pp. 79–94. New York: Cambridge University Press.

39. Noell-Neumann, E. 1974. The spiral of silence: A theory of public opinion. *Journal of Communities* 24:43–51.

40. Pentz, M.A. 1993. Comparative effects of community-based drug abuse prevention. Pp. 69–87. in *Addictive Behaviors Across the Lifespan; Prevention, Treatment, and Policy Issues*, eds. J. S. Baer, G. A. Marlatt, and R.J. McMahon, California: Sage.

41. Dryfoos, J.G., and Dryfoos, G. 1993. Preventing substance use: Rethinking strategies. *American Journal of Public Health* 83(6):793–795.

42. Dryfoos, J.G. 1991. Adolescents at risk: A summation of work in the field: Programs and policies. Special issue: Adolescents at risk. *Journal of Adolescent Health* 12(8):630–637.

43. Council on Scientific Affairs, 1990. Providing medical services through school-based health programs. *Journal of School Health* 60(3):87–91.

44. Jackson, S.A. 1994. Comprehensive school health education programs: Innovative practices and issues in standard setting. *Journal of School Health* 64(5):177–179.

45. Nader, P.R. 1990. The concept of "comprehensiveness" in the design and implementation of school health programs. *Journal of School Health* 60(4):133–138.

46. Kolbe, L.J. 1993. An essential strategy to improve the health and education of Americans. *Preventive Medicine* 22(4):544–560.

47. Perry, C.L., and Kelder, S.H. 1992. Models for effective prevention. *Journal of Adolescent Health* 13(5): 355–363.

48. Shamai, S., and Coombs, R.B. 1992. The relative autonomy of schools and educational interventions for substance abuse prevention, sex education, and gender stereotyping. *Adolescence* 27(108):757–770.

49. U.S. Centers for Disease Control. 1994. Guidelines for school health programs to prevent tobacco use and addiction. *Journal of School Health* 64(9):353–360.

50. Connell, D.B., Turner, R.R., and Mason, E.F. 1985. Summary of findings of the school health education evaluation: Health promotion effectiveness, implementation, and costs. *Journal of School Health* 55(8):316–321.

51. Tobler, N.S. 1986. Meta-analyses of 143 adolescent drug prevention programs: Quantitative outcome results of program participants compared to a control or comparison group. *Journal on Drug Issues* 17:537–567.

52. Hansen, W.B., Johnson, C.A., Flay, B.R., Graham, J.W., and Sobel, J. 1988. Affective and social influences to the prevention of multiple substance abuse among seventh grade students: Results from Project SMART. *Preventive Medicine* 17:135–154.

53. Perry, C.L. 1987. Results of prevention programs with adolescents. *Drug Alcohol Dependency* 20(1):13–19.

54. Hansen, W.B. 1992. School-based substance abuse prevention: A review in curriculum, 1980–90. *Health Education Research* 7(3):403–430.

55. Lavin, A.T., Shapiro, G.R., and Weill, K.S. 1992. Creating an agenda for school-based health promotion: A review of 25 selected reports. *Journal of School Health* 62(6):212–228.

56. Gensheimer, L.K., Ayers, T.S., and Roosa, M.W. 1993. School-based preventive interventions for at-risk populations. *Evaluations and Program Planning* 16:159–167.

57. Kirby, D., Short, L., Collins, J., Rugg, D., Kolbe, L., Howard, M., et al. 1994. School-based programs to reduce sexual risk behaviors. *Public Health Reports* 109(3):339–360.

58. Walter, H.J., and Vaughan, R.D. 1993. AIDS risk reduction among a multiethnic sample of urban high school students. *Journal of the American Medical Association* 270(6):725–730.

59. Ellickson, P.L., Bell, R.M., and McGuigan, K. 1993. Preventing adolescent drug use: Long-term results of a junior high program. *American Journal of Public Health* 83(6):856–861.

60. Flay, B.R., Koepke, D., Thompson, S.J., Santi, S., Best, J.A., and Brown, K.A. 1989. Six-year follow-up of the first Waterloo School smoking prevention trial. *American Journal of Public Health* 79(10):1371–1376.

61. Murray D.M, Perry, C.L, Griffin G., et al. 1992. Results from a state-wide approach to adolescent tobacco use prevention. *Preventive Medicine* 1992(21):449–472.

62. Botvin, G. J., Baker, E., Dusenberry, L., Botvin, E.M., and Diaz, T. 1995. Long-term results of a randomized drug-abuse prevention trial in a white middle-class population. *Journal of the American Medical Association* 273(14):1106–1112.

63. Gingiss, P.L., and Basen-Engquist, K. 1994. HIV education practices and training needs of middle school and high school teachers. *Journal of School Health* 64(7):290–295.

64. Gingiss, P.L., Gottlieb, N.H., and Brink, S.G. 1994. Increasing teacher receptivity toward use of tobacco prevention education programs. *Journal of Drug Education* 24(2):163–176.

65. McGovern, J.P., and DuPont, R.L. 1991. Student assistance programs: An important approach to drug abuse prevention. *Journal of School Health* 61(6):260–264.

66. Swisher, J.D., Baker, S.B., Barnes, D. Gebler, M.K., Hadleman, D.E., and Kophazi, K.M. 1993. An evaluation of student assistance programs in Pennsylvania. *Journal of Drug and Alcohol Education* 39(1):1–18.

67. Dryfoos, J.G. 1994. Medical clinics in junior high school: Changing the model to meet demands. *Journal of Adolescent Health* 15:549–557.

68. Jones, M.E., and Mondy, L.W. 1994. Lessons for prevention and intervention in adolescent pregnancy: A five-year comparison of outcomes of two programs for school-aged pregnant adolescents. *Journal of Pediatric Health Care* 8(4):152–159.

69. Olson, C.M., Devine, C.M., and Frongillo, E.A., Jr. 1993. Dissemination and use of a school-based nutrition education program for secondary school students. *Journal of School Health* 63(8):343–348.

70. Perry, C.L., Parcel, G.S., Stone, E., Nader, P., McKinlay, S.M., Luepker, R.V., and Webber, L.S. 1992. The Child and Adolescent Trial for Cardiovascular Health (CATCH): Overview of the intervention program and evaluation methods. *Journal of Cardiovascular Risk Factors* 2(1):36–44.

71. Stone, E.J., Perry, C.L., and Luepker, R.V. 1989. Synthesis of cardiovascular behavioral research for youth health promotion. *Health Education Quarterly* 16(2):155–169.

72. Simons-Morton, B.G., Parcel, G.S., and O'Hara, N.M. 1988. Implementing organizational changes to promote healthful diet and physical activity at school. *Health Education Quarterly* 15(1):115–130.

73. Parcel, G.S., Simons–Morton, B.G., O'Hara, N.M., Baranowski, T., and Wilson, B.S. 1989. School promotion of diet and physical activity: Impact on learning outcomes and self-reported behavior. *Health Education Quarterly* 16(2):181–199.

74. Simons-Morton, B.G., Parcel, G.S., Baranowski, T., Forthofer, R., and O'Hara, N.M. 1991. Promoting physical activity and healthful diet among children: Results of a school-based intervention study. *American Journal of Public Health* 81(8)986-91.

75. Nader, P.R., Sallis, J.F., Patterson, T.L., Abramsen, I.S., Rupp, J.W., Senn, K.L., Atkins, C.J., Roppe, B.E., Morris, J.A., and Wallace, J.P. 1989. A family approach to cardiovascular risk reduction: results from the San Diego Family Health Project (Reaching Families Through the Schools). *Health Education Quarterly* 16(2):229–244.

76. Resnicow, K., Cross, D., and Wynder, E. 1991. The role of comprehensive school-based interventions: The results of four "Know Your Body" studies. *Annals of the New York Academy of Sciences* 623:285–298.

77. Errecart, M.T., Walberg, H,J., Ross, J.G., Gold, R.S., Fiedler, J.L., and Kolbe, L.J. 1991. Effectiveness of teenage health teaching models. *Journal of School Health* 61(1):26–30.

78. Bruininks, R.H., Frenzel, M., and Kelly, A. 1994. Integrating services: The case for better links to schools. *Journal of School Health* 64(6):242–248.

79. Cleary, M.J. 1991. Restructured schools: Challenges and opportunities for school health education. *Journal of School Health* 61(4):172–175.

80. Elder, J.P., Schmid, T.L., Dower, P., and Hedlund, S. 1993. Community heart health programs: Components, rationale, and strategies for effective interventions. *Journal of Public Health Policy* 14(4):463–479.

81. Community Intervention Trial for Smoking Cessation (COMMIT). 1995. II. Changes in adult cigarette smoking prevalence. *American Journal of Public Health* 85(2):193–200.

82. Community Intervention Trial for Smoking Cessation (COMMIT). 1995. I. Cohort results from a four-year community intervention. *American Journal of Public Health* 85(2):183–192.

83. Schinke, S.P., Orlandi, M.A., and Cole, K.C. 1992. Boys and girls clubs in public housing development: Prevention services for youth at risk. *Journal of Community Psychology (Special Issue)*:118–128.

84. St. Pierre, T.L., Kaltreider, D.L., Mark, N.N., and Aikin, K.J. 1992. Drug prevention in a community setting: A longitudinal study of the relative effectiveness of a three-year primary prevention program in boys and girls clubs across the nation. *American Journal of Community Psychology* 20(6):673–706.

85. Lear, J.G., Foster, H.W., Jr., and Baratz, J.A. 1989. The High Risk Young People's Program. A summing up. *Journal of Adolescent Health Care* 10(3):224–230.

86. Jones, M.E., and Mondy, L.W. 1990. Prenatal education outcomes for pregnant adolescents and their infants using trained volunteers. *Journal Adolescent Health Care* 11(5):437–444.

87. Gottlieb, N.H., Brink, S.G., and Gingiss, P.H. 1993. Correlates of coalition effectiveness: The Smoke Free Class of 2000 program. Special issue: Community coalitions for health promotion. *Health Education Research* 8(3):375–384.

88. Allensworth, D.D. 1993. Health education: State of the art. *Journal of School Health* 63(1):14–20.

89. Dhillon, H.S., O'Byrne, D.K., Kolbe, L., Baldo, M., and Jones, J.T. 1993. Mobilizing support to strengthen the role of schools in preventing HIV infection, STD and other significant health problems. *Hygiene* 12(3):20–21.

90. Nader, P.R., Ray, L., and Brink, S. 1981. The new morbidity: Use of school and community health care resources for behavioral, educational, and social–family problems. *Pediatrics* 67(1):53–60.

91. Mittlemark, M.B., Hunt, M.K., Heath, G.W., and Schmid, T.L. 1993. Realistic outcomes: Lessons from community-based research and demonstration programs for the prevention of cardiovascular diseases. *Journal of Public Health Policy* 14(4):439–462.

92. Kaufman, J.S., Jason, L.A., Sawlski, L.M., and Halpert, J.A. 1994. A comprehensive multi-media program to prevent smoking among black students. *Journal of Drug Education* 24(2):95–108.

93. Flynn, B.S., Worden, J.K., Secker-Walker, R.H., Badger, G.J., Geller, B.M. and Constanza, M.C. 1992. Prevention of cigarette smoking through mass media intervention and school programs. *American Journal of Public Health* 82(6):827–834.

94. Flay, B.R., Miller, T.Q., Hedeker, D., Siddequi, O., Britton, C.F., Brannon, B.R., Johnson, C.A., Hansen, W.B., Sussman, S., and Dent, C. 1995. The television, school and family smoking prevention and cessation project. *Preventive Medicine* 24:29–40.

95. Murray, D.M., Prokhorov, A.V., and Harty, K.C. 1994. Effects of a statewide anti-smoking campaign on mass media messages and smoking beliefs. *Preventive Medicine* 23(1):54–60.

96. Lagana, L., and Hayes, D.M. 1993. Contraceptive health programs for adolescents: A critical review. *Adolescence* 28(110):347–359.

97. Collingwood, T.R., Reynolds, R., Kohl, H.W., Smith, W., and Sloan, S. 1991. Physical fitness effects on substance abuse risk factors and use patterns. *Journal of Drug Education* 21(1):73–84.

98. Rosenbaum, D.P., Flewelling, R.L., Bailey, S.L., Ringwalt, C.L., et al. 1994. Cops in the classroom: A longitudinal evaluation of drug abuse resistance education (DARE). *Journal of Research in Crime and Delinquency* 31(1):3–31.

99. Wiener, R.L., Pritchard, C., Frauenhoffer, S.M., and Edmonds, M. 1993. Evaluation of a drug-free schools and community program: Integration of qualitative and quasi-experimental methods. *Evaluation Review* 17(5):488–503.

100. Carlson, K.A. 1994. Identifying the outcomes of prevention: results of a longitudinal study in a small city school district. *Journal of Drug Education* 24(3):193–206.

101. Carlson, C.E. 1990. HIPP: A comprehensive school-based substance abuse program with cooperative community involvement. Special issue: The Virginia experience in prevention. *Journal of Primary Prevention* 10(4):289–302.

102. Perry, C.L., Kelder, S.H., Murray, D.M., and Klepp, K.I. 1992. Communitywide smoking prevention: Long-term outcomes of the Minnesota Heart Health Program and the Class of 1989 Study. *American Journal of Public Health* 82(9):1210–1216.

103. Prokhorov, A.V., Perry, C.L., Kelder, S.H., and Klepp, K.I. 1993. Lifestyle values of adolescents: Results from Minnesota Heart Health Youth Program. *Adolescence* 28(111):637–647.

104. Carleton, R.A., Sennett, L., Gans, K.M., Levin, S., Lefebvre, C., and Lasater, T.M. 1991. The Pawtucket Heart Health Program: Influencing adolescent eating patterns. *Annals of the New York Academy of Sciences* 623:322–326.

105. Barthold, J., Pearson, J, Ellsworth, A., Mason, C., Hohensee, T., McLaud, B., and Lewis, C. 1993. A cardiovascular health education program for rural schools. *Journal of School Health* 63(7):298–301.

106. Shea, S., Basch, C.E., Lantigua, R., and Wechsler, H. 1992. The Washington Heights-Inwood Healthy Heart Program: A third–generation community-based cardiovascular disease prevention program in a disadvantaged urban setting. *Preventive Medicine* 21(2):203–217.

107. Havas, S., Heimendinger, J., Damron, D., Nicklas, T.A., Cowan, A., Beresford, S.A.A., Sorensen, G., Buller, D., and Bishop, D. 1995. 5-A-Day for better health: 9 community research projects to increase fruit and vegetable consumption. *Public Health Reports* 110(1):68–79.

108. Puczynski, M., and Marshall, D.A. 1992. Helmets: All the pros wear them. *American Journal of Diseases of Children* 146(12):1465–1467.

109. Stevens, M.M., Freeman, D.H., Mott, L.A., Youells, F.E., and Linsey, S.C. 1993. Smokeless tobacco use among children: The New Hampshire Study. *American Journal of Preventive Medicine* 9(3):160–167.

110. Kantor, G.K., Caudill, B.D., and Ungerleider, S. 1992. Project Impact: Teaching the teachers to intervene in student substance abuse problems. *Journal of Alcohol and Drug Education* 31(1):11–27.

111. Kalnins, I.V., Hart, C., Ballantyne, P., Quartaro, G., Love, R., Sturis, G., and Pollack, P. 1994. School-based community development as a health promotion strategy for children. *Health Promotion International* 9(4):269–279.

112. Perry, C.L., Williams, C.L., Forster, J.L., Wolfson, M., Wagenaar, A.C., Finnegan, J.R., Mcgovern, P.G., Veblenmortenson, S., and Komro, K.A., et al. 1993. Background, conceptualization and design of a community-wide research program on adolescent alcohol use: Project Northland. *Health Education Research* 8(1):125–136.

113. Vincent, M.L., Clearie, A.F., and Schluchter, M.D. 1987. Reducing adolescent pregnancy through school and community-based education. *Journal of the American Medical Association* 257(4):3382–3386.

114. Eggert, L.L., Seyl, C.D., and Nicholas, L.J. 1990. Effects of a school-based prevention program for potential high school dropouts and drug abusers. *International Journal of the Addictions* 25(7):773–801.

115. Peine, H.A., and Terry, T. 1990. Family co-operation program description. *Medicine and Law* 9(4):1036–1042.

116. Johnson, C.A., Pentz, M.A., Weber, M.D., Dwyer, J.H., MacKinnon, D.P., Flay, B.R., Baer, N.A., and Hansen, W.B. 1990. The relative effectiveness of comprehensive community programming for drug abuse prevention with risk and low risk adolescents. *Journal of Consulting and Clinical Psychology* 58(4):447–456.

117. Pentz, M.A. 1993. Benefits of integrating strategies in different settings. in American Medical Association State-of-the-Art Conference on Adolescent Health Promotion: Proceedings, A. Elster, S. Panzarine, and K. Holt, eds. *Research Monographs. NCEMCH* 15–34.

118. Manger, T.H., Hawkins, J.D., Haggerty, K.P., and Catalano, R.F. 1992. Mobilizing

communities to reduce risks for drug abuse: Lessons on using research to guide prevention practice. *Journal of Primary Prevention* 13(1):3–22.

119. Peterson, P.L., Hawkins, J.D., and Catalano, R.F. 1992. Evaluating comprehensive community drug risk reduction interventions: Design challenges and recommendations. *Evaluation Review* 16(6):579–602.

120. Pentz, M.A. 1994. Adaptive evaluation strategies for estimating effects of community-based drug abuse prevention programs. *Journal of Community Psychology (Monograph Series CSAP Special Issue)*:26–51.

121. Koepsell, T.D., Wagner, E.H., Cheadle, A.C., Patrick, D.L., Martin, D.C., Diehr, Ph.D., and Perrin, E.B. 1992. Selected methodological issues in evaluating community-based health promotion and disease prevention programs. *Annual Review of Public Health* 13:31–57.

122. Rothman, M.L. 1995. The potential benefits and costs of a comprehensive school health education program. Unpublished manscript.

123. Pentz, M.A. In press. Costs, benefits, and cost-effectiveness of comprehensive drug abuse prevention. NIDA Research Monograph.

APPENDIX
B
Guidelines for Comprehensive School Health Programs

Adapted from the American School Health Association
Kent, Ohio
Second Edition, November 1994

INTRODUCTION

"What is very clear, is that education and health for children are inextricably entwined. A student who is not healthy, who suffers from an undetected vision or hearing deficit, or who is hungry, or who is impaired by drugs or alcohol, is not a student who will profit optimally from the educational process. Likewise, an individual who has not been provided assistance in the shaping of healthy attitudes, beliefs and habits early in life, will be more likely to suffer the consequences of reduced productivity in later years."

—J. Michael McGinnis, Director
Disease Prevention and Health Promotion
U.S. Public Health Service

School can be one of the primary sites through which children and youth learn about the factors that influence their health. It also can be the site that provides or coordinates some or all of the needed health care services. It has been said that youth are one-third of our population and all of our future. As such, their care and nurture within the school setting is of concern to the American School Health Association (ASHA).

These guidelines address the eight separate components of the comprehensive school health program: school environment; health education; health services; physical education; counseling, guidance and mental health; school food and nutrition services; worksite health promotion; and integration of school and community health activities. Developed by the American School Health Association, the guidelines provide an operational set of practices and outcomes that may serve local school districts as the basis for developing needs assessment tools, defining staff development needs, improving program planning and evaluating the efficacy of local comprehensive school health programs. The guidelines are descriptive rather than prescriptive. They will be re-examined periodically by the ASHA Board of Directors and updated as appropriate.

—Rosemary K. Gerrans
Past President
American School Health Association

COMPREHENSIVE SCHOOL HEALTH PROGRAM

The health and well-being of children and youth must be a fundamental value of society. Urgent health and social problems have underscored the need for collaboration among families, schools, agencies, communities and governments in taking a comprehensive approach to school-based health promotion.

Health scientists have established that 50 percent of premature illness, injury and death is due to an unhealthy lifestyle. Experience and research evidence suggest that a comprehensive school health approach can improve the health-related knowledge, attitudes and behaviors of students.

It is also recognized, however, that other major determinants of health status such as genetics, the health care delivery system and socioeconomic, cultural and environmental factors require a multifaceted approach to the maintenance and improvement of health status.

A comprehensive school health approach includes a broad spectrum of activities and services which take place in schools and their surrounding communities that enable children and youth to enhance their health, develop to their fullest potential and establish productive and satisfying relationships in their present and future lives. The goals of a comprehensive approach are to:

- promote health and wellness.
- prevent specific diseases, disorders and injury.
- prevent high risk social behaviors.
- intervene to assist children and youth who are in need or at risk.
- help support those who are already exhibiting special health care needs.
- promote positive health and safety behaviors.

Attainment of these goals requires an integrated approach that coordinates multiple programs and provides multiple strategies. Work teams in collaboration with a coordinating council should involve families, students and community members in the program planning process. Further, professional staff development is necessary to effectively address specific health-related issues. A comprehensive school health program focuses on priority behaviors that contribute to the health, safety and well-being of students, staff and families, while assuring a supportive and healthy environment that nurtures academic growth and development. The successful implementation of this comprehensive approach necessitates leadership from health and education agencies and elected and appointed officials, adequate funding, trained personnel, administrative support, appropriate policy, quantitative and qualitative evaluation, legislation and regulations.[1]

SCHOOL ENVIRONMENT

Policy and Administrative Support

• District policies and administrative guidelines reflect a commitment to maintaining an open and positive psychosocial climate and a healthy physical environment that are conducive to high student achievement and the long-term health of students and staff.

• Policies, rules and regulations are consistently enforced.

• The chief administrator, the school board and the school health coordinating council receive, at least annually, a report on the psychosocial climate of the school and a report on the physical environment, along with an action plan for continuous improvement of the school environment.

• A uniform process for reporting injuries and health problems in the school environment should be in place and analyzed for the purpose of monitoring risk factors, trends and patterns and suggesting possible preventive measures.

• Effort should be made to compare the progress in the psychosocial and physical health arenas with relevant educational goals.

• Policies that assure safe transport of students to and from school (e.g., bus, bicycle, walking) are enforced.

Psychosocial Environment

• Administrative support for a healthy psychosocial environment is evidenced by district and campus policies and procedures.

• The school environment is friendly, nurturing, respectful of differences, physically and emotionally safe and conducive to learning with high expectations for academic success.

• School climate problems are addressed directly, in a timely manner and discussed openly within the limits of privacy.

• Effective instructional plans and techniques are used with all students to foster learning, self worth and mental health.

• Students, families and staff work as a team in planning and implementing programs and activities to affirm all cultural, linguistic and socioeconomic backgrounds.

• Students, families and staff are regarded as valuable and are involved in school governance.

• Students are empowered to take a leadership role in the development and implementation of programs to promote a healthy school.

• Focus is placed on people's feelings and needs as well as tasks and duties.

• Strong encouragement is given for students and staff to cooperatively solve problems and resolve conflict in an open and respectful manner.

• A crisis response system has been established to support students and staff in the event of violence, suicide, unintentional injury, death and other schoolsite incidents.

• Family involvement and support is encouraged.

Physical Environment

• The quality of air, water and other environmental elements is monitored to ensure the safety and well-being of students and staff.

• The district/school has a tobacco-free, drug-free and violence-free policy for students, staff and visitors on all school-owned property and vehicles.

• The structure of, or adaptations to, school buildings ensure access by persons with disabilities.

• District and school emergency disaster plans are established and emergency drills held periodically.

• Staff and students are trained in and practice emergency, first aid and infection control procedures including universal precautions.

• All schools have and maintain equipment and supplies needed to implement first aid and universal precautions for infection control.

• Buildings, equipment, playgrounds and athletic fields are clean, kept in good repair, free of hazards and meet all safety standards.

• Student and staff comfort is maintained by adherence to appropriate standards for heating, cooling, ventilation, lighting, space, safety glass and noise.

• The cafeteria facility creates an environment that encourages students to participate in the meal service.

• Safe, clean, appropriately equipped bathrooms, including facilities for hand washing, are available.

HEALTH EDUCATION

Policy and Administrative Support

• District policies and administrative guidelines reflect a commitment to attain desired student outcomes essential to optimal physical and mental health.

• The chief administrator, the school board and the school health coordinating council receive, at least annually, reports on actions taken and results achieved related to desired student outcomes, along with the action plan for continuous improvement in health education.

• At the intermediate and secondary level, certified health education specialists with teacher certification teach the health courses. Coordination and team teaching with related professionals is encouraged.

• At the elementary level, teachers have professional preparation in elementary health education.

• Educators are given opportunities for effective professional training when implementing a new curriculum.

Goals and Objectives

• District/school goals and objectives for health education are clear, based on assessed needs and stated in terms of student outcomes expected at each grade level and for each course.

Student Outcomes

• Entry and exit-level performances are defined for each grade level or health education course along with adaptations for students with special needs.

• Formative evaluations are conducted to monitor the implementation process and to determine the response of administrators, teachers, other staff, families and students to the curricular materials.

• Summative evaluations are conducted to measure changes in students' knowledge, attitudes, behaviors, skills and social action related to health.

• Congruence exists between the evaluation measures used, the district's health education curriculum, teaching strategies and the critical health objectives for student learning.

• Students demonstrate competence in essential health education objectives established for each grade level or course.

Curriculum

• Health education curriculum content is targeted at priority areas appropriate for developmental stage and potential risks.

• Health education includes integration of the physical, intellectual, social, emotional and spiritual dimensions of health as a basis of study in the ten content areas suggested by the 1990 Joint Committee on Health Education Terminology: community health, consumer health, environmental health, family life, growth and development, nutritional health, personal health, prevention and control of disease, safety and injury prevention and substance use and abuse.

• Health education occurs as a regularly scheduled component of the curriculum at each grade level. The successful completion of health education is required for graduation.

• Health and safety issues are infused regularly into the curriculum of various subject areas (e.g., home economics, science, language arts, social studies, vocational education).

• Healthy decision making and psychosocial health are reinforced through guidance and counseling curricula and other pupil services prevention plans. Health-enhancing messages are promoted via the media, social clubs, community service, extra-curricular activities and all school programming, including school nutrition services.

• Opportunities to practice generic personal and social skills (e.g., problem solving, decision making, communication) are provided to students at all levels.

Teaching Methods

• Appropriate instructional strategies are chosen to achieve instructional goals.

• Peer instruction is used to solicit active student involvement in instruction.

• Active family involvement with health lessons is planned and implemented.

Teaching/Learning Materials

• Current, research-based, instructional materials for regular and special needs students as well as for students with limited English proficiency are available to teachers.

• Health education resources from appropriate agencies and organizations are coordinated and used (e.g., state, county or city health departments, state departments of education, American Cancer Society, American Heart Association, American Lung Association, American Red Cross).

Health Educator Standards

Responsibilities and competencies for those providing health and safety education include:[2]

• Assessing individual and community needs for health education.
• Planning effective health education programs.
• Implementing health education programs.
• Evaluating effectiveness of health education programs.
• Coordinating provision of health education services and acting as a resource person in health education.
• Communicating health and health education needs, concerns and resources.

Professional Development

• Teachers are involved in: (1) identifying staff-development needs and (2) working with school leaders to implement staff-development programs to ensure achievement of standards.
• Staff development and inservice programs related to current health and safety issues and instructional strategies are provided at the district level and from professional organizations.

HEALTH SERVICES

Policy and Administrative Support

• Policies and administrative guidelines promote, protect and improve the health and safety of students, staff and the community.
• Policies and administrative guidelines reflect quality assurance and accountability for an effective health services component.
• A plan exists to coordinate health services with other school and community programs.
• The chief administrator, the school board and the school health coordinating council review, at least annually, reports on actions taken and results achieved by the health services component, along with an

action plan for continuous improvement in the delivery of health services.

• The director of the school health services may be a physician trained in school or child/adolescent health or a registered nurse with a minimum of a baccalaureate degree in nursing (BSN) and relevant experience in school, child/adolescent or community health.

• The planning, management and delivery of school health services are provided by a school health professional (e.g., at least a registered nurse or physician).

• School nurses are registered nurses with a baccalaureate degree who have met specific school nurse requirements.

Goals, Objectives and Program Outcomes

• Goals and objectives for the health services component are clear, based on assessed needs and stated in terms of expected outcomes.

Student Services

• All school health services are conducted as required by law or as defined by the school health services plan (e.g., dental, hearing, vision and spinal screenings, sports participation physicals).

• School nurses assess the health status of students, plan appropriate interventions and evaluate the care provided.

• Nursing interventions include case finding, direct care, health counseling, health education, referral and follow up.

• School nurses provide students with direct, one-on-one health instruction as needed and deliver classroom instruction in collaboration with teachers and administrators.

• Students with special health care needs have a written, individualized health care plan and, when appropriate, the plan is incorporated into the individualized education plan (IEP), 504 modification plan or individual family service plan (IFSP).

• The minimum standards for ratios of school nurses to students are:

— 1:750 for the general school population.
— 1:225 for special needs students mainstreamed within the general school population.
— 1:125 for severely/profoundly disabled students.
(Students with complex medical needs may require lower ratios and must be decided on a case-by-case basis.)

• According to state law and district policy, and upon proper medical authorization, the delegation of nursing activities to other school personnel requires that the school nurse provide training and ongoing supervision for the designated personnel regarding the delegated care.

• Educational programs that empower students and families to effectively access and utilize health care services are provided.

• All school health records are maintained as required by law or as defined by the school health services plan.

• School policies include provisions for the protection of confidential health/mental health records as defined by federal and state law.

• School illness, injury and violence reports are analyzed to facilitate prevention.

Coordination of Services

• Services are provided in each school in a health room or clinic with appropriate facilities and adequate equipment and supplies.

• School health services are coordinated with related in-school professionals and with students' primary care providers, as well as with community, city, county and state agencies and organizations.

• School health services make use of available school-based resources and community-based resources including professional and volunteer health organizations.

• The director collaborates with community primary care providers to ensure that every student has continuous access to comprehensive primary health care services.

• The plan to coordinate health services with other school programs is monitored by the district school health coordinating council.

Physician Standards

• A qualified consulting physician is available to consult with school health professionals and the school administration.

• The school health physician is familiar with laws, regulations, policies and programs (e.g., federal, state and local) related to comprehensive school health programs.

• The school physician assures efficient linkages and liaisons with the medical community; provides timely medical consultation on individual students, health procedures, curriculum and program issues; and regularly reports on consultation activities to the district administration.

Nursing Standards

The health services component employs standards of school nursing practice.[3] Accordingly, the school nurse:

- Utilizes a distinct clinical knowledge base for decision making in nursing practice.
- Uses a systematic approach to problem solving in nursing practice.
- Contributes to the education of the student with special health needs by assessing the student, planning and providing appropriate nursing care and evaluating the identified outcomes of care.
- Uses effective written, verbal and nonverbal communication skills.
- Establishes and maintains a comprehensive school health program.
- Collaborates with other school professionals, families and caregivers to meet the health, developmental and educational needs of the students.
- Collaborates with members of the community in the delivery of health and social services and utilizes knowledge of community health systems and resources to function as a school-community liaison.

Professional Development

- Contributes to nursing and school health through innovations in practice and participation in research or research-related activities.
- Identifies, delineates and clarifies the nursing role; promotes quality of care; pursues continued professional enhancement; and demonstrates professional conduct.

PHYSICAL EDUCATION

Policy and Administrative Support

- District policies and administrative guidelines reflect a commitment to students' physical development, motor skills acquisition and knowledge to support lifetime health and physical activity practices.
- The chief administrator, school board and the school health coordinating council review, at least annually, a report on the actions taken and results achieved in relation to students' physical fitness (muscular strength, cardiovascular endurance, body composition, muscular endurance and flexibility) and other desired outcomes as well as the action plan for continuous improvement in the physical education program.
- Certified teachers with specialization in physical education teach physical education at all levels.

Goals and Objectives

- District/school goals and objectives for physical education, based on state frameworks and national standards, are clear, and are based on assessed needs and stated in terms of student outcomes expected at each grade level.

• Supervision and positive role modeling occur during physical education activities.

Student Outcomes

• Entry and exit-level performances for physical development are defined for grade levels and physical education courses; adaptations are made for all students, particularly those with special physical, intellectual or emotional needs.[4]

• Evaluations are conducted to appropriately measure students' knowledge of physical development and physical activity skills, as well as the amount of participation in moderate to vigorous physical activity.[4]

• Students demonstrate appropriate levels of health-related fitness (for age and development as defined by American Alliance for Health, Physical Education, Recreation and Dance, American College of Sports Medicine, etc.) and physical competence related to satisfying and safe physical activity participation.[4]

Curriculum

• Instruction includes integration of the intellectual, social and emotional dimensions of participation in physical activity and its relationship to physical health.

• Students are involved daily in quality, health-related physical activity and motor skills instruction at the elementary and secondary level taught by a qualified physical education specialist.

• The curriculum is developmentally and instructionally appropriate in that it is suitable for the specific students being served.

• The physical education program provides instruction in a variety of movement forms and devotes time to instruction about lifetime physical activities.

• The physical education program includes instruction relating to physiological and biomedical principles that support safe participation in physical activity to minimize the risk of injury.

• In addition to class time for skills instruction, the physical education program provides opportunities for all students to have a minimum of 60 minutes of moderate to vigorous health-related activity per week. Programs to promote development of muscular strength, endurance and flexibility are provided three times a week.

• Students in third grade and above participate annually in a health-related physical fitness testing program using an accepted set of measures to test body composition, muscular strength and endurance, cardiorespiratory endurance and flexibility. Individualized exercise prescriptions are provided based upon the assessment.

• Athletic and playing fields are well maintained and free of hazards.

• Proper and correctly fitted equipment to prevent injury is worn or in place for all athletic practices and events (e.g., mouth guards, break away bases, mats on concrete gym walls, etc.).

• Injury data should be collected and reviewed regularly to identify remedial measures that could prevent future incidents and avoid litigation.

• A policy for transport of injured students should be developed with specific and appropriate guidelines for various types of injuries.

• Equipment for emergencies is accessible and available at practice and competitions.

• Coaches receive continuing education to upgrade their skills in recognizing, treating and preventing injuries.

• Congruence exists between state intramural and interscholastic association recommendations and the sports activities sponsored by the district in order to ensure safety of all players at practice and during competition.

Teaching Methods

• Effective teaching methods are used to achieve the desired student outcomes related to physical development and lifetime physical activity.

• Ongoing individual assessments of students are performed and serve as the basis for teacher decisions regarding individualization of instruction, curriculum planning, communication with families and evaluation of program effectiveness.

• Class size is equal to the size of other classes.

Professional Development

• The district level administration of physical education staff is involved in identifying staff-development needs and working with school leaders to implement goals that assure achievement of guidelines.

• Staff development provided for the physical education staff is ongoing and effective.

• All physical education staff are trained in appropriate emergency procedures.

COUNSELING, GUIDANCE AND MENTAL HEALTH

Policy and Administrative Support

- District policies and administrative guidelines reflect a commitment to and accountability for the social and psychological health of students.
- The chief administrator, school board and the school health coordinating council review, at least annually, status reports on the extent to which students demonstrate social and psychological growth and the extent to which identified student needs are met, along with action plans for continuous improvement in guidance, counseling, social and psychological services.
- School policies include provisions for the protection of confidential health/mental health records as defined by federal and state law.
- Mental health services must be directed by a certified or licensed school psychologist or school social worker with a minimum of an advanced professional degree and related national/state certificate.
- A plan to coordinate services with health and other school programs is monitored by the district and used to improve program effectiveness.
- Certified/licensed counselors, school psychologists and school social workers, along with school physicians and nurses, are available to meet the needs of students.
- The counseling and mental health staff is effective in achieving the program objectives.

Goals, Objectives and Outcomes

- The goals of the counseling, guidance and mental health program are clear, based on assessed needs and stated in terms of student outcomes.

Direct Services to Students

- The minimum standard for counselors to students is 1:250; school psychologists to students 1:1000; and school social workers to students is 1:800.
- Counseling, guidance and psychosocial service activities are provided to reduce inappropriate and unhealthy student behavior, promote optimal mental and emotional health and identify and address problems that impede learning.
- Programming with students promotes problem solving, social

skills, decisionmaking, self-esteem building, academic guidance and transitions.

 • Peer programs are organized to address health, safety and social issues.

 • Coordination of confidential health/mental health records is required.

 • The counseling, guidance and mental health staff use available resources from health agencies and other community resources, including volunteers, to facilitate achievement of student and staff mental health needs.

Professional Development

 • Effective in-service education is provided by and to the counseling, guidance and mental health staff addressing the multitude of mental health issues of children and adolescents (e.g., multicultural sensitivity, dysfunctional family systems, disability awareness, developmental learning, etc.).

 • In-service programs are provided to assist with the implementation of experiences that promote interpersonal development in students.

 • Consultation services are available to teachers, administrators, families and others on student and system levels to improve learning and psychosocial developmental outcomes.

SCHOOL FOOD AND NUTRITION SERVICES

Policy and Administrative Support

 • District policies reflect a commitment to meeting the nutritional needs of all students in an environment fostering positive attitudes and social skills.

 • The chief administrator, the school board and the school health coordinating council, including the school food service professional, review at least annually, reports on the status of the food and nutrition services and progress toward achieving annual objectives, along with the action plan for continuous improvement of school nutrition.

 • Nutrition education is an integral part of the cafeteria experience, complementing the classroom curriculum in comprehensive school health.

 • The planning, management and delivery of the nutrition services are directed by a qualified food service/nutrition professional, preferably with a baccalaureate degree in food service systems management.

- The local food service manager has the appropriate training and experience in institutional food service management, including courses in nutrition.
- All food service staff are certified according to their level of practice, meeting state requirements or professional standards.
- Food items available to students during school hours (fund raisers, vending machines, snack bars) that compete for student monies or replace their consumption of regular school meals provide adequate nutrition.

Goals and Objectives

- The goal of the school food and nutrition services is to provide nutritionally appropriate meals to students at a reasonable price in an environment that is pleasant, comfortable and conducive to the practice of positive nutrition behavior.

Program Components

- School food and nutrition personnel support teachers and students by offering their services, technical expertise and resource materials to enhance nutrition and health education curricula and activities.
- Pleasant eating environments are provided. This includes adequate time and space to eat school meals, cafeterias that are well lighted, at comfortable temperature and sound levels; walls and ceilings in good repair; positive supervision; and role modeling at meal time.
- School staff are recognized as role models promoting nutrition and eating competence.
- Students are taught to make responsible, healthy choices in their meals at school.
- Students eligible for free or reduced-priced meals are receiving these at school. Confidentiality of status is maintained to protect the dignity of students.
- Students with special dietary needs have a written individualized food plan as part of their individualized education plan (IEP). Meals served at school are consistent with the nutritional goals established by the USDA [U.S. Department of Agriculture].
- Meals offered to students include a variety of foods, particularly fresh fruit, fresh vegetables and whole grain products.
- Meals served at school contain the appropriate levels of sodium, calcium and iron.
- Meals are planned with the goal of meeting the recommended 30

percent or less of total calories from fat; and 10 percent or less of total calories from saturated fat.

• Fund raisers, vending machines and sale of foods by organizations other than the school food and nutrition service offer foods that provide appropriate nutrition.

• Menu planning practices reflect the ethnic and cultural food preferences of students.

• Students and families are involved in menu planning, menu evaluation and taste testing.

• Nutrition messages are included on printed menus for students and families.

Professional Development

• Staff development programs are ongoing and effective.

• The staff development program includes training in food service management; the procurement, preparation, planning and promotion of foods/meals; and nutrition education to achieve the goal of providing nutritious meals.

WORKSITE HEALTH PROMOTION

Policy and Administrative Support

• District policies and administrative guidelines reflect a philosophical and financial commitment to employee health and safety, including support for staff health promotion programs.

• At least annually, the worksite health promotion program is evaluated and a status report is compiled and presented to the chief administrator and the school health coordinating council, along with an action plan for continuous improvement in worksite health promotion for school employees.

• An individual with appropriate training and skills is designated to coordinate the worksite health promotion program and is provided administrative support, including decision-making authority and release time to coordinate the program.

• Staff are encouraged to model a healthy life-style.

Goals and Objectives

• The goals and objectives of the district's staff health promotion program are clear, based on assessed needs and stated in terms of expected outcomes.

Program Components

- The health promotion programs offered are based upon health assessment and employee preferences.
- Staff are provided access to health assessments, screenings, health education and appropriate referrals.
- School facilities are made available for health promotion activities during non-instructional time.
- Staff are given adequate opportunities and incentives to participate in health promotion activities.
- Health promotion activities offered to school employees include employee assistance programs, smoking cessation, nutrition education, weight management and aerobic activity.
- Confidentiality is maintained regarding all staff assessments.

INTEGRATION OF SCHOOL AND COMMUNITY HEALTH ACTIVITIES

Policy and Administrative Guidelines

- District policies and administrative guidelines reflect a commitment to effective school/community relationships.

Goals and Objectives

- The goals and objectives of the school–community component of comprehensive school health are clear, based on assessed needs and stated in terms of intended outcomes.

Program Components

- An interdisciplinary/interagency school health coordinating council that includes school staff, families who represent all segments of the community, students and community resource personnel is organized at the community level to coordinate programs among agencies that promote the health and safety of youth.
- Interdisciplinary school health teams (committees) that include teachers, families, students, school nurses, physicians, health educators, school psychologists, coaches, social workers/counselors and community resource personnel are organized at the school level to address priority school health and safety issues that interfere with the learning process.
- Interdisciplinary school health teams and the interdisciplinary/interagency coordinating council achieve identified goals by implement-

ing the program planning model (assessment; planning; setting of goals,
objectives and strategies; implementation; and evaluation).

- A systematic means for sharing information and resources and
coordinating programs is established
- Periodic meetings of the interdisciplinary/interagency coordinating council are held to assess needs, initiate recommendations and evaluate programs.
- Integrated efforts to eliminate illegal use of alcohol and other drugs,
use of tobacco, motor vehicle injuries, sports injuries, sexually transmitted diseases, suicide, child abuse, violence, teen pregnancies and other
health and safety-related concerns are implemented.
- Evaluations are conducted at least annually to assess the level of
satisfaction with the comprehensive school health program.
- Continuing education programs are offered for families and community members.
- Efforts are made to encourage family and other community member attendance and involvement with school and academic programs (e.g.,
health education, child care, evening meetings, coordination with other
school activities).
- A two-way communication system is established between school
and homes to encourage maximum involvement in areas of mutual interest.
- Families, after receiving the results of health-related fitness tests,
encourage their child to complete an individualized activity plan.
- Programs are provided to assist families and community members
in building communication and other family skills, as well as understanding child growth and development.

DEFINITIONS

Health[5]

- A state of complete physical, mental and social well-being and not
merely the absence of disease, injury and infirmity.
- A quality of life involving dynamic interaction and independence
among the individuals' well-being, their mental and emotional reactions
and the social complex in which they exist.
- An integrated method of functioning which is oriented toward
maximizing an individual's potential. It requires that the individual maintains a continuum of balance and purposeful direction with the environment where he or she is functioning.
- A set of health-enhancing behaviors, shaped by internally consistent values, attitudes, beliefs and external social and cultural forces.

Comprehensive School Health Program[5]

- An organized set of policies, procedures and activities designed protect and promote the health and well-being of students and staff which has traditionally included health services, health school environment and health education. It should also include, but not be limited to physical education; food and nutrition services; counseling, psychological and social services; health promotion for staff; and family/community involvement.

School Health Coordinating Council

- An organization that supports and monitors the implementation of the comprehensive school health program. Members include families, students, teachers, school nurses, physicians, health educators, a child nutrition director and other school health and mental health professionals, as well as community members, including but not limited to representatives from the health district, social services, juvenile justice, voluntary health agencies, business and mental health agencies.

ENDNOTES

1. Adapted from Consensus Statement on School Health. Canadian Association for School Health.

2. Responsibilities and competencies for entry-level health educators. Provider Designation Handbook. New York, NY: National Committee for Health Education Credentialing, Inc; 1991.

3. Proctor ST, Lordi SL, Zaiger DS. School Nursing Practice Roles and Standards. National Association of School Nurses, Inc., Scarborough, ME: 1993;18. These standards for school nursing practice are based upon Standards of Clinical Nursing Practice. Washington, DC: American Nurses' Publishing; 1991.

4. Outcomes of Quality Physical Education Programs. National Association for Sport and Physical Education: 1992.

5. Adapted from the Report of the 1990 Joint Committee on Health Education Terminology. J Sch Health 1991;61(6):251-254.

APPENDIX
C
Health Behavior Change
alth Education Programs

Ken Resnicow, Ph.D.

Health education programs have been informed by several theoretical models of health behavior change including the Health Belief Model, the Theory of Reasoned Action, and the Operant Learning Theory (Skinner, 1974). Over the past 10 years, however, one model, the Social Cognitive Theory (SCT) (Bandura, 1986; Bandura, 1995; Perry et al., 1990) has become perhaps the dominant theoretical framework for health education. The emergence of SCT as the preeminent model within health education can be attributed to several factors. First, whereas the Health Belief Model (Rosenstock, 1988; Rosenstock, 1990) and the Theory of Reasoned Action/Planned Behavior (Ajzen and Fishbein, 1972; Ajzen and Madden, 1986) focus primarily on cognitive factors, SCT extends beyond knowledge and attitude domains to include behavioral elements, such as social skills, and environmental influences. Second, whereas the Health Belief Model, the Theory of Reasoned Action, and the Operant Learning theory focus essentially on individual-level behavior (Rosenstock, 1988; Skinner, 1974), SCT addresses the behavior of social groups and the dynamic interaction of the individual within the larger social context. Consequently, SCT may be a more appropriate model for designing comprehensive school health programs (CSHPs), which include both individual and environmental interventions. Given the predominance of SCT in the current health education paradigm, a brief overview, including a discussion of how this model can guide the development of health education programs, is provided.

SOCIAL COGNITIVE THEORY: AN OVERVIEW

At the core of Social Cognitive Theory is the triadic model comprising person, behavior, and environment. This model addresses the behavior of individuals and social groups, and their dynamic interaction, referred to as reciprocal determinism, is an essential element of SCT (Bandura, 1986; Bandura, 1995). To illustrate, individual person-level factors, such as outcome expectations and self-efficacy, may increase the likelihood of an individual's executing a behavior; conversely, the behavior of an individual within a defined social group (e.g., school) can shift norms among others within that shared social environment, which in turn may influence personal motivation (e.g., outcome expectations) and subsequent behavior. Environmental factors can also influence behavior (e.g., availability of healthful foods in the school cafeteria), serving either to enhance or to suppress individual motivation. Comprehensive school health education programs similarly include both individual and environmental intervention. Specifically, health education curricula tend to focus on person-level factors, whereas other elements of the CSHP program, such as healthy environment or school policy, foodservices, and community involvement, largely address environmental factors.

Self-Efficacy

Self-efficacy (SE) plays a central role in SCT. SE is defined broadly as the confidence in one's ability to execute a specific behavior or set of behaviors. In other words, if a student does not feel confident in his or her ability to resist peer appeals to use drugs, the likelihood of employing appropriate communication skills is diminished; similarly, low efficacy regarding athletic performance may inhibit involvement in physical activity. Two fundamental assumptions regarding SE are critical to understanding its importance in SCT. First, Bandura (1986) posits SE as a *cause* of behavior, not simply as the *result* of reinforcement, as operant learning theorists may contend. Second, SE is task specific, as distinguished from more global, largely immutable personality attributes such as self-esteem, self-concept, and locus of control. Individuals are not self-efficacious in general, but instead, their sense of efficacy is tied to specific behaviors and tasks, which are amenable to change. For example, an adolescent may have high SE regarding his or her ability to perform well on standardized tests, but little efficacy regarding ability to dance or play sports. Although SE is conceptualized as task specific, when tasks are similar in their cognitive and behavioral demands, as well as in the context in which they occur, crossover or generalizability of SE can occur. For example, a high school student, because of positive experiences in high school mathematics, may have high efficacy regarding his or her ability to perform well in college math courses, despite having low efficacy regarding his or her ability to perform well in college language courses. Additionally, within tasks, the degree of SE that an individual may possess is not absolute. Instead, a gradient of SE can be plotted, with levels of SE generally decreasing as the complexity or difficulty of the task increases. Thus, an adolescent may report high SE that he or she can resist an appeal to try marijuana from a casual acquaintance but may report low SE if the appeal is from a popular peer opinion leader. Similarly, an adolescent may be highly self-efficacious with regard to asking a long-time partner to use a condom, but less efficacious with a new partner (Maibach and Murphy, 1995).

Efficacy can develop through four sources: performance mastery experience, vicarious observation, verbal persuasion, and physiologic or psychologic states. Performance mastery experiences are considered the most influential source, producing the strongest and most enduring efficacy effects. Performance success raises efficacy beliefs, whereas failure lowers them. Of considerable theoretical and clinical import is the fact that the perception of successful performance, rather than performance per se or subsequent external reinforcement, predicts future behavior. Thus, independent of actual performance, individuals who are convinced (through either their own appraisal or the assessment of others) that they performed well on a task develop stronger efficacy beliefs and are more likely to continue efforts than do individuals who perform well but perceive their performance as unsuccessful. This points to the need for health teachers to reinforce successful performance—for example, to praise even small positive changes in dietary, exercise, or safety habits.

Vicarious observation involves seeing (or visualizing) individuals under comparable demand parameters successfully perform the target behavior. This can include vicarious observation of simulated performance in clinical settings or instructional media or in vivo observation of peers and family members. Observing adult or peer role models successfully perform positive behaviors represents an important potential source of efficacy that is often lacking in disadvantaged populations. The absence of positive role models can then be recast as an absence of positive observational learning situations and, therefore, as a problem of low personal efficacy rather than low self-esteem. In addition to affecting efficacy directly, positive role models can also influence behavior by altering outcome expectations and normative beliefs.

Verbal persuasion, encouraging an individual to attempt a behavior change and providing assurance he or she has the skills necessary to do so, can be an effective motivational strategy, although encouragement must be titrated to the behavioral and cognitive capacity of the individual. Determining "how high to aim" requires considerable understanding of an individual's talents, interests, motivation, and baseline efficacy. Finally, physiologic and affective states, such as excessive arousal, anxiety, and depression, can diminish efficacy and discourage continued efforts, whereas positive states, such as stimulation, euphoria, and physical enjoyment, can encourage future effort. Pressuring an adolescent to attempt a new behavior or modify an existing one when that person is not prepared or sufficiently motivated to do so can create dysphoric levels of anxiety, arousal, anger, or resentment that, even with successful performance, can result in diminished motivation to continue efforts. Efficacy operates through four processes: choice behavior, effort expenditure and persistence, thought patterns, and emotional reactions. The first two are reflected in the behavioral domain; the last two are largely cognitive in nature. Individuals with high SE are more likely to attempt to perform a behavior (i.e., choice) and more likely to continue their efforts in the face of initial setbacks or frustration (i.e., expenditure and persistence). On the cognitive level, highly self-efficacious individuals tend to visualize and dwell on their successes more than their failures (i.e., thought patterns) and to process positive affective aspects of their performance more than the negative (i.e., emotional reactions).

Outcome Expectations

Outcome expectations include the perceived positive and negative results of a behavior (i.e., pros and cons). Initial and continued behavioral efforts are more likely when perceived positive outcomes (i.e., benefits) outweigh the perceived negatives (i.e., costs). This dimension of SCT includes much of what operant learning theorists classify as reinforcement, although SCT differs in its emphasis on the cognitive, conscious expectations of environmental contingencies rather than on the conditioned (and largely unconscious) responses resulting from reward or punishment. SCT delineates three categories of outcome effects: physical, social, and self-evaluative. Physical effects include anticipated positive and negative sensory experiences (pleasure or pain), as well as assumed short- and long-term health consequences resulting from a behavior. This may include achieving of positive physical effects (e.g., by losing weight) or avoiding negative effects (e.g., by reducing the risk of heart disease). It is within this domain that health knowledge operates. Knowledge regarding what behaviors improve or impair health, as well as the resources and options at one's disposal, are necessary though insufficient precursors of outcome expectations. As first described by Rosenstock (1988) in his delineation of the Health Belief Model, awareness of the connection between behavior and health generally does not spur action unless the individual feels personally susceptible to the potential risks (or rewards)—that is, the person believes the potential outcomes of a behavior are likely on a personal not only an abstract (i.e., to "others") level. Social effects include approval from friends and family, recognition, monetary reward, and improved status, as well as inhibiting factors such as disapproval, rejection, censure, or ostracization. Social effects are particularly influential among school-age youth, since their identity is determined largely through peer relationships and normative comparison. Studies on substance use, diet, and sexual habits have demonstrated that perceptions regarding peer behaviors and group norms are strong predictors of behavior (Botvin et al., 1992; Botvin and Dusenbury et al., 1993; Wulfert and Wan, 1993). The third class of outcome expectations, self-evaluation, includes the positive and negative internal reactions resulting from behavior. Although related to perceived social effects, insofar as personal values are largely derived from peer standards and social mores, self-evaluative expectations refer more to the perceived intrapersonal or intrapsychic consequences of behavior—that is, how one will feel about him- or herself morally and emotionally as a result of engaging in a behavior, beyond its external, social contingencies. During adolescence, moral development is largely under construction and contingent more on external than on internal reference (Kohlberg, 1977; Kohlberg et al., 1983). As a result, self-evaluative effects are seen as less influential than social effects in this age group.

Modifying outcome expectations is an important component of many health education programs. For example, substance use programs often include information regarding the positive and negative physical health effects of tobacco, marijuana, and alcohol use, while nutrition education programs address the consequences of consuming foods high or low in fat. Given the "present" orientation of most adolescents, saliency of health information for this population is enhanced by focusing on immediate rather than delayed consequences of behavior. For example, substance use prevention programs that place greater emphasis on concurrent or short-term physical effects, such as impaired stamina and athletic performance, appear more effective than those emphasizing long-term health effects such as cancer, cirrhosis, or heart disease (Glynn et al., 1990).

Modifying perceived social effects may have an even greater impact on health behavior than does improving knowledge of physical consequences. Social effects include perceptions of how engaging in a behavior will alter social status. For example, decisions regarding substance use are influenced by how the individual perceives these behaviors will alter his or her social image. Based on the observation that many adolescents overestimate the prevalence and therefore the normalcy of substance use, researchers have developed programs aimed at correcting erroneous perceptions regarding prevalence and acceptability, and initial results of these interventions appear promising (Hansen and Graham, 1991; Sussman et al., 1993). Although most "normative influences" programs have focused on substance use behaviors, this approach may be applicable to other health habits, such as sexual behavior and diet (Baranowski,1989–1990; Jemmot and Jemmot, 1992; Maibach and Murphy, 1995).

Goals

Setting discrete, realistically ambitious goals and then attaining them can significantly increase performance motivation. Setting goals can establish a hierarchy of behavioral tasks that is sequential and reinforcing. Attainment of goals that are too easily achieved produces little motivation, while setting unrealistic goals, though initially motivating, can eventually take its toll, resulting in low efficacy states if not helplessness and depression. The relation between "attainability" and motivation may differ for short- and long-term goals. Ambitious long-term goals can be useful if the short-term goals needed to achieve them are divided into realistic, hierarchical steps and sequentially attained. Individuals, rather than hinging all sense of their success on glamorous future goals, can be taught to gain satisfaction from progressive mastery of "minigoals" and can then learn to use these short-term successes as stepping stones toward their ultimate ambition. Specifically, it may be appropriate to encourage youth to set their sights on high achievement, wealth, or fame, as long as appropriate, progressive proximal goals, such as completing high school, doing well on the SATs, and applying to college, are established and attained. SCT-based health education programs help youth establish positive goals, such as eating five servings of fruit and vegetables per day, regularly wearing a seat belt or safety helmet, or exercising three times per week. Similar to shaping techniques used in operant conditioning, goals are hierarchical and sequential—for example, starting with an increase of one serving of fruits, then adding one serving of vegetables, and gradually building toward the final goal of five servings a day.

According to SCT, personal goals mediate motivation in three ways. First, anticipated self-satisfaction from achieving performance standards can stimulate initial efforts and continued persistence (i.e., expectations of accomplishment can stir one to action). Second, successful performance and goal attainment can enhance personal efficacy, motivating heightened efforts and progression to more complex tasks and hierarchical goal achievement. The third type of influence involves adjustment of standards in response to performance attainment. Individuals who readjust their goals upward after successful performance are more likely to continue efforts, whereas those who are satisfied with simply attaining the same standard again invest little subsequent effort. In other words, individuals who continue setting their sights on new heights are often those who achieve greatness. The relationship among expectations, goals, and motivation can be somewhat complex. In the face of initial failure, some individuals become demoralized while others persist. Motivation is best maintained by a strong sense of efficacy not only to succeed but to withstand failure. In applying this principle to youth, it may be important to provide them with motivation not only to attempt new behaviors but also to prepare them to regroup and try again if initial efforts are not entirely successful. This strategy—encouraging realistic expectations for success and preempting defeatist interpretations of failure—is an essential element of *relapse prevention* (Brownell et al., 1986; Marlatt and Gordon, 1985). The challenge again lies in providing realistic expectations without injecting a self-fulfilling prophecy of failure.

Skills

For some behaviors, high SE and motivation (i.e., strong positive outcome expectations) are insufficient to produce successful behavior change. Task-specific social and motor skills are often needed. For example, to resist appeals from peers to use alcohol, tobacco, and other drugs, specific skills, decisionmaking, stress management, and communications may be needed. Younger children may require skills to request that parents purchase and serve healthier foods. Motor skills include athletic skills and condom use skills or, for youth with chronic illnesses, proper use of an asthma inhaler or insulin injection.

The Interaction of Self-Efficacy, Outcome Expectations, Skills, and Goals

As discussed earlier, SCT delineates multiple determinants of behavior change. Self efficacy is, however, seen as occupying a central role in this model. As such, it is important to understand how SE interacts with other personal and environmental determinants, as well as how a comprehensive school health program can employ SCT. Individuals with high SE are more likely to attempt a behavior if they have strong positive outcome expectancies and possess the skills necessary to accomplish the task. Possessing requisite skills is also likely to increase opportunities to attain mastery experiences, which will instill increased efficacy and promote continued behavioral effort. Additionally, if realistic goals are set, performance is more likely to be perceived as successful and efficacy beliefs will be strengthened. If unattainable goals are set, performance may be perceived as failure, which will decrease efficacy and thereby discourage persistence. On the environmental level, excessive levels of family stress, chaotic living conditions, lack of positive peer and adult models, and insufficient access to preventive services can suppress positive outcome expectations and initial effort, as well as reduce the likelihood of experiencing positive mastery experiences, which in turn can decrease efficacy and persistence.

REFERENCES

Ajzen, I, and Fishbein, M. 1972. Attitudes and normative believes as factors in influencing behavioral intentions. *Journal of Personality and Social Psychology* 21(1):1-9.

Ajzen, I., and Madden, T.J. 1986. *Understanding attitude and predicting social behavior.* Englewood Cliffs, N.J.: Prentice-Hall.

Bandura, A. 1986. *Social Foundations of Thought and Action: A Social Cognitive Theory.* Englewood Cliffs, N.J.: Prentice-Hall.

Bandura, A. 1995. *Self-Efficacy: The Exercise of Control.* New York: Freeman.

Baranowski, T. 1989–1990. Reciprocal determinism at the stages of behavior change: An integration of community, personal and behavioral perspectives. *International Quarterly of Community Health Education* 10(4):297–327.

Botvin, G.J., Baker, E., Botvin, E.M., Dusenbury, L., Cardwell, J., and Diaz, T. 1993. Factors promoting cigarette smoking among black youth: A causal modeling approach. *Addiction and Behavior* 18(4):397–405.

Botvin, G.J., and Dusenbury, L. 1992. Smoking prevention among urban minority youth: assessing effects on outcome and mediating variables. *Health Psychology* 11:290–299.

Brownell, K.D., Marlatt, G.A., Lichtenstein, E., and Wilson, G.T. 1986. Understanding and preventing relapse. *American Psychologist* 7:765–782.

Glynn, T.J., Boyd, G.M., and Gruman, J.C. 1990. Essential elements of self-help/minimal intervention strategies for smoking cessation. *Health Education Quarterly* 17:329–345.

Hansen, W.B., and Graham, J.W. 1991. Preventing alcohol, marijuana, and cigarette use among adolescents: Peer pressure resistance training versus establishing conservative norms. *Preventive Medicine* 20:414–430.

Jemmott, L.S., Spears, H., Hewitt, N., and Cruz-Collins, M. 1992. Self-efficacy, hedonistic expectancies, and condom-use intentions among inner-city black adolescent women: A social cognitive approach to AIDS risk behavior. *Journal of Adolescent Health* 13:512–519.

Kohlberg, L. 1977. Moral development: A review of the theory. *Theory into Practice* 16(2): 53–59.

Kohlberg, L., Levine, C. and Hewer, A. 1983. Moral stages: A current formulation and a response to critics. *Contributions to Human Development* 10:174.

Maibach E., and Murphy, D.A. 1995. Self-efficacy in health promotion research and practice: Conceptualization and measurement. *Health Education Research* 10(1):37-50.

Marlatt, G.A., and Gordon, J.R. 1985. *Relapse Prevention Maintenance Strategies in Addictive Behavior Change.* New York: Guilford.

Perry, C.L., Baranowski, T and Parcel, G. 1990. *How Individuals, Environments, and Health Behavior Interact: Social Learning Theory in Health Behavior and Health Education: Theory, Research, and Practice.* Glanz, K., Lewis, F.M. and Rimer, B., eds., San Francisco, CA, Jossey-Bass.

Rosenstock, I. 1988. Social learning theory and the Health Belief Model. *Health Education Quarterly* 15:175–183.

Rosenstock, I. 1990. *The Health Belief Model: Explaining Health Behavior Through Expectancies in Health Behavior and Health Education: Theory, Research, and Practice*, Glanz, K., Lewis, F.M. and Rimer, B., eds., San Francisco, CA, Jossey-Bass.

Skinner, B.F. 1974. *About Behaviorism*. New York: Knopf.

Sussman, S., Dent, C.W., Stacy, A.W., Sun, P., Craig, S., Simon, T.R., Burton, D., and Flay, B.R. 1993. Project towards no tobacco use, 1-year behavior outcomes. *American Journal of Public Health* 83(9):1245–1250.

Walter, H.J., Vaughan, R.D., Gladis, M.M., Ragin, D.F., Kasen, S. and Cohall, A.T. 1993. Factors associated with AIDS-related behavioral intentions among high school students in an AIDS epicenter. *Health Education Quarterly* 20(3):409–420.

Wulfert, E., and Wan, C.K. 1993. Condom use: A self-efficacy model. *Health Psychology* 12:346–353.

APPENDIX
D
New Approaches to the Organization of Health and Social Services in Schools

Joy Dryfoos, M.A.

SUMMARY

The current state of organization of health and social services in schools does not lend itself to orderly description. In any given school, one might find a complex program that includes a mental health team, a school-based clinic, case management, and a family resource center. In another school a nurse may be carrying the full responsibility with only part-time visits from a school district social worker, counselor, and/or psychologist. Out of this broad landscape, several major trends are discernible. In many communities where the school system serves primarily disadvantaged students who lack access to health services, community agencies are relocating their services into schools to augment the work of school staff. In a few places, school health efforts have been integrated with school reform initiatives to create a completely different kind of community or full-service school that is responsive to the needs of the local population. Both school systems and community agencies are open to making new administrative arrangements that will improve the status of child and family health.

Research and evaluation findings demonstrate that low-income families and their children do indeed gain access to needed health services through school-based programs. Among adolescents, those with the greatest needs (measured by high-risk behaviors) are using the services the most. Users of school-based health services are less likely than others to have health insurance. Mental health and dental services are particularly in demand in communities with marginal resources; however, clinics in schools are also finding many previously undocumented cases of chronic diseases (asthma, heart problems) and illnesses. Use of hospitals and emergency rooms has declined in a few places with school-based health services. It has been more difficult to document the impact of these school-based services on high-risk behaviors, such as substance abuse, unprotected sexual intercourse, or violence. School attendance and achievement have improved in some schools with support programs. The data suggest that intense and targeted programs produce the most measurable effects.

Broad replication of comprehensive health and social service programs in schools will require many systemic changes in both the educational establishment and community agencies that supply the services. A number of issues must be addressed, such as financing, governance, turf, staffing, controversy, community input, and parent involvement. A strong movement is under way to create new kinds of arrangements for the delivery of primary health care and social services in schools in conjunction with upgrading the quality of education. States and foundations have taken the lead and will probably have to continue to do so. Leadership at the federal level, as well as opportunities for technical assistance in planning, training, evaluation, and research, would contribute to the growth of this emerging field.

ORGANIZATION OF SERVICES IN SCHOOLS

Traditionally, when we think of school health services, we remember the school nurse who was on hand to take temperatures of sick children, call their families, and keep reports on absences. The nurse also measured students' heights and weights every year and examined their posture for signs of scoliosis.

Today's picture of school health services is vastly changed. First of all, the domain of "health" has stretched to include mental health, social services, and social competence—whatever is needed to enhance the lives of children and families. As a result, the number of different health, mental health, and social services available on school property has greatly increased and the organizational arrangements have become much more complex. Tyack (1992) has shown that despite the growing shift toward academic concerns in recent years, the proportion of school staff who are not teachers has grown significantly, from 30 percent in the 1950s to 48 percent in 1986. He believes that schools are increasingly becoming "multipurpose agencies" despite the push toward academic testing and standards.

Just how complex this picture of school health services has become can be seen in the vast array of issues that are being addressed by different kinds of interventions. Table D-1 displays the diverse goals and components of current programs based in schools. Table D-2 reveals that at least 40 types of personnel enter into schools to provide services; some are employed by the school districts, others by community agencies. Table D-3 presents the assortment of organizations that bring services into schools, including local public health departments, voluntary agencies, businesses, and foundations.

TABLE D-1 Goals and Components of School-Based Programs

Categorical (single) Goals
Improve school readiness
Improve academic achievement
Improve attendance
Improve classroom behavior
Improve graduation rate
Improve health and nutrition
Prevent depression and suicide
Prevent substance abuse
Prevent teen pregnancy
Prevent violence

Special Target Groups
Physically handicapped
Behavioral problems
Language problems, immigrants
Children of alcoholics
Children of divorced parents
Depressed or stressed
"At-risk" students (many definitions)
Pregnant and parenting teens
African-American males
Hispanics
Asians
Rural or isolated populations

Program Components
Parent involvement, leadership
  training, literacy
Case management, home visiting
Crisis intervention
Social skills, resistance, assertiveness
"Self-esteem", self-efficacy, competency,
  life skills
Basic cognitive skills
Job skills or placement
Counseling: psychosocial, alcohol
  and drugs
Community outreach
Transportation
Food, clothes, housing
Health and mental health care,
  immunization, dental care
Family planning, condom distribution
AIDS education, information, testing
After-school recreation, culture
Head Start, childcare
Eligibility establishment, immigration services
Hot line
Incentives

Comprehensive (multiple) Goals
Collaborative dropout, substance use, teen
  pregnancy, depression prevention
Comprehensive services to pregnant and
  parenting teens
Alternative schools
School reorganization
"One-stop" services for children, youth
  and families
Full-service school

TABLE D-2 Personnel Involved in School-Based Programs

Registered nurse	Program coordinator
Nurse practitioner	General youth worker
Physician	General family worker
Physician's assistant	Eligibility worker
Health aide	Job trainer
Dentist	Legal adviser
Dental hygienist	Recreation specialist
Optometrist	Arts and culture specialist
Audiometrist	Volunteer
Social worker	Parent
Case manager	Senior citizen
Psychologist	Business mentor
Psychosocial counselor	College student
Substance abuse counselor	University researchers
Parent advocate	Psychology
Community worker	Education
Outreach worker	Health or Medicine
Tutor or mentor	Justice
Resource teacher	Police
Classroom aide	Law professors
Mediation trainer (nonviolence)	Court officers
	Clergy

This section reviews the various ways in which health and other services are made available in schools, ranging from the simplest categorical models to quite complex comprehensive delivery systems (Dryfoos, 1994a, 1994b, 1994c). As the models become more complicated, personnel from outside the school system enter the picture (and the school building), bringing their protocols, liability coverage, and financing with them.

In the many source documents that report on school-based services, no two models are alike in regard to organizational framework. According to a discussion of school-based or school-linked service models in Maryland, "recognizing the diversity of communities and school systems across the state, it is important to realize that each service model may look different in terms of selected location and management style. The determination of which model will work better in a given situation must be a local decision based on an analysis of that community" (State of Maryland, 1994).

The section starts with a description of programs and models and provides examples (and costs where known). It also includes a summary of major findings from research and evaluation, and discusses major issues as they apply to organizing comprehensive school health programs.

TABLE D-3 Organizations That Bring Services into Schools

Local

County-city government
  Mayor's office
  County administrator
  Youth bureau
  Local education agency (school board)
  Public health department
  Mental health department
  City or County hospital
  Community health center
  Public welfare department
  Department of human resources
  Police department
  Probation office
  Court office
  Extension service
  Parks and recreation
  Child protective services, foster care

Private or nonprofit
  Hospital, medical or nursing school
  Health maintenance organization
  Medical or dental society
  Mental health center
  Women's health center, Planned
    Parenthood
  Community-based neighborhood
    organization
  Cities in Schools
  Senior citizen group
  Service club (Kiwanis, Elks, Lions)
  United Way, local planning councils
  Youth council
  Youth organization (Girls, Inc.;
    Girls and Boys Clubs; 4H; YWCA and
    YMCA)
  Social services agency

Colleges and universities
  Education, graduate school
  Social work
  Psychology
  Public health
  Medical and nursing school
  College (general)
  Community college
  Specialized research center
Business
Labor union
Bar association
Local foundations

State
  Governors office initiative
  Legislative initiative
  Health department
  Education department
  Human resources department

National
  Special governmental initiatives
    Center for Substance Abuse Prevention
    Maternal and Child Health Adolescent
    Initiative
    Division of School and Adolescent
    Chapter 1
    Drug Free Schools
  Foundation initiative
  "Think tank" research and development
    organizations

The following typology has been used here:

- pupil personnel teams,
- student assistance programs,
- school-based health centers,
- school-based dental clinics,
- mental health centers,
- family resource centers,
- case management and cities in schools,
- school-based youth service centers,
- teen parent programs,
- comprehensive multicomponent programs,
- school reorganization, and
- community or full-service schools.

Pupil Personnel Teams

Many schools organize their pupil personnel staff by teams with various configurations. The school social worker, guidance counselor, nurse, and psychologist meet with the principal and selected teachers. Team members review "cases" and work together to make sure that the needs of the students and their families are being met. The major pupil personnel agencies have joined together to form the National Alliance of Pupil Services Organizations (NAPSO), with a mission of promoting interdisciplinary approaches to their professions and supporting integrated service delivery processes (National Alliance of Pupil Services Organizations, 1992). The group's statement spells out significant roles for its 2.5 million professional constituents: "School-based pupil services personnel, who are responsible for delivering education, health, mental health, and social services within school systems, comprise a critical element which forms a natural bridge between educators and community personnel who enter schools to provide services. They are of the schools as well as in the schools. They can serve to mediate, interpret, and negotiate between other school personnel and persons entering the school from the outside."

Taylor and Adelman promote the creation of a resource coordinating team that would focus on identifying resources rather than on individual cases. Such a team "provides a necessary mechanism for enhancing systems for coordination, integration, and development of intervention . . . ensures that effective referral and case management systems are in place, [works on] communication among school staff and with the home, . . . [and] explores ways to develop additional resources" (Taylor and Adelman, in press). The resource coordinating team reaches beyond pupil personnel and adds special education and bilingual teachers, dropout counselors, and representatives from any community agency that is involved at the school.

In actual practice, many school systems do not have the funds to employ pupil personnel staff. Budget cuts, particularly in disadvantaged communities, have made huge dents in these categories. If social workers and psychologists are employed by school systems, they are often shared between schools and cannot possibly work in teams because of the demands on their time. One solution to this problem in needy areas has been for outside agencies to put together teams and relocate them in schools.

In Catawba County, North Carolina, the county government has assumed responsibility for providing school services through a team. The Public Health Department contributes a nurse, the Department of Social Services provides a social worker, and the Department of Mental Health supplies a psychologist (Moore, 1992). Placed in an office in a school, this team serves elementary, middle, and high schools. A second team has been organized to serve three elementary schools and one middle school. The lead team member is the psychologist; the team does intensive work with individual children, conducts home visits, follows up on attendance problems, refers students to the health department for medical care, and works closely with teachers singly and in groups. The program is managed by the Public Health Department, which acts as the home base where records are kept, supervision is maintained, and a health clinic is located. This program was created jointly by the county manager and the school superintendent and is supported by county tax dollars. Its success has been attributed to starting with what the school system perceived as the problem—in this case, head lice. The first component was the implementation of a "no-nit" policy whereby health department staffs screened and treated all students. After that, the team was free to work on other problems identified by the school staff, particularly teen pregnancy, truancy, and smoking.

The Travis County (Texas) Health Department, in conjunction with the Austin City School District, has organized a school services team in high-risk elementary schools: the team consists of a nurse, mental health counselor, social worker, and community outreach worker (Maternal and Child Health Bureau, 1993). The team provides screenings, case management, home visits, and health promotion activities. Initial agency–school communication problems were overcome by inviting the principals and counselors in the pilot schools to be part of the interview team and involved hiring decisions. The annual cost is $150,000 per school, which is provided by city and county funds (EPSDT [Early Periodic Screening, Detection, and Treatment] funding is being accessed).

In Florida, an analysis of data from sites supported by the Supplemental School Health Program reported that the team approach cost $55 per student (Eimhovich and Herrington, 1993).

Student Assistance Programs

Student assistance programs (SAPs) are another genre of school-based programs that tend to be categorical in that they are aimed at specific behaviors, but they also provide services that are more comprehensive than the categorical classroom-based prevention programs. One example is the Student Assistance Model developed and implemented in Westchester County (New York) almost a decade ago. This program brings full-time professional counselors (social workers) into schools to provide alcohol and drug abuse intervention and prevention services targeted at students and their families. This program, one of five selected by the National Institute of Alcohol Abuse and Alcoholism as a model, has four basic components (National Institute of Alcohol Abuse and Alcoholism, 1984):

1. group counseling sessions (eight to 20 sessions) for students with alcoholic parents, focusing on increased self-efficacy and improved academic, behavioral, social, and emotional functioning;
2. individual, family, or group counseling services for students who are using alcohol or drugs dysfunctionally; (referral to community treatment program if available);
3. counseling services for students who exhibit poor school performance (and are therefore at high risk for alcohol or drug abuse); and
4. collaboration with parent and community groups to develop ways of dealing with substance abuse problems.

Although based in schools, the counselors are all employed and supervised by, and receive intensive training from, an outside corporation, such as a county mental health department, and therefore do not operate under the same constraints as school guidance counselors (e.g., they can maintain confidentiality, and they have more time for individual attention). However, schools and their principals must be heavily committed to the program and provide space, equipment, open communication with the staff, and other supportive policies. An important aspect of this program is training teachers, parents, and other gatekeepers to be sensitive to student problems and to refer the students appropriately to counselors. Mandatory referral is required if students are found under the influence of alcohol or drugs on school grounds.

Teen Choice is another targeted program operated by outside professionals in public schools, this one focused on pregnancy prevention. It is operated by Inwood House, a voluntary social service agency, in the New York City public schools (Inwood House, 1987). Specially trained professional social workers staff three components: small groups, individual counseling and referral, and classroom dialogues. The small groups meet once a week for a semester and cover issues of sexuality, birth control, values clarification, peer pressure, and similar issues. The workers are assigned to a school and are on-site three to five days per week in seven schools. The most common problems that arise in counseling sessions include pregnancy scares (25 percent of cases), birth control, relationship and family issues, and general mental health evaluation.

School-Based Health Centers

One response to the growing health needs of students has been the development of school-based health centers (SBHC), most frequently in inner city high schools but increasingly in middle and elementary schools (Lear et al., 1991). No one knows exactly how many SBHCs are up and running. My own estimate is that there are about 650 SBHCs, and they operate in almost all parts of the country. However, the recent School Health Policies and Programs Study states that 11.5 percent of school districts reported at least one school-based clinic. Applying this proportion to the 13,169 school districts yields an estimate of more than 1,400 school-based clinics, twice the number usually given (Small et al., 1995).

A school-based health center is defined here as one or more rooms located within a school building or on school property and designated as a place where students can go to receive primary health services. This center or clinic is more than a school nursing station; students are also able to receive health services not generally available in school, such as physical examinations, treatment for minor injuries and illnesses, screening for sexually transmitted diseases, pregnancy tests, and psychosocial counseling. Services are provided by nurse practitioners, health aides, outreach workers, social workers, and physicians. Most of these practitioners are employed by one or more local agencies, such as health departments, hospitals, medical schools, or social service agencies.

Most SBHCs also provide health education and health promotion in the clinic, the classroom, for staff, and even for the community; 86 percent of providers offer health education in classrooms in clinic schools (Hauser-McKinney and Peak, 1995). Most run group counseling sessions in reproductive health care, family problems, asthma control, depression, and other relevant subjects.

In some communities, a school-based health services program provides care for more than one school. A mobile van is equipped to go from school to school, allowing workers to provide physical examinations, ambulatory services, immunizations, and referrals for more comprehensive medical and dental care. These functions can also be provided on-site if a room can be appropriately equipped and privacy ensured.

The average expenditure reported by school-based clinics in 1993 was about $150,000, plus about $30,000 in in-kind or matching funds (Hauser-McKinney and Peak, 1995). State public health-sponsored clinics reported the lowest budgets (about $100,000) and mental health agencies the highest (more than $200,000). In 1994, states reported that they provided $37 million for SBHCs: $25 million in state initiatives and $12 million from Maternal and Child Health (MCH) block grants. Also, some funds are received from Medicaid, Title XX (social services), Drug Free Schools, and Title X (family planning). A few states (Colorado, Delaware, Florida, Illinois, Louisiana, Massachusetts, Michigan, New York, and Texas) account for most state funds. It is estimated that about $100 million is currently being spent on SBHCs—half from states, a small amount from federal sources, some from foundations, lots of in-kind contributions, and very little coming directly from education budgets. Although many students are eligible for Medicaid, only about 7 percent of costs for school-based primary care is being reimbursed by this source.

Practitioners from across the country have recently organized a National Assembly for School-Based Health Care to promote this model and encourage the provision of high-quality care. State coalitions of providers in New York, California, and Connecticut are actively involved in working on such issues as managed care and information systems. The Robert Wood Johnson Foundation has given grants to 10 states to develop coordination mechanisms at the state level and create model district-wide school-based health care demonstrations.

The Jackson-Hinds Comprehensive Health Center in Jackson, Mississippi, currently operates school-based health services in four high schools, three middle schools, and one elementary school. In 1979, when the program was first initiated at Lanier High School, the staff found many conditions that demonstrated the extensive unmet needs of the students, including urinary tract infections, anemia, heart murmurs, and psychosocial problems. In a student body of 960, more than 90 girls either were pregnant or already had a child. Some 25 percent of the pregnancies had occurred while the youngsters were in junior high, which prompted the program to extend resources to an inner city junior high school and to a second high school the following year. The other clinics were added in the late 1980s.

Clinics are located in whatever rooms schools can make available. At Lanier High School, two small rooms near the principal's office are equipped as clinics. Group counseling and health education classes are provided in a large classroom that has been outfitted with private offices for individual counseling. The infant care center is located in a mobile unit attached to the school. The staff includes a physician, nurse practitioner, licensed practical nurse, two nurse assistants, and an educator or counselor, all part-time workers.

The school-based clinic protocol includes a medical history and routine lab tests of hematocrit, hemoglobin, and urinalysis. Each enrolled student completes a psychosocial assessment to provide information about risk levels for substance abuse, violence, suicide, pregnancy, sexually transmitted diseases (STDs), accidents, and family conflict. Depending on indications from the health history and the assessment tool, the student is scheduled for a visit with the physician and/or counselor. However, the clinic is always open from 8:00 a.m. to 5:00 p.m. for walk-in visits for emergency care and crisis intervention.

Clinic staff conduct individual and group counseling sessions. Students who are sexually active are given birth control methods, including condoms, and are followed up bimonthly. Staff members also dispense formal health instruction about such specific issues as compliance with medication protocols or treatment of acne, and conduct informal "rap sessions" on parenting, the reproductive health system, birth control methods, sexual values, STDs, and substance abuse. The counseling and clinic services are closely coordinated. Enrollees in the school clinic are referred to the primary community health center for routine dental screening, cleaning, and fluoride application. This facility is always open to students after school hours, on weekends, and on holidays.

Arrangements for early prenatal care are made through the obstetrical department of the health center. Teen mothers are carefully monitored throughout their pregnancies, with special attention paid to keeping the young women in school as long as possible and getting them back within a month after delivery. Day care is provided at the school. Young mothers are counseled and instructed about child development and parenting skills. The day care center is also used for teaching child psychology to high school students.

School-Affiliated Dental Services

Earlier in the century, many schools had established dental clinics, but very few such clinics remain in existence. Yet school-based health staff frequently report dental health needs as pressing; many disadvantaged youth have no access to a family dentist. A few school-based clinics have added dental services to their protocols. The clinic in Pinkston High School in Dallas, Texas, incorporates a fully equipped dental suite and a full-time dentist on staff. A new elementary school in Bridgeport, Connecticut, incorporates a large medical suite, with one of its offices equipped and used solely for dentistry.

In what may be the most exemplary dental program in the nation, the Board of Health in the city of Beverly, Massachusetts, has maintained a school-based dental clinic for underprivileged children for 76 years. Each child is expected to pay 10 cents a visit. If the clinic exam reveals more complex needs (extractions, orthodontia), the student is referred to local dentists who complete the work for free or at a reduced fee. The clinic also supports dental health education presented by a dental hygienist who visits 135 classrooms annually. The clinic has a singing group called "The Merry Molar Singers" and a "Clean Tooth Club."

A 1992 survey conducted by the National School Boards Association of 87 school districts selected as models for comprehensive health programs revealed that about half provided some type of dental services (Poehlman, 1992). A follow-up survey (with a 35 percent response rate) showed that most of the programs were located in elementary schools. Some three-fourths of those with dental services provided screening on school sites; about one-fourth also offered teeth cleaning, and one in ten gave fluoride rinses or sealants for prevention of tooth decay. Actual treatment was provided in more than one-third of the schools with dental programs: education for dental health was offered in two-thirds. Toothbrushes and toothpaste were distributed in several schools. Local dentists gave presentations, contributed their services at schools, or accepted referrals at low or no fee. In some communities, the Kiwanis Club was active in providing funds.

Mental Health Centers

When school-based clinic providers are asked what the largest unmet need is among their clients, they most frequently mention mental health counseling. Students come to the medical clinics with a litany of complaints about stress and depression, their typical adolescent problems exacerbated seriously by the deteriorating and unsafe social environment in which they live. The demand for mental health counseling has led to the development of school clinics that have a primary function of screening and treating for psychosocial problems, but mental health interventions in schools take many forms. In some communities, a mental health worker, either a psychologist or a social worker, is placed in a school by a community agency. A number of universities have collaborative arrangements with schools for internship experiences with mental health counseling. Within a broader framework of training young people to enhance their social skills, many university-based social psychologists have been busy designing and implementing school-based curricula.

A mental health center in a school transfers the functions of a community mental health center to a school building. In this model, a room or group of rooms in a school building is designated as a services center. This center is not usually labeled a "mental health" facility but rather is presented as a place where students can go for all kinds of support and remediation. The staff typically includes clinical psychologists and social workers. Depending on the range of additional services, other staff might be youth workers, tutors, and mentors. The goals of school-based mental health centers are to improve the social adjustment of students and to help them deal with personal and family crises.

A network of school-based mental health programs has been organized by the School Mental Health Project at the University of California at Los Angeles, a national clearinghouse that offers training, research, and technical assistance (Adelman and Taylor, 1991). This project works in conjunction with the Los Angeles Unified School District's School Mental Health Center. Based on this experience, the project is in the process of developing a guidebook for practitioners who want to follow a mental health model. Howard Adelman and Linda Taylor, directors of the project, believe that the major challenge for school-based mental health centers is to identify and collaborate with programs that are already going on in the school district. Many schools have programs focused on substance abuse and teen pregnancy prevention, crisis intervention (suicide), violence reduction, self-esteem enhancement, and other kinds of support groups. However, these efforts lack cohesiveness in theory and implementation, often stigmatize students by targeting them, and suffer from the common bureaucratic problem of poor coordination between programs. One of the most demanding roles for the mental health center is to establish working relationships with key school staff members.

The oldest mental health center in a school appears to have been operating within the Memphis City Schools since 1970. The Memphis City Schools Mental Health Center (MCSMHC) is a private, nonprofit corporation that also acts as an administrative arm of the school system. It is funded largely through contracts with the Tennessee Department of Human Services, the Department of Health, and a grant from Drug Free Schools and Communities. MCSMHC is a state-licensed center with a staff of 161, including psychologists, social workers, alcohol and drug counselors, and homemakers. The programs focus is to provide the overall school environment with many different components that have powerful preventive interventions affecting all children and their families, rather than to concentrate on providing specific services for individuals. The core program consists of 36 mental health teams that are housed in two school centers and rotate through all 160 schools, providing assessments, consultation, faculty inservice, crisis intervention, and counseling.

The teams work closely with School Support Teams, which make sure that interventions are actually carried out in the classroom, with families, and with individual students. The center organizes prevention groups in such areas as social skills, divorced families, grief issues, and anger control. In 1992–1993, the teams provided more than 9,000 hours of treatment to students and their families and 7,500 hours of consultation.

The Mental Health Center also takes responsibility for implementing drug abuse prevention, including training teachers in a K–12 curriculum. MCSMHC counselors are assigned to the schools and coordinate the programs, including Student Leadership Training, Just Say No clubs, and Parent to Parent Training. The mental health staff train school teams to work with community groups to address neighborhood issues. A Student Assistance Program specially trains teachers to identify high-risk students. School students suspended for a drug incident are required to attend nine sessions as part of an Early Intervention Group, a requirement that has resulted in a decline in school problems.

The center's most recent initiatives have sought to reduce conflict and violence. Its staff members have organized prevention groups in conflict resolution, using officers from the Memphis police department as co-facilitators. One school is involved in a firearms eradication program. Students and their parents who have received firearms suspensions are seen by a center psychologist and receive more in-depth services if appropriate. One mental health team is located at the Adolescent Parenting Program and works on this issue throughout the school system. Counseling is available, and workshops are offered on stress management, personal goal setting, and African-American issues. MCSMHC also offers services for abused and neglected children, including a Homemaker Program for families that have experienced abuse problems.

An exemplary school-based mental health program was initiated in New Brunswick, New Jersey, in 1988, funded by the New Jersey School-Based Youth Services Program (Reynolds, personal communication). It is operated in the high school and five elementary schools by the local Community Mental Health Center of the University of Medicine and Dentistry of New Jersey. Grantees of the New Jersey School-Based Youth Services Program receive $250,000 to $400,000 per year through the state's Department of Human Resources. The New Brunswick program is funded at the higher end because it covers more than one school. The program has ten full-time core staff members, including eight clinicians (psychologists and social workers), one of whom serves as the director. Staff members conduct individual, group, and family therapy and serve as consultants to school personnel and other agencies involved with adolescents. An activities or outreach worker plans and supervises recreational activities and contacts at the high school. Specialized part-time staff include a pregnancy or parenting counselor, substance abuse counselor, and consultants in suicide prevention, "social problems," and medical care.

The facility at New Brunswick High School is located in the old band room, which has been fixed up to resemble a game room in a settlement house, with television, Ping-Pong and other active games, comfortable furniture, and books and tapes on loan. The center offers tutoring, mentoring, group activities, recreational outings, and educational trips. A number of "therapeutic" groups have been organized in such areas as problem-solving, substance abuse, children of alcoholics, and coping skills for the gifted and talented. Students are referred and provided with transportation to the local neighborhood health center for health services and treatment. During the past two years, one in four of the enrolled students has been involved in active mental health counseling with a clinician. According to Gail Reynolds, the program director, the demand for services is overwhelming, requiring immediate and time-consuming interventions with the family, school, and other social agencies.

The South Tama County (Iowa) Partnership Center is an example of a rural school-linked mental health program focused on dropout and substance use prevention (STC Partnership Center, 1994). Located in a rented building in "downtown" Tama, this school-operated center contracts with 14 public and nonprofit agencies, including the local mental health clinic, public health department, juvenile court, and Job Corps. School buses provide transportation for students and their families to the center, where they receive a variety of human services, employment services, education, and recreation. Full-time staff include a social worker and an employment specialist. This program has been funded until recently by a state grant of $200,000 and an in-kind matching grant of $50,000. The current budget is approximately $150,000, which is obtained from various categorical sources.

Family Resource Centers

An unknown number of Family Resource Centers (FRCs) are located in school buildings, while other FRCs are community-based. A few states, including California, Connecticut, Florida, Kentucky, North Carolina, and Wisconsin, have passed legislation that appropriates funds for FRCs (Kagan, 1991). Kentucky's legislation mandates that every elementary school with more than 20 percent of its students eligible for free lunch must have a Family Service Center (Illback, 1993). These programs offer parent education and refer parents to infant and child care, health services, and other community agencies. Grants average $75,000, a minimal amount to cover the cost of a full-time coordinator and other part-time staff. In other states, FRCs supported various state initiatives and federal grants to deliver comprehensive services on school sites, including parent education, child care, counseling, health services, home visiting, and career training. The Chicago-based Family Resources Coalition acts as a clearinghouse for the development of family support programs that can deliver preventive, coordinated, community-based services. Nationwide, some 2,000 programs have been identified that provide the three "Rs": resources, referrals, and relationships. Many of these family and child centers are located in school buildings.

The Family Resource Center in Gainesville, Florida, consists of seven portable units situated between an elementary and a middle school. This program includes a health clinic, experimental nursery, parent education, GED (General Educational Development) preparation and literacy classes, case management, economic services (Aid for Dependent Children, Medicaid, and Food Stamps eligibility establishment), job training and computer education, toy lending library, and family liaison. In a pattern that is typical of multiservice programs, the funding for this effort derives from many sources, including a state Full-Service Schools grant, Chapter I, College of Nursing and Medicine, Even Start, Head Start, Community College, Mental Health Services, School Board, state health grants, and Medicaid reimbursements. The state has awarded the program $2.5 million to build a new center that will have 2,500 square feet of space (currently it has 750 square feet).

Nashville, Tennessee, has a project called "One-Stop-Shopping in a Northeast Nashville Community," which consists of a family resource center and clinic located at a school devoted to serving preschool and kindergarten children. Regular services include home visiting, case management, GED classes, a family literacy program, help with welfare eligibility, year-round school nursing, counseling, job training, and referral. "The unique nature and effectiveness of the project is evidenced by the cooperative relationship in one location of state and local social services, health, literacy, housing and transportation, job training, and public education" (Maternal and Child Health Bureau, 1993). The annual budget is $675,000, which is obtained from local government funds, United Way, MCH Sprans grants, and general state funds.

Case Management

Another variant of school-based health or social services places social workers from community agencies into schools to act as case managers. Cities in Schools (CIS), a national nonprofit organization founded by William Milliken in Washington, D.C., has promulgated this model for prevention of school dropout. CIS operates in more than 122 communities with 384 school sites to facilitate a process of collaboration to bring health, social, and employment services into schools to help high-risk youngsters (Leonard, 1992). Each local entity has its own version but, in general, the program involves "brokering" community social service agencies to provide case management services within the school building. Local businesses are involved in arranging for mentoring and apprenticeship experiences (Cities in Schools, 1988).

In most CIS programs, a case manager is assigned to each high-risk child. Communities vary in program design; some operate alternative schools, and some offer special life skills classes and other forms of remediation and tutoring. A wide array of partnerships has been established through the CIS processes; these include involving Girls and Boys Clubs of America, VISTA, United Way, and Junior League. Several CIS programs have achieved national prominence. For example, Rich's Academy in Atlanta (one of six CIS schools in that community) is an alternative school created in partnership with a department store. CIS has joined with the Iacocca Institute and the Lehigh University College of Education in Pennsylvania to create the National Center for Partnership Development, designed to address the dropout problem by meeting the multiple needs of youth. The CIS strategy has been translated into formal curriculum and training materials and uses computer-based interactive multimedia sessions.

One CIS spin-off is the Pinal County (Arizona) Prevention Partnership, which involves 13 middle and high schools in a collaborative effort of the Department of Human Services, the county school superintendent's office, and a nonprofit agency (Pinal County Human Services, 1990). According to director Charles Teagarden, the strategy calls for "a school-based, integrated delivery system of networking service providers connecting at-risk youths through diligent case management to targeted prevention programs, then to job and career opportunities created by economic development, all monitored by a data system evaluation." More than 100 different human service providers are brought into the schools to conduct these activities, or referrals are arranged. Family Resource Centers in eight of the schools allow parents to interact and work in support groups.

CIS has developed a concept paper calling for schools to create a Teen Health Corps. These programs would include peer education and leadership training centered around preventive health issues, starting with STDs and HIV (Human Immunodeficiency Virus). School-based activities, such as health fairs and class presentations to lower grades, will be organized with involvement by local health department staff (Teen Health Corps Project, undated).

School-Based Youth Service Centers

Some school-based centers focus more on coordination and referral than on providing services in schools. Kentucky's major school reform initiative in 1988 called for the development of youth service centers in high schools that have more than 20 percent of their students eligible for free school meals. In this case, small grants (under $75,000) were given to school systems to set up a designated room in the school and to appoint a full-time coordinator to oversee referrals to community agencies for health and social services and to provide on-site counseling related to employment, substance abuse, and mental health.

In New York City, the Beacons Program, created by the city youth agency, supports community-based agencies to develop "lighted school houses" that are open from early morning until late at night, as well as on weekends and during the summer. These "Beacons" offer a wide range of activities depending on neighborhood needs; the activities include after-school recreation, educational remediation, community events, and health services. Grants are in the $300,000 range. Beacons were used as the prototype for the Family and Community Endeavors part of the 1994 Crime Bill, based on the belief that offering after-school activities in high-risk communities would help prevent delinquency.

Comprehensive Multicomponent Programs

A number of school-based interventions have been initiated that address an array of interrelated issues, based on the observation that prevention approaches must be more holistic if they are to be successful. Many of the components discussed above are integrated into these efforts. These programs are put together by an outside organization that provides a full-time coordinator and other services to the school in order to implement all the separate pieces of the package.

The Walbridge Caring Community (Missouri) is one of the most sophisticated models that includes many components and many agencies. An initiative of the Missouri Department of Mental Health, this effort brings together the St. Louis City Public Schools and the Danforth Foundation in a collaborative effort with the state's Departments of Health, Social Services, and Education (Mathtech and Policy Studies Associates, 1991). The center created in this program provides an array of intensive services to the children and families of the Walbridge Elementary School; the center is also open to other community residents. Services include family counseling, case management, substance abuse counseling, student assistance, parenting education, before- and after-school activities, youth programs, health screening, and pre-employment skills. The family counseling and case management component, directed at the families at highest risk, may involve a home therapist. Most of the funding for the intensive individual services (for 14 positions) is provided by the state's Department of Mental Health, while the Department of Social Services supports the after-school program (5 positions). Health services are provided by a school nurse, and the state's Department of Health supports the activities of a home health visitor and a clerical assistant. Funds from the Danforth Foundation and the state offices jointly support the director. One of the unique qualities of this program is its use of an Afrocentric concept in developing self-help, community empowerment, and rites-of-passage ceremonies.

The Schools of the Future Project is a large-scale foundation effort to help schools evolve into primary neighborhood institutions for promoting child and family development (Holtzman, 1992). The Texas-based Hogg Foundation for Mental Health is supporting major programs in four cities (Austin, Dallas, Houston, and San Antonio) by providing five-year grants of $50,000 per year to use elementary and middle schools as the locus of delivery of services. An equal amount of funding has been set aside for evaluation and monitoring. The foundation is interested in creating and testing an intervention that combines the latest models, including the Comer School Development Program, Zigler's Schools of the 21st Century, school-based clinics, programs for community renewal, and family preservation. Each program has a full-time project coordinator (a social worker) to establish links and partnerships between the schools and the providers of health and human services and to involve parents and teachers in program activities. For example, at San Antonio's three school sites, 11 graduate student interns were providing family, group, and individual therapy and 10 graduate social worker students were providing crisis intervention, home visits, and AFDC (Aid to Families with Dependent Children) and Food Stamp certifications, and were working with child protective services. Parent education, parent volunteer activities, after-school recreation, gang prevention programs, and other efforts were developed that involve many local organizations.

San Diego's New Beginnings is frequently cited as a model for providing integrated services in a nonfragmented services. Located in an inner city middle school, this program grew out of a partnership formed by the City (police, parks, recreation) and the County (health, social services, and probation) of San Diego, the school district, the community college, and the San Diego Housing Commission. These collaborators spent two years planning a school-based center to house a score of local agencies who were "expected to leave behind their parochial origins and become family service advocates" (Melaville and Blank, 1993). Workers relocated from the participant agencies (family service advocates) serve all families with children between the ages of 5 and 12 who attend that school. Services include case management; preventive health care, screening, and immunizations; drug, alcohol, and mental health treatment; adult education and school tutoring; and other community services as needed, such as day care, translation, transportation, and extended library and park hours. In order to link school and center staff, a Task Force was formed of administrative, clerical, and front-line workers to iron out the difficult process of changing roles and relationships. The New Beginnings model is being replicated in other communities and schools, with the stated mission being "a tearing down of barriers, a giving up of turf, and a new way of doing business."

Teen Parent Programs

Not so many years ago, schools were permitted to expel students who were pregnant. Since 1975, however, with the implementation Title IX of the Education Amendments, publicly supported educational programs have been prohibited from discriminating on the basis of pregnancy status. Schools are required to provide equal educational opportunities to pregnant teens and young parents, though not necessarily in the same building as the other students. In a number of communities, alternative schools for teen parents have been organized with funding from foundations and government grants. The model that has been used builds on concepts of comprehensive services, putting together an array of health services, social services, educational remediation, childcare components, and a lot of individual attention.

The New Futures School, Inc., in Albuquerque, New Mexico, is an alternative school run by the local school system in conjunction with a community-based organization (Goetz, 1992). It offers educational, health, counseling, vocational, and childcare services to pregnant adolescents and adolescent parents, including young fathers. Over the past 21 years, 5,000 parents have received services from this school. New Futures is one of four program models used as a basis for federal legislation on adolescent pregnancy and has been widely replicated throughout the United States. Its operating budget is about $1.1 million, 79 percent of which comes from the school system and the rest from state and federal grants and private sources.

The New Vistas High School is an alternative program for pregnant teens and teen mothers in the Minneapolis (Minnesota) public school system. The facility is located in the headquarters of the Honeywell Corporation (Rigden, 1992). The corporation provides the facility as well as funds for equipment and special projects, food, a staff liaison, and volunteers and mentors. The Minneapolis school system provides academic instruction and support services. Other corporations have donated computers and software. Health services are provided on-site by the Minneapolis Children's Medical Center and the Health Department. A fully equipped day care center is located next door and staffed by County Community Services, and a social worker is supported by the Big Brothers/Big Sisters organization.

School Reorganization

Many of the examples discussed so far are aimed at categorical problems: that is, they are single-component programs that attempt to prevent substance abuse, delinquency, teen pregnancy, or school dropout, or they are multicomponent programs that put together packages of health and social services. Yet many authorities believe that these separate programs serve only to "patch up" a few of a child's and a family's problems, and that what young people need in order to succeed requires making more sweeping changes in the way children are educated. In the educational domain, this means altering the ways in which children are taught and designing schools that are responsive to the needs of contemporary families and students. School quality is perceived as the ultimate intervention to ensure the long-term "health" of the child.

Several major authorities have emerged, each with a different view of what has to be done to change the environment in schools. None of these educational leaders is currently attached to a school system, but all of them are heavily involved in shaping school systems of the future through their academic centers. Henry Levin, of Stanford University, has proposed "accelerated schools" in reaction to the continuing failure of the schools to educate high-risk children. "The premises of the remediation approach are demonstrably false," according to Levin, "and the consequences are debilitating" (Colvin, 1988). Levin's group has initiated elementary school demonstration projects that are rich in curriculum content relevant to students' lives. The goal is to accelerate learning prior to sixth grade so that disadvantaged students catch up while they still can. Children are exposed to literature, problem-solving, and a range of cultural experiences, rather than simply being exposed to drill lessons. Techniques such as cooperative learning, peer tutoring, and community outreach are incorporated. Parents, staff, and students enter into contractual relationships that define the obligations of each party.

The School Development Program, a school-based management approach to making school a more productive environment for poor minority children, is an important example of how outside expertise can be utilized to influence the total school environment (Comer, 1984). This process, developed by James Comer from the Yale University Child Study

Center, has been implemented successfully in several inner city elementary schools in New Haven and is being replicated in at least 165 schools throughout the country. The program attempts to strengthen and redefine the relationships among principals, teachers, parents, and students. Representative management and governance is implemented through an elected School Advisory Council that includes the principal, teachers, teacher aides, and parents. A Mental Health Team that include the school psychologist and other support personnel provides direct services to children and advises school staff and parents. An innovative Parent Participation Program calls for a parent to work in each classroom on a part-time basis. In addition to serving as representatives to the Advisory Council, parents are encouraged to volunteer as teacher aides and librarians, publish newsletters, and organize social activities. A social skills curriculum has been developed that integrates the teaching of basic skills with the teaching of "mainstream" (middle-class) arts and social skills. According to Comer, the strength of this project is its focus on the entire school rather than on any one particular aspect and its attention to institutional rather than individual change. This is one of the few models that has successfully engaged parents in school programs.

Success for All is a demonstration program for elementary schools that was initiated by Robert Slavin and colleagues at the Johns Hopkins University Center for Research on Elementary and Middle Schools (Center for Research on Elementary and Middle Schools, 1989). The program restructures the entire school to do "everything" necessary to ensure that all students will be performing at grade level by the end of the third grade. Interventions include a half-day preschool and full-day kindergarten, a Family Support Team, an effective reading program, reading tutors, individual academic plans based on frequent assessments, a full-time program facilitator and coordinator, training and support for teachers, and a school advisory committee that meets weekly. The Family Support Team works full-time in each school and consists of social workers, attendance workers, and a parent-liaison worker. The team provides parenting education and support assistance for day-to-day problems, such as nutrition, getting glasses, attendance, and problem behaviors. Family Support Teams are responsible for developing linkages with community resources. Success for All is currently being replicated in seven schools in Baltimore and one school in Philadelphia. One program has a public health nurse practitioner who provides on-site medical care, while another school is connected with a family counseling agency that provides some school-based services. One Success for All school has worked with a community agency to have a food distribution center at the school, and another houses a clothes bank.

The Coalition of Essential Schools is a consortium of schools that have reorganized to incorporate the principles derived from the work of Theodore Sizer of Brown University (Sizer, 1984). Based on his experience studying American high schools, he has concluded that the most important task for schools is to teach students mastery of their school work. Sizer believes that it is more important for children to learn a few important ideas "deeply" than to be exposed to fragmented and ineffectual teaching. In a model Coalition school, Central Park East in New York City, Principal Deborah Meier intensely exposes students in grades 7 through 10 to a classical curriculum in the arts, sciences, and humanities. The last two years of high school serve as an "institute," with each student following individual program—such as courses in other places, field work, and projects. Teachers act as coaches and counselors for the students; each day begins with a meeting of an advisory group of 15 students, at which time any subject may be brought up and shared with other students.

Community or Full-Service Schools

In the past, the phrase "community school" has been applied mainly to adult education classes held in school buildings. The new generation of community schools begins to follow the broader construct of full-service schools and includes the integration of quality education with support services (see Table D-4). Several schools have been identified as potential models (IS 218, PS 5, and Children's Aid Society in New York City; Robertson and Hanshaw in Modesta, California; Farrell School System in Pennsylvania; Turner School in Philadelphia). What these community schools have in common are restructured academic programs integrated with parent involvement and services for parents; health centers and family resource rooms; after-school activities; cultural and community activities; and around-the-clock operation. Mental health services are provided by contract with community mental health agencies and by using interns from schools of social work. Each of these community schools is striving (in different ways) to become a village hub; by combining in joint efforts with community agencies to create as rich an environment as possible for children and their families.

IS 218, a middle school in Washington Heights, New York, was created through a partnership between the school system and the nonprofit Children's Aid Society (CAS) (Peder Zane, 1992). With this unique arrangement, CAS has created a "settlement house" in a school, located in a new building with air-conditioning for summer programs, outside lights on the playground, and an unusually attractive setting indicative of a different kind of school. It offers students a choice of five self-contained "academies": Business; Community Service; Expressive Arts; Ethics and

TABLE D-4 Full-Service Schools: One-Stop, Unfragmented
Collaborative Institutions

Quality Education Provided by Schools	Support Services Provided by Community Agencies
Effective basic skills	Primary health services
Individualized instruction	Health screening
Team teaching	Immunizations
Cooperative learning	Dental services
School-based management	Family planning
Healthy school climate	Individual counseling
Alternatives to tracking	Group counseling
Parent involvement	Substance abuse treatment
Effective discipline	Mental health services
	Nutrition or weight management
	Referral with follow-up
Services Provided by Schools or Community Agencies	Basic services: housing, food, clothes
	Recreation, sports, culture
	Mentoring
Comprehensive health education	Family welfare services
Health promotion	Parent education, literacy
Social skills training	Child care
Preparation for the world	Employment training or jobs
of work (life planning)	Case management
	Crisis intervention
	Community policing
	Legal aid
	Laundry

Law; or Mathematics, Science and Technology. The school opens at 7:00
a.m. for breakfast and classes in dance, Latin band, and sports, and stays
open after school for educational enrichment, mentoring, sports, computer lab, music, arts, trips, and entrepreneurial workshops. In the
evening, teenagers are welcome to use the sports and arts facilities and to
take classes along with adults who come for English, computer work,
parenting skills, and other workshops. A Family Resource Center provides parents with social services such as immigration, employment, and
housing consultations. Twenty-five mothers have been recruited to work
in the center as family advocates; they receive a small stipend for their
services. A primary health and dental clinic run by the Visiting Nurses
Association is also located in the lobby of the school. Services include
food and nutrition programs, health screening, dental care, treatment and
specialist referrals, drug and teen pregnancy prevention, immunization,
and developmental testing. School-supported and CAS-supported social

workers and mental health counselors work together to serve students and families. The school stays open weekends and summers, offering the Dominican community many opportunities for cultural enrichment and family participation. This full-service program adds about $1,000 per student to the budget (over and above the average amount of $6,500 spent in New York City). These additional costs are paid by Medicaid reimbursements and grants to the Children's Aid Society from foundations.

RESEARCH FINDINGS ON SCHOOL SERVICES MODELS

Research on the utilization of school-based health and social services has advanced well, and has documented the use of services by needy and high-risk youth. Conducting impact studies has been more problematic because of the difficulties of surveying, tracking, and establishing control groups for school populations (Gomby, 1993; Support Center for School-Based and School-Linked Health Care, 1995). Over the past decade, a few significant studies of school-based clinics have been conducted. Several recent summaries of these studies have confirmed the consistent finding that clinics could be implemented successfully in schools, enrolling substantial percentages of students (Dryfoos et al., in press; Kirby, 1994). Clinic users were reported to have received adequate care that was provided in a cost-effective manner and to be very satisfied with both the quality of the services and the caregivers.

Utilization Studies

This section focuses on studies that have been conducted since 1990. In general, the studies offer further evidence of high utilization rates.

Enrollment

A basic measure of program utilization is how many of the students in a school enroll in the clinic. Typically, enrollment involves the submission of a form indicating parental consent. Non-enrolled students can be treated for emergencies, but they must then go through the enrollment process. Clinics start out with low enrollments and gradually build over the years, with a high proportion of the students eventually signing up. A related measure is the percentage of enrollees who actually use the facility.

Advocates for Youth (AFY) reports that in 1993, about two-thirds of the students in respondent schools were enrolled in their school-based health centers and 75 percent of them utilized the program over the reporting year (Hauser-McKinney and Peak, 1995). A survey of 19 schools supported by the Robert Wood Johnson (RWJ) Foundation showed identical proportions (Kisker et al., 1994).

A study of a sample of students from nine Baltimore school-based clinics compared enrollees with non-enrollees and found that those who enrolled are significantly more likely to have had health problems, are in families receiving medical assistance (Medicaid), are in special education, and are African American. Those who did not enroll in the clinic reported a variety of reasons, primarily being satisfied with their current provider (Santelli et al., in press).

Client Characteristics

Among the respondents to the AFY survey, clinics reported that about 60 percent of enrolled students were female. One-third of the enrollees were African American, one-third white, 20 percent Latino, and the rest were Asian, Native-American, and other (Hauser-McKinney and Peak, 1995). Most reports show that although clinic users tend to mirror the student population in regard to race and ethnicity, females are more likely to use clinics (especially if reproductive health care is offered). However, the fact that 40 percent of the users are male is significant and demonstrates that when services are conveniently located, young men will use them.

Enrollees show very different patterns of use. In one school-based clinic in Los Angeles, within a one-year period, 5 percent of enrollees had made no visits, 41 percent had visited once, 39 percent had made two to five visits, 8 percent made six to ten visits, and 6 percent had used the clinic more than ten times (Adelman et al., 1993). Users reported ease of access as the most important reason for using the facility in the school, and they perceived the care provided as helpful and confidential. Nonusers stated that they did not use the clinic because they did not need it or they were concerned about lack of confidentiality. In this sample, frequent clinic users were more likely to score high on indices of psychological stress. The authors concluded that "an on-campus clinic can attract a significant number of students who otherwise would not have sought out or received such help."

Students who report higher rates of high-risk behaviors, such as substance abuse and early initiation of sexual intercourse, appear to be more likely than other students to use school-based clinics . A study of students in four schools in Oregon showed a consistent and significant association between number of clinic visits and number of preexisting high-risk health behaviors (Stout, 1991). Only one-third of those students who reported no risk behaviors used the clinics, as compared to more than two-thirds of the highest-risk students. Frequent users (three or more times) of School

Wellness Centers in Delaware were more likely than nonusers to report having engaged in such high-risk behaviors as suicide attempts, substance abuse, unprotected sexual activity, and eating-related purging (National Adolescent Health Resource Center, 1993).

Users of Denver's three high school clinics made an average of three visits per year (Wolk and Kaplan, 1993). However, a small number of students (11 percent) made 15 or more visits per year, accounting for 40 percent of all patient visits. These frequent visitors were significantly more likely to be females and to have lower grade point averages. Some 23 percent of the frequent visitors were diagnosed with mental health problems at the time of their initial visit, compared to 4 percent of the average users. By the end of the school year, 61 percent of all visits by frequent users were for mental health-related issues, compared to 10 percent of all visits by the average users. High-risk behaviors were significantly more prevalent among frequent users, particularly unprotected sexual activity and use of alcohol and drugs (but not tobacco). It is of some consequence that most of the frequent users initially presented acute medical problems, at which time they were identified as students in need of mental health counseling. Many practitioners believe that the provision of comprehensive services offers a means for troubled students to enter into counseling and treatment for psychosocial problems. Youth are concerned about the stigma of attending a program specifically labeled mental health.

Surveys in Florida schools with school-based services showed that students who engaged in high-risk behaviors were more likely to visit the health room than were other students. Students reported high levels of satisfaction with the program, as did school administrators and parents. "Principals seemed very accommodating [of school based health services staff] because their presence relieved other staff from dealing with students with various health needs: calling parents for pick up, delivering first aid, and at least in one site, delivering a baby in the school parking lot" (Eimhovich and Herrington, 1993).

The Robert Wood Johnson Foundation evaluation describes the characteristics of the population of students in schools with SBCHCs (rather than of students who used the clinics) (Kisker et al., 1994). In these 19 schools, 15 percent of students were non-Hispanic white, 44 percent were Hispanic, and one-third were African American. One-fourth of the youths stated that their parents had not completed high school and another third said their parents had no post-secondary education. One in five families was on welfare, and one-third received free or reduced-price school lunches. In the 1992 follow-up survey, 30 percent of the health center school students reported that their families had no health insurance, 20 percent were covered by Medicaid, 31 percent had private insurance or belonged to a health maintenance organization (HMO), and the remaining 19 percent did not know what type of coverage they had. As would be expected, health insurance coverage varied widely by school, ranging from 1 percent to 48 percent for families that had no coverage at all.

Brindis and coworkers (1995) found in a study of three urban schools that students with private insurance or HMO coverage had the highest rates of SBHC utilization (67 and 66 percent, respectively) and students without insurance or with Medicaid had the lowest (57 and 59 percent, respectively). Use of medical services did not differ by insurance status; however, clinic-enrolled students with Medicaid coverage were more likely to use SBHC mental health services than were others (30 percent compared to 22 percent).

Outcome Data

In the early 1980s, interest in incorporating school-based clinics as an important part of a strategy for pregnancy prevention was stimulated by the publication of data from St. Paul, Minnesota, that showed a decline in pregnancy rates in schools with clinics (Edwards et al., 1980). However, a later examination of birth rates showed that there were large year-to-year fluctuations and that the clinics had little or no impact (Kirby et al., 1993). In fact, a review of the earlier studies showed mixed results for an array of behavioral impact measures (Kirby, 1994). Studies that found positive effects on high-risk behaviors were offset by those that found negative effects or more likely, no effects. Recent studies also contain a mix of results.

Pregnancy-Related Outcomes

Pregnancy-related outcomes include delaying the onset of intercourse, consistent use of contraception among those who are sexually active, lower birth rates, and lower pregnancy rates. In general, studies have confirmed that the presence of a school-based clinic has no effect on the rate of sexual intercourse and has little effect on contraceptive use unless the clinic offers a pregnancy prevention program. A study of two schools with clinics that dispensed contraceptives on-site found few differences in contraceptive use compared to two schools where contraceptives were prescribed and not dispensed. The only significant variable related to use was the higher number of contacts that the students had with the clinic staff (Brindis et al., 1994).

When Florida created a Supplemental School Health Services Program, the legislation mandated evaluation to study how effectively the program met its objectives of pregnancy prevention and the promotion of student health (Emihovich and Herrington, 1993). The report on the first year, produced by Florida State University, was based on student surveys and site visits to 12 counties. All of the grantees had a designated health room in the school and the evaluation found heavy utilization rates, primarily for physical complaints, physical examinations, and minor injuries. The evaluation also stated that school-reported pregnancy rates had declined in some of the schools, but the data presented appeared to be estimates and were not validated. However, one comment from the report is interesting: "The most dramatic shift occurred at Glades Central High School in Palm Beach where the pregnancy rate dropped almost 73 percent. This project is also the only one where students can obtain prescriptions for contraceptives at the school and where there is a family practice physician available three days a week" (Emihovich and Herrington, 1993).

The first evaluation of the California Healthy Start initiative presents data on 40 different grantees, including eight youth service programs, five of which are school-based clinics. The report showed that adolescent clients of programs with the explicit goal of reducing teen pregnancy had significant reductions in the rate of initiation of sexually activity and an increase in the rate of reliable contraceptive use (Wagner et al., 1994). Among teenagers in pregnancy prevention programs, about 45 percent were sexually active at the end of the first six-month follow-up period, a significant 23 percent decrease from the proportion at intake (77 percent). Youth service programs showed large gains in linking clients to sources of health care.

An evaluation of the Teen Choice program showed that students were generally at high risk of pregnancy (Inwood House, 1987). In addition to demonstrating positive changes in knowledge and attitudes, participants were shown to have significantly improved their use of contraception following their group experiences and to have maintained these practices over time. Strengths of the program cited by the evaluators included that the program was convenient, students are respected, and although abstinence is encouraged, contraceptive use is recommended for those who choose not to abstain.

Other High-Risk Behaviors

At Lincoln High School in Denver, Colorado, a student who commits a drug offense can enter into a treatment contract for seven sessions at the school-based clinic rather than be suspended from the school. This component has resulted in an 80 percent reduction in suspensions (Bureau of Primary Health Care, 1993).

The Healthy Start data from California showed that in school-based youth programs aimed at reducing violence, a significant reduction in gang activity was reported at the six-month follow-up (from 7 to 2 percent) (Wagner et al., 1994).

The Student Assistance Program, a school-based substance abuse program, was evaluated by an outside contractor in the early years of the program (Moberg, 1988). The summary report stated that the program was very effective in preventing nonuser students from taking up alcohol and marijuana use and in reducing or stopping the prevalence among users. Alcohol users improved their attendance at school. There was some evidence that the larger the number of individual counseling sessions, the greater the success. No effect was shown for users of hard drugs. This evaluation did not include data from control schools.

Mental Health

The evaluation of California's Healthy Start clients included examining families as well as students. Six months after the initiation of the program, the proportion of core clients who reported some level of depression dropped from 28 to 22 percent, and when depression did occur, it was significantly less likely to be reported as a major problem at follow-up (32 versus 23 percent of those who were depressed) (Wagner et al., 1994).

Health System Related

Students attending the nine school-based clinics in Baltimore were compared with students in four matched schools in regard to their access to medical and social services and their hospitalizations and use of emergency rooms (Santelli et al., in press). Students in schools with health clinics were more likely to report seeing a social worker (11 percent) than were students in schools without clinics (8 percent). Those in schools with clinics were more likely to have received specific health services (physicals, acute health care, family planning, counseling) and reported significantly lower rates of hospitalization. In regard to use of emergency rooms, rates were reduced only for those students who had been enrolled in the schools with clinics for more than a year.

Decreases in the use of emergency rooms by students in schools with clinics were reported in San Francisco (from 12 to 4 percent over two years) and San Jose (from 9 to 4 percent). At the same time, significant increases were shown in the percentage of students who said that they were able to access health services when needed, presumably through the school-based clinics (Center for Reproductive Health and Policy Research, 1993). The school-based clinic in San Fernando, California, specifically targets students with little or no access to health care—93 percent of its enrollees report no other source of medical care and no health insurance (Bureau of Primary Health Care, 1993). A unique finding was the high level of use of mental health services in school-based clinics among students with HMO and private insurance. According to the Center for Reproductive Health and Policy Research (1993), the extensive use of the school clinic by students with other health care options "implies that the clinic is able to provide mental health services in a manner that is more acceptable to the adolescents, and that the integration of this service with a comprehensive array of health services may help diminish the stigma often associated with this kind of service . . . (it) may also reflect the relative unavailability . . . of these services as provided through HMO or private insurance coverage" (Center for Reproductive Health and Policy Research, 1993).

In a survey of 500 users of school-linked Teen Health Centers in Michigan, 21 percent of the respondents indicated that they would not have received health care if the centers did not exist (Anthony, 1991). The main reasons given were lack of transportation and lack of a family physician. Some 38 percent reported learning of new health problems during the visit (the problems included cancer symptoms, penicillin allergy, ear trouble, and high cholesterol), and 65 percent indicated that their behavior had changed as a result of their contact with the Teen Health Centers.

The RWJ evaluation found that students in schools with health centers received significantly more health care during the year before the follow-up survey and were more likely to have a usual place of health care than they would have if their health care use had followed the same pattern as that of urban youths nationally (Kisker et al., 1994). Students in schools with SBHCs reported greater increases in treatment for illnesses and injuries. Students who used the Healthy Start youth service programs reported significant gains in access to medical care and a marked improvement in having a regular source of care.

School-based health centers have been shown to identify students with serious physical or mental health problems. The survey of students in two Delaware schools with Wellness Centers in showed that during a year, center users were more likely than nonusers to have had physical exams (72 versus 55 percent) gynecological exams (24 versus 19 percent), psychological counseling (21 versus 14 percent), and eye exams (73 percent versus 60 percent). Little difference between users and nonusers was shown in whether they had their hearing checked or whether they had seen a health provider at least once (National Adolescent Health Resource Center, 1993). Users of the centers were more likely to have sought a health professional for advice about friends or family members. Students who did not use the centers reported that they had been healthy and did not need any services or had another source of care. Students who used the services cited convenience in scheduling, transportation, and confidentiality as their main reasons.

The recent focus on immunization suggests another important role for school-based clinics—the ability to respond rapidly to epidemics and crises in the health system. The New York State Department of Health recently created a pilot immunization project involving outreach efforts by three state-funded school health centers in New York City elementary schools (Bosker, 1992). Many immunizations were provided at low cost, not only to school children but also to their younger siblings. However, the highest-risk families failed to respond, which prompted the providers to recommend a better-orchestrated annual immunization campaign, more appropriate educational materials, and central coordination and support.

When the California Healthy Start evaluation looked at all clients, including adults, it found an increase from 19 to 26 percent in the number of core families who had children participating in the California Health and Disability Program within six months of enrolling in a Healthy Start intervention (Wagner et al., 1994). A reduction in health care due to illness or injury (from 36 to 29 percent) was also reported.

Parents at the Walbridge Caring Community school reported fewer problems with health care access. They also were more likely than parents in a comparison school to report that it was easy for students to get help with health problems (96 versus 59 percent) and that the school helped a lot with their own health care needs (47 versus 25 percent) (Philliber Research Associates, 1994).

School Related

Advocates of SBHCs assert that achievement and graduation rates should increase when health services are made accessible. Washington Senator Brock Adams claimed at a Senate hearing that a school clinic in Seattle's Ranier Beach High School "prevented 40 students from dropping out of school and significantly reduced the number of youth sent home from school" (Adams, 1992). In the San Fernando (California) High School, school-based clinic users were half as likely to drop out of school as were nonusers (9 versus 18 percent) (Bureau of Primary Health Care, 1993). A study of a clinic located in an alternative school and run by a health department is a unique example of an evaluation that focuses entirely on school performance (McCord et al., 1993). Students who used the clinic were twice as likely to stay in school and nearly twice as likely to graduate or be promoted than non-registered students. The more visits that students made to the clinic, the higher their graduation or promotion rates. The researchers found this relationship "particularly striking" among black males and attributed these successful outcomes to the trust and support provided by the clinic staff to help students function better in school.

Results from California's Healthy Start program showed that children who received intensive services in school-based programs made a significant improvement in grade point average, particularly among younger students and those who were performing least well before participating in the programs (Wagner et al., 1994). Teacher ratings of student behavior also improved significantly for those who received intensive services.

Evaluation of the Walbridge Caring Community program showed that students who received intensive services had a 27 percent increase in how their teacher rated their work habits, a 16 percent improvement in their social–emotional growth, and a 23 percent improvement in grade point average (Philliber Research Associates, 1994).

The Children's Aid Society reported "overwhelmingly positive results" after the first two years that IS 218 Community School had been opened: "student scores are up 15 points in both math and reading, attendance is the highest in the district; there has been no incidence of violence . . . [and] no destruction of property or even graffiti" (Children's Aid Society, 1994). At least 1,000 parents have been involved and the schools have become a central meeting place in the community.

The Partnership Center in Tama, Iowa, claims an increase in attendance and grade point averages as a result of its program, but the center cites no significant decreases in dropout rates (STC Partnership Center, 1994).

The study of school-based health programs in Florida showed a high percentage of students who were returned to class after being seen in the health room (Eimhovich and Herrington, 1993). Only 10 percent of elementary students and 18 percent of high school students were unable to return, much lower rates than those typically found in routine school nursing practices. In the Baltimore study, absenteeism because of illness was not significantly different between schools with SBHCs and other schools, where 51 percent of the sample of students reported having been absent in the past 30 days (Santelli et al., in press).

Although it is difficult to locate evaluations that specifically look at the effect of the provision of medical services on long-term outcomes, some success stories are emerging from an array of other kinds of school-based interventions. Several of the Success for All elementary schools in Baltimore that included Family Support Teams (social worker, school nurse, facilitator) and Integrated Human Services (on-site health clinic run by the health department or services from family counseling or mental health agency) showed significant improvements in attendance and reductions in the numbers of students retained (left back) to close to zero (Dolan and Haxby, 1992). A strong school-based case management program in Fresno, California, conducted in conjunction with the county department of social services, showed a 40 percent reduction in unexcused absences, a decrease of 70 percent in referrals for misbehavior, and a substantial increase in parental involvement (Center for Future of Children, 1992).

The Metropolitan Health Department of Nashville, Davidson County, Tennessee, reported that its One Stop Shopping Family Resource Center provided easier access to prenatal care, pediatric services, and school health (Maternal and Child Health Bureau, 1993). The immunization rate for enrolled 4- to 5-year-olds was 98 percent in 1993, and 150 families were in intensive case management.

Organizational Research

A few studies have been conducted to document the design and implementation of SBHCs. A unique survey of 90 clinics in 1991 focused on planning strategies and barriers to implementation (Rienzo, 1994). Key variables that influenced the capacity of SBHCs to offer comprehensive services (number of clinical and outreach services provided) included the presence of a strong coordinator, the use of information such as needs assessments for gaining support in the community, and obtaining funding from national sources, particularly foundations. The ideal coordinator was described as a "workaholic," with the ability to acquire funding and expertise in adolescent care. The more successful programs carefully organized planning committees and community advisory boards, and relied on committed school administrators to facilitate "navigation" through the approval process. Barriers to implementation included insufficient funding (66 percent) and problems with staff training and turnover (33 percent), issues that are related at least in part to the matter of funding. Many programs initially confronted organized opposition and dealt with controversy through public hearings. As a result, several changed their policies in regard to birth control and abortion counseling; birth control was limited in 28 percent of the cases and abortion counseling proscribed in 9 percent.

One study documented the importance of providing services on school property (school based) rather than nearby (school linked). A health center was removed from school grounds in Quincy, Florida, during the tenure of a conservative governor, who refused to allow public funds to be used for school-based clinics (Center for Human Services Policy and Administration, 1990). The level of service activity declined immediately, with a drop of 30 percent during the year, particularly among males and younger students. The largest decline (66 percent) was in students using the clinic for first aid. According to the staff, the implementation of more complicated, less private procedures for obtaining permission to visit the center during the school day tended to reinforce the negative effect of the relocation. Students had to go through the central office in order to leave the campus and walk across the street to the clinic. Almost the first act of the new governor, Lawton Chiles, in 1990 was to inform county officials of his intent to return the center to the school grounds. A new building was dedicated in early 1991 on the campus, and utilization immediately climbed back to its previous level.

The RWJ evaluation attempted to conduct a "dose–response" analysis to determine the effect of "stronger" health centers versus "weaker" ones. The 19 sites were scored on a composite index that included staffing, turnover, location, integration into school, and relationship to school establishment (Kisker et al., 1994). "Erratic results" were reported. Only a few significant findings were plausible: stronger SBHCs, particularly those that were well staffed, did produce higher enrollment and visit rates.

Research has shown that although the emerging school-based models—centers, community schools, clinics—have many differences, there are a number of common components of successful programs, as measured by utilization. Key factors include the following:

• School and community people join together to develop a shared vision of new institutional arrangements. Open communication is essential at every stage. The planning process starts with a needs assessment to ensure that the design is responsive to the requirements of the students and their families. An advisory board includes school and agency personnel, parents, and community leaders (and, in some places, students). Parental consent is required for receipt of services.

• The principal is instrumental in the implementation and smooth operation of school-based programs. Schools provide space, maintenance, and security. School doors are open before and after school, on weekends, and during the summer. Classrooms, gyms, playgrounds, music rooms, and computer facilities are open for community use.

• A special space is designated within the school as a center for individual and group counseling, parent education, career information, offices for case managers, kitchen, play space, clothes or food distribution, and arrangements for referrals. If primary health care is provided, adequate space is designated in or near a school for a medical clinic with examining rooms, a lab, an area for confidential counseling, and arrangements for recordkeeping and referrals.

- The configuration of services brought in by community agencies depends on what already exists in the school. School personnel have to participate in the process from the beginning.

- A full-time coordinator or program director runs the support services in conjunction with school and community agencies. Personnel are trained to be sensitive to issues related to youth development, cultural diversity, and community empowerment.

- Staff recruitment requires time and attention. It is difficult to locate certified youth workers with appropriate language skills (Spanish, Asian, etc.) in many areas.

- Parents are involved at many program levels, as users of services, volunteer aides, paid program workers, and advisory board members.

- A data system is in place, preferably a computerized management information system that can process records, update needs assessments, and be used for evaluation.

- The process of program development is greatly enhanced by the availability of technical assistance. State and foundation staffs have played a major role in extending these models, especially in rural areas.

- A designated space, such as a center in a school, acts as an anchor for bringing in other services from the community.

Cost–Benefit Studies

Several studies have estimated costs and benefits. One study estimated that if young people in New York State received early preventive care through school clinics, $327 million could be saved annually in hospitalizations for delivery of teen pregnancies, low-birthweight babies, and chronic diseases such as asthma (New York State Department of Health, 1994). A cost–benefit analysis of three California school-based clinics compared the costs for the school services with the estimated cost in the absence of the school clinic (Center for Reproductive Health and Policy Research, 1993). Variables used included reduced emergency room use, pregnancies avoided, early pregnancy detection, and detection and treatment of chlamydia, a prevalent sexually transmitted disease. The ratios of savings to costs ranged from $1.38 to $2.00 in savings per $1.00 in costs, suggesting that the school clinic services were a good investment for the health system.

Igoe and Giordano (1992) reported that "cumulative evidence over the past decade shows that nurses have delivered cost-effective care (in school clinics) that can be substituted for physician's services in many situations (with) outcomes as good as or better than those physicians achieve in primary care—and at lower cost."

DISCUSSION

What's Going on Here?

This paper has reviewed a number of examples of service delivery arrangements that bring health, mental health, and social services to young people in schools. Preliminary research on utilization and outcomes has been summarized, showing great gains in access for high-risk students but only scattered returns in regard to outcomes. During the past decade, we have clearly experienced a significant movement of personnel into schools from outside agencies to assist the schools' personnel in dealing with growing demands for services. The new programs appear to be more complex, creative, and innovative than in the recent past. Many of the new interventions are based on contemporary research on child and adolescent behaviors, and they represent an attempt to design more effective programs. As a result, school-based efforts are more comprehensive and holistic, and are framed to approach the total needs of the child and the family in the context of the community. Many components have been put together that have proven impact in the prevention field; these components include individual attention, sustained attention, respect for confidentiality, and outreach and home visiting to involve parents (Dryfoos, 1990).

What's Driving All This Activity?

Why the accelerated movement toward comprehensive school-based services? The plight of young people growing up in inner cities or poor rural areas has been well documented. The "new social morbidities"—such adverse effects of the modern age as unsafe sex, drugs, violence, depression, and stress—account for a vast number of youth who will never make it without immediate intervention. These disadvantaged young people live in run-down, resource-poor communities; attend decaying schools; lack nurturing and caring; and cannot overcome the odds unless they receive substantial assistance. Many observers maintain that the existing systems for providing services to disadvantaged families and their children are fragmented and ineffective. Both the human services agencies and the educational system are called upon to respond to these social deficiencies. Thus, the rationale for creating new kinds of institutional arrangements crosses several domains: health, education, and social services integration. Consensus is building among educators about the importance of bringing support services into schools that will strengthen their efforts at restructuring. Service integration—the establishment of linkages between agencies—is a "hardy perennial" that reappears whenever there are a plethora of categorical programs and over-whelming needs, but little new money to address the problem. The subject is of interest to advocates of school-based programs because of the necessity for welding together fragmented health and social service agencies with educational systems. This is often a challenging experience because of the fragmentation that has resulted from the development of specialized programs to address each category of need as it gains visibility in a very competitive funding and media environment.

The fact that these categorical programs have only limited and short-term effects has fed the demand for "integration" of services, reducing the fragmentation of existing service systems for families. Many of the new "family-centered" programs are being placed in schools to facilitate one-stop-shopping for whatever families and their children need to overcome the enormous odds with which they are confronted in disadvantaged communities. Much of the service integration rhetoric calls for "systems changes," new ways of organizing administrative structures so they will be more responsive to consumers. In this literature, considerable attention is being directed toward the involvement of the community and the importance of a sense of "ownership" by parents and other residents, which recalls the language of the community action programs of the 1960s.

Issues in the Development of
Comprehensive School-Based Programs

Funding

Much of the impetus for school-based centers and community-schools has come from state initiatives and foundation demonstration projects. Although the current federal administration has evidenced an interest in adolescent health issues, educational restructuring, and service integration, all that has come through in the way of tangible support for direct services has been a new small grants program in the Bureau of Primary Health Care, along with some new funds for training in the Bureau of Maternal and Child Health. For the first time, about $3 million in grants has been awarded to 27 new school-based clinics around the country. In what some observers see as an era of budget cutting, we cannot anticipate much new action at the federal level, even though the concept of full-service schools has emerged in many different domains, including health reform, revision of Chapter 1 (now Title 1, support for schools with high numbers of disadvantaged youth), welfare reform, crime prevention, and positive youth development.

Until the law changes, all state Medicaid programs were required to cover hospitalization, physician services, laboratory and x-ray services, family planning, and Early and Periodic Screening, Diagnostic, and Treatment services for children under age 21. The EPSDT component of Medicaid was originally designed to provide comprehensive health screening for poor children, as well as subsequent diagnosis and treatment services for conditions found during the screening exams. Comprehensive screening included not only basic health, vision, hearing, and dental components but "anticipatory guidance" that could include counseling services, case management, and health prevention. Although federal law mandated EPSDT services for Medicaid-eligible children and adolescents, states have not provided sufficient outreach and follow-up to ensure that those eligible are actually screened.

The potential of EPSDT as a funding source for school-based services is ambiguous. Currently, Medicaid enrollees are being required to obtain coverage through managed care. Many HMOs and other managed care providers may not include preventive services, mental health services, and health screening as part of the package. In some places, school health service providers may have to negotiate with multiple plans for students in their schools. As Brindis (1995) points out, there are "conflicting priorities of SBHCs which seek to increase access to care and . . . managed care programs which must find ways to contain costs." Many other barriers stand between SBHCs and this form of health financing, not the least of which is the assurance of confidentiality. One proposal has been to create "school health resource partnerships" between districts, health providers, and other community agencies to address the financial viability of school health service programs in a managed care environment (Brellochs, 1995). States would require that managed care plans participate as a condition of licensure.

The recent revision of Chapter 1 will make it possible for schools to use some of the funds for social services in partnerships with community agencies. The various crime bills called for many millions for Beacon-type programs, but those funds have disappeared. Finally, the Division of Adolescent and School Health (DASH) at the Centers for Disease Control Prevention (CDC) is supporting many state and local HIV prevention initiatives, and recently began funding 12 states to strengthen their offices of health and education to provide more comprehensive school health services and health education.

In some states, including Florida, California, and Kentucky, competitive grants have been awarded to school districts that must then seek partners in collaboration. In other states, such as New Jersey, a community-based agency may be the lead grantee and seek partnerships with a school. More than $30 million is being spent each year in Florida on the state's innovative full-service schools program, supporting collaborative school-based projects of varying service mixes, including family resource centers, case management, recreational programs, and school-based clinics. The expectation is that all schools will participate in this program in a few years and that child care, vocational education, and mental health services will gradually be phased in.

California's Healthy Start Support Services for Children Act was launched in 1991 with high ideals: "to be a catalyst in a revolution that will fundamentally change for the better the way organizations work together, the way resources are allocated for children and families, the nature and location of services provided, and ultimately, the outcomes experienced by children and families" (Wagner et al., 1994). The $20 million initiative directly funds 40 service projects and 200 planning projects. School districts have created four types of collaborative programs: school site family resource centers, satellite school-linked family service centers, family service coordination teams involving school personnel with project staff, and youth service programs that include school-based clinics. Since 1987, New Jersey's Department of Human Resources has committed more than $6 million annually for its School-Based Youth Services Program.

Foundations have played an important role in creating demonstration projects of many descriptions. In 1987, the Robert Wood Johnson Foundation awarded grants to launch health centers in 24 schools; building on that experience, RWJ has created the Making the Grade initiative, supporting 10 states to create state-level offices for school-based services and model clinics in local school districts. The Carnegie Corporation is supporting states in its Turning Point initiative to help middle schools link students to comprehensive health and social services as one component of middle school reorganization. The Hogg Foundation for Mental Health has been instrumental in creating the Schools of the Future, changing schools into primary neighborhood institutions for promoting child and family development, building on the Comer School Development Program, Zigler's Schools of the 21st Century, school-based clinics, programs for community renewal, and family preservation.

Funding is definitely a major issue in the future development of school-based services. My own estimates call for 16,000 schools to be "full serviced" within the near future (Dryfoos, 1994a). This encompasses one in five schools in the nation, including all of those in which more than half of the students are eligible for free lunches. If start-up costs of $100,000 to $200,000 per school are assumed, the amount of money needed to replicate these models is around $1.6 to $3.2 billion per year, about the same amount being spent for Head Start and half of the appropriation for Chapter 1.

The advent of managed care greatly complicates the fiscal arrangements for providing on-site health care in schools, but practitioners are working hard to overcome the bureaucratic and policy barriers to using managed care contracts to fund these programs. Although financing is a barrier to the expansion of full-service schools, it is not the only hurdle faced by program developers. Other factors such as governance, turf, responsiveness to the community, staffing and training, and controversy must also be addressed.

Governance

Much of the rhetoric in support of developing health and social services in schools has been presented in the language of systems change, calling for radical reform of the way educational, health, and welfare agencies provide services (Knitzer, 1989; Melaville and Blank, 1993). Consensus has formed around the goals of one-stop, seamless, service provision, whether in a school or in a community-based agency, along with empowerment of the "target population." A review of current models reveals that little systems change has taken effect. Most of the new wave of programs have moved services from one place to another; for example, a medical unit from a hospital or health department relocates into a school through a contractual arrangement, or staff of a community mental health center is reassigned to a school, or a grant to a school creates a coordinator in a center. As the program expands, the center staff work with the school to draw in additional services, fostering more contracts between the schools and community agencies. Yet few of the school systems or the agencies have changed their governance. The outside agency is not involved in school restructuring or school policy, nor is the school system involved in the governance of the provider agency. Partners—schools and community agencies—have agreed on goals and signed contracts or memoranda of understanding that leave the status quo of the organizations entirely intact. The agreements may specify policies regarding fiscal responsibility, client–student data collection, confidentiality, and other administrative issues.

The first evaluation of New Beginnings in San Diego, a multiagency program that operates a family resource center in Hamilton School, warns that it is "difficult to overestimate the amount of time collaboration takes" (Barfield et al., 1994). The participants discovered that it was easier to get agencies to make "deals" (sign contracts to relocate workers) than to achieve major changes in delivery systems. Staff turnover, family mobility, fiscal problems, and personality issues were cited as some of the barriers to change. Most school-based health centers are funded by grants made directly from state health departments to local health agencies, which then contract with school systems to provide services. This is a matter of policy for some state health departments and foundations, which believe that the school system should not be burdened with the responsibility for providing primary health and social services to the students. At the same time, the local education agencies are the grant recipients for the largest state programs (California, Florida, and Kentucky), and these systems may either provide services themselves or, more typically, contract them out.

Although few school services models have been able to overcome the barriers to the formation of new kinds of governance, this should not be perceived as a deterrent to further service integration efforts. Past attempts at systems reform have shown that it is much more difficult to alter the way in which entrenched administrators operate across agencies than it is to make incremental changes in the existing systems they run. The movement toward service integration as exemplified in full-service schools has clearly had an effect on cutting red tape in some programs, but practitioners are still confronted with the conflicting eligibility criteria and restrictions that go along with categorical programs.

Turf

Bringing outside health or social services into a school building under the auspices of an outside agency is an invitation to turf wars. Two or more different staffs operate under separate jurisdictions in terms of unions, policies, pay schedules, hours of work, and direction. Without careful planning and negotiation, the school staff can be very threatened by the appearance of a new group of workers. School nurses have been particularly vulnerable because they feel replaced by a differently trained nurse (nurse practitioner), who is allowed to conduct complete physical examinations, prescribe and administer medication, suture wounds, and perform other hands-on activities. However, school social workers, psychologists, and guidance counselors often have similar initial negative responses. Who is responsible for the children and their families? Some teachers oppose school-based services if students leave their classes for clinic appointments. Custodians resent keeping buildings open so families can use them. A significant area for potential conflict is discipline. The school has its own practices, such as suspension and other forms of punishment, that may be antithetic to the ethos of the newcomers.

Competition between community agencies can also arise in the development of full-service schools. Agencies begin vying for scarce resources when states or foundations issue requests for proposals (RFPs) that call for proposals that stress collaboration. Who represents the "community"?

One key to successfully overcoming these situations appears to be a sensitive principal who, right from the planning stage, involves his school personnel along with outside personnel in creating a team approach. Serious and ongoing in-service training involving both the existing staff and the staff of the outside agency will be needed to negotiate areas of tension and to learn to understand where each side is "coming from." Experience shows that within a short period of time, most schools find more than enough crises to go around. School personnel become major supporters of school-based services when attendance improves and behavioral problems are addressed by practitioners. For their part, practitioners come to recognize how difficult it is to maintain order in today's schools.

Initial planning that anticipates school–agency friction is more successful. In a new elementary school in Bridgeport, Connecticut, which has a built-in public health department-sponsored clinic, the school nurse (paid school funds) was placed in the central position in the clinic as traffic director, to screen all students and direct them to the appropriate clinic staff member—nurse practitioner, dentist, outreach worker, or counselor. In restructured middle schools, outside social workers have been assigned to houses or academies, in keeping with the new design of the school. Clinic coordinators from around the country report that when the principal expresses ownership and refers to "my clinic," the staff know that they have it made.

School-Based Versus Community-Based

Questions have also been raised about placing the locus of full-service programs in schools in communities that are distrustful of the educational establishment (Chaskin and Richman, 1992). In some locations, community leaders feel that the school systems are so resistant to change that the leaders have little confidence that the quality education component of the full-service vision will ever materialize. Human resource planners have proposed an alternative model that places services in buildings run by community-based organizations, in which families feel comfortable and are assured of greater roles in decisionmaking. This service integration theory still holds, but the locus of services is placed firmly in the neighborhood, with the services operated directly under local control. The school board has no place in this model, obviating the difficult negotiations that can be stressful and time-consuming. Michigan's experience with its 19 teen health centers (11 school based or school linked and 8 in the community) suggested that community-based centers had greater flexibility, especially in regard to the provision of family planning; could more easily ensure confidentiality; could serve more dropouts; were free to set their own parental consent protocols; and avoided the (unfounded) suspicion that school funds were being used for nonacademic services. However, the school-based centers were found to have reduced the necessity for outreach; they more readily involved school personnel, could serve students on-site, were perceived to have more direct access to teens;

were more likely to obtain foundation support; took on the function of health promotion in the schools; and were able to garner in-kind resources from the school system, such as space, maintenance, utilities, and supplies.

Concern has been raised about the viability of full-service schools as sites for dealing with young people who no longer attend school. Some of the existing school-based centers do serve out-of-school youth as well as siblings and parents of current students. Others do not. For two major youth-serving organizations in New York City (El Puente and the Door), the transformation into full-service schools started with community organizations that added basic educational components to their rosters of services and obtained certification as part of the public school system. This community youth center–school model offers an approach for working with school dropouts who are often youth agency clients. The disaffected youth are drawn back into the school system through the efforts of trusted youth service agency staff.

Transportation

Program reviews in both Florida and Kentucky cited transportation as a major issue for people who used their centers. Those who relied on school-linked services found that referrals to community agencies were not carried out because the students and families were not able to get to those places. School-based models that were open after school hours or wanted to bring parents into school during school hours also encountered transportation problems. School buses are usually run by contractors with inflexible schedules. Few programs have the necessary resources to offer van service to families, particularly those that live in outlying rural areas.

Issues such as transportation can be dealt with through the planning process. School systems may be willing to alter contracts with bus companies or negotiate with their own bus driver unions to schedule bus runs for the convenience of the families rather than the convenience of the system. Buses can be scheduled for late afternoons, evenings, and weekends. In many places, the precedent exists if the destination involves a competitive athletic event.

Staffing and Training

If programs are already experiencing difficulty hiring nurse practitioners and social workers, where will the staff for 16,000 full-service schools come from? If the concept catches on and schools are seen as the locus for new kinds of institutional arrangements that cut across categorical lines, almost every category of professional worker will need to be retrained and new professionals will need to be cross-trained. Educators will have to better understand youth and family development issues, become more culturally sensitive, and further master their own specialties. Human service workers will have to learn how to function in schools and understand the culture of educational institutions. New types of coordinators and directors for school-based services will have to be able to interrelate with both schools and community agencies and help everyone bridge the gap. In addition, they will need strong fiscal management skills to handle the complexities that go along with multiple funding sources and accountability.

Even when staff can be identified, turnover rates are often high. Working with disadvantaged children and families is labor intensive and can lead to burn out if the management does not address personnel issues with care and grace. In addition, practitioners in some areas report that the greatest difficulty is recruiting trained professionals who are bilingual.

The need for appropriately trained personnel stands as a major barrier to replication. This issue is already being addressed on a small scale in a few university settings, where there are efforts to change curricular offerings and coordinate master's level requirements. The major professional organizations for pupil personnel services (school nurses, school psychologists, school social workers, guidance counselors) are already working together to define the roles of their constituencies in new program models.

Controversy

It has been observed that the phrase "school-based clinic" is like a red flag for those waiting to raise community tensions over sexuality issues. The most highly publicized school-based health programs in the early 1980s were heralded as pregnancy prevention programs, leading to attacks from the opposition that schools were opening "sex clinics" and "abortion mills." When later replications of these models were shown to have little effect on pregnancy rates because they did not include family planning services, the attack shifted and the opposition organized against bringing any kind of services into school buildings, even elementary schools. For example, at the time that the Kentucky Youth and Family Centers were first proposed, the Eagle Forum put out brochures referring to the proponents as "child snatchers."

In reality, few programs have been stopped in their tracks because of organized opposition. Accounts of these events are elucidating. Parents invariably surface as the most articulate and credible advocates for school-based services. National and local polls have documented the high level of support for these concepts. The 1992 Gallup Poll reported that 77 percent of respondents favored using public school buildings in their communities to provide health and social services to students, administered and coordinated by various government agencies. A majority of respondents (68 percent) approved of condom distribution in their local public schools, although one in four of them would require parental consent (Elam et al., 1992). A 1993 sample survey of North Carolina registered voters showed that 73 percent believed that health care centers offering prevention services should be located at high schools. There were no differences by gender, religion, or parental status, although the strongest support came from African Americans between the ages of 18 and 34. More than 60 percent favored providing birth control at the centers.

Many state programs were authorized by legislation that prohibited the distribution of contraceptives and referral for abortions on school premises. Other "comprehensive" programs developed during the school–community planning process omitted the distribution of birth control, suggesting that the expectation of controversy has a cooling effect on service provision. State officials have also been articulate on these issues. When Joycelyn Elders (former Surgeon General of the United States) was Director of Health in Arkansas, she strongly supported the concept of school-based services, always emphasizing that the decision about how to provide family planning was strictly up to the local school and community. Several local school boards voted to provide contraception when given the option. In recent years, school systems have been changing such policies to allow the distribution of condoms in schools, as long as parents do not object. Typically, the local health department comes into the school to hand out the condoms, relieving the school system of the responsibility.

State initiatives offering grants to communities that develop collaborative projects have engendered some negative responses from local practitioners. One group of representatives from a remote rural area expressed concern about "Big Brother." The group did not want the state to tell its members how to organize services in their community. It feared that a school-based collaborative project that placed social services along with health and child protective services might "inflict help" on people who didn't want it. Concern was expressed that one-stop services might make families more dependent, rather than empowering them to act for themselves. In some communities, objections have been raised to the provision of mental health services and substance abuse counseling in the schools because they are too "personal."

Experience across the nation has shown that the response to requests for proposals from state governments and foundations has been overwhelming. Fear of controversy appears to be secondary to the need for support for innovative services in schools. The media could play a more positive role in emphasizing the comprehensive scope of full-service schools and their potential to create better institutions for children and families.

Too Little, Too Late

Perhaps the most powerful argument that can be made, however, is that all of this program development will not make much difference in the lives of disadvantaged youth. Many very troubled young people, no matter what goes on behind the schoolhouse door, must still return to dangerous households or the streets after school. Few would quarrel with the point that early intervention is essential, but this should not be used as a justification for ignoring the millions of teenagers who can still be assisted. At the same time, in communities with school-based services, attention is turning toward the development of more sites in elementary schools. The preferred arrangement is the "cluster," tracking youngsters from kindergarten (or even preschool) through high school and providing related support services at each school along the way. In the new RWJ initiative, states are being asked to support school districts with the capacity for creating district-wide plans for comprehensive school-based health and social services.

The development of new forms of organizational arrangements to enhance delivery systems and improve educational experiences is an optimistic enterprise. It represents the aggregate energies of hundreds of practitioners, youth workers, educators, and advocates who plow ahead despite the obstacles to try to create more responsive institutions for the twenty-first century. Indisputably, the budget crisis is having a cooling effect. Yet this movement will continue to expand because it fits with the times, is certainly needed, uses resources rationally, puts significant program components together, and is enthusiastically supported by both the consumers and the providers.

REFERENCES

Adams, B. (Senator) 1992. Washington in helping America's youth in crisis. Testimony presented at Hearing of the Committee on Labor and Human Resources, U.S. Senate, Washington, D.C. July 28.

Adelman, H., and Taylor, L. 1991. Mental health facets of the school-based health center movement: Need and opportunity for research and development." *Journal of Mental Health Administration* 18:272–283.

Adelman, H., Barker, L., and Nelson, P. 1993. A study of a school-based clinic: Who uses it and who doesn't? *Journal of Clinical Child Psychology* 22(I):52–59.

Anthony D. 1991. Michigan Department of Public Health: Remarks to support center for school-based clinics annual meeting, Dearborn, Michigan, October.

Barfield, D., Brindis, C., Guthrie, L., McDonald, W., Philliber, S., and Scott, B. 1994. The evaluation of New Beginnings. First Report. San Francisco: Far West Laboratory.

Bosker, I. 1992. A school-based clinic immunization outreach project targeting measles in New York City. Paper presented at the Annual Meeting of the American Public Health Association, Washington, D.C., November.

Brellochs, C. 1995. School health services in the United States: A 100-year tradition and a place for innovation. Paper prepared by the School Health Policy Initiative, Montefiore Medical Center, N.Y.

Brindis, C., Kapphanhn, C., McCarter, V., and Wolfe, A. 1995. The impact of health insurance status on adolescents' utilization of school-based clinic services: Implications for health reform. *Journal of Adolescent Health Care* 16:18–25.

Brindis, C., Starbuck-Morales, S., Wolfe, A.L., and McCarter V. 1994. Characteristics associated with contraceptive use among adolescent females in school-based family planning program. *Family Planning Perspectives* 26:160–164.

Brindis, C. 1995. Promising approaches for adolescent reproductive health service delivery: The role of school-based health centers in a managed care environment. *Western Journal of Medicine* 163(Suppl.):50–56.

Bureau of Primary Health Care. 1993. *School-Based Clinics That Work.* Washington D.C.: Division of Special Populations, Health Resources and Services Administration, HRSA 93-248P.

Center for the Future of Children. 1992. *The Future of Children: School Linked Services* 2(1), Appendix A.

Center for Human Services Policy and Administration. 1990. Shanks Health Center Evaluation. Final report: Third year of program operation. Tallahassee: Florida State University.

Center for Reproductive Health and Policy Research. 1993. Annual Report to the Carnegie Corporation of New York and the Stuart Foundations: July 1, 1991–June 3, 1992. San Francisco: Institute for Health Policy Studies, University of California.

Center for Research on Elementary and Middle Schools. 1989. *Success for All.* CREMS Report. Baltimore: Johns Hopkins University.

Chaskin, R., and Richman, H. 1992. Concerns about school-linked services: Institution-based versus community-based models. *The Future of Children: School Linked Services.* 2(1):107–117.

Children's Aid Society. 1994. Handout prepared for the Invitational Conference of the U.S. Department of Education and the American Educational Research Association: School-linked comprehensive services for children and families, Leesburg, Va., September 28 to October 2.

Cities in Schools. 1988. "Fact sheet" and "Questions about cities in schools." Washington D.C.: Cities in Schools.

Colvin, R. 1988. California researchers "accelerate" activities to replace remediation. *Education Week* November 30.

Comer, J. 1984. Improving American education: Roles for Parents. Hearing before the Select Committee on Children Youth and Families, June 7. Washington D.C.: U.S. Government Printing Office.

Dolan, L., and Haxby, A. 1992. The role of family support and integrated human services in achieving success for all in the elementary school. Baltimore: Johns Hopkins University, Center for Research on Effective Schooling for Disadvantaged Students. Report No. 31, April.

Dryfoos, J. 1990. *Adolescents-at-Risk: Prevalence and Prevention.* New York: Oxford University Press.

Dryfoos, J. 1994a. *Full-Service Schools: A Revolution in Health and Social Services for Children, Youth, and Families.* San Francisco: Jossey-Bass.

Dryfoos J. 1994b. Medical clinics in junior high school: Changing the model to meet demands. *Journal of Adolescent Health* 15(7):549–557.

Dryfoos, J. 1994c. School-linked comprehensive services for adolescents. Paper commissioned for the Invitational Conference of the U.S. Department of Education and the American Educational Research Association: School-linked comprehensive services for children and families, Leesburg, Va., September 28 to October 2.

Dryfoos, J., Brindis, C., and Kaplan, D. In press. Research and evaluation in school-based health care. In *Health Care in Schools, A Special Edition of Adolescent Medicine: State of the Art Reviews,* ed. L. Juszak and M. Fisher.

Edwards, L.E., Steinman, M.E., Arnold, K.A., and Hakanson, E.Y. 1980. Adolescent pregnancy prevention services in high school clinics. *Family Planning Perspectives* 12(1):7.

Elam, S., Rose, L., and Gallup, A. 1992. The 24th Annual Gallup/Phi Delta Kappa Poll of the public's attitudes toward the public schools. *Phi Delta Kappan* (Sept. 1992): 41–53.

Eimhovich, C., and Herrington, C.D. 1993. Florida's Supplemental School Health Services Projects: An evaluation. Tallahassee: Florida State University.

Goetz, K., ed. 1992. *Programs to Strengthen Families: a Resource Guide.* 3rd ed. Chicago: Family Resource Coalition.

Gomby, D.S. 1993. Basics of program evaluation for school-linked service initiatives. Working Paper No. 1932. Los Altos, Calif. David and Lucille Packard Foundation, Center for the Future of Children, February.

Hauser-McKinney, D., and Peak, G. 1995. Update 1994. Washington D.C..: Advocates for Youth, Support Center for School-Based and School-Linked Health Care.

Holtzman, W. ed. 1992. *School of the Future.* Austin, Tex.: American Psychological Association and Hogg Foundation for Mental Health.

Igoe, J., and Giordano, B. 1992. *Expanding School Health Services to Serve Families in the 21st Century.* Washington D.C.: American Nurses Publishing.

Illback, R. 1993. Formative evaluation of the Kentucky Family Resource and Youth Service Centers: A descriptive analysis of program trends. Louisville: REACH of Louisville.

Inwood House. 1987. Community outreach program: Teen choice. A model program addressing the problem of teenage pregnancy. Summary report.

Kagan, S.L. 1991. *United We Stand: Collaboration for Child Care and Early Education Services.* New York: Teachers College Press.

Kirby, D. 1994. Findings from other studies of school-based clinics. Presentation given at meeting on evaluation sponsored by the Robert Wood Johnson Foundation, Washington, D.C., September 23.

Kirby, D., Resnick, M.D., and Downes, B. 1993. The effects of school-based health clinics in St. Paul on school-wide birth rates. *Family Planning Perspectives* 25:12–16.

Kisker, E.E., Brown, R.S., and Hill, J. 1994. *Healthy Caring: Outcomes of the Robert Wood Johnson Foundations's School-Based Adolescent Health Care Program.* Princeton, N.J.: Mathematica Policy Research.

Knitzer, J. 1989. *Collaborations Between Child Welfare and Mental Health: Emerging Patterns and Challenges.* New York: Bank Street College of Education.

Lear, J., Gleicher, H., and St. Germaine, A. 1991. Reorganizing health care for adolescents: The experience of the School-Based Adolescent Health Care program. *Journal of Adolescent Health* 12(6): 450–458.

Leonard, W. 1992. Keeping kids in school. *Focus* (June 4-5).

Maternal and Child Health Bureau (MCH). 1993. Briefing sheet from 1993 Urban MCH Leadership Conference Profile. Washington, D.C.

Mathtech and Policy Studies Associates. 1991. Selected collaborations in service integration. Report for the U.S. Department of Education and U.S. Department of Health and Human Services, ED Contract LC89089001, February.

McCord, M.D., Klein, J.D., Foy, J.M., and Fothergill, K. 1993. School-based clinic use and school performance. *Journal of Adolescent Health* 14:91–98.

Melaville, A.I., and Blank, M.J. 1993. *Together We Can: A Guide for Crafting a Profamily System of Education and Human Services.* Washington, D.C.: U.S. Government Printing Office.

Moberg, D. 1988. Evaluation results for a student assistance program. Paper presented at Annual Meeting of the American Public Health Association, Boston, Mass., November 14.

Moore, B. 1992. Maternal and Child Health Nursing Supervisor, Catawba County Health Department. Interview, March.

National Adolescent Health Resource Center. 1993. Evaluative review: Findings from a study of selected high school wellness centers in Delaware. University of Minnesota, Division of General Pediatrics and Adolescent Health.

National Alliance of Pupil Services Organizations. 1992. Mission Statement. Washington, D.C.: National Alliance of Pupil Services Organizations, December.

National Institute on Alcohol Abuse and Alcoholism. 1984. *Prevention Plus: Involving Schools, Parents, and the Community in Alcohol and Drug Education.* Washington, D.C.: U.S. Department of Health and Human Services.

New York State Department of Health. 1994. Unpublished data from School Health Division. Albany, N.Y.

Peder Zane, J. 1992. Teacher, doctor, counselor in one. *New York Times,* February 26, p. B-1.

Philliber Research Associates. 1994. An evaluation of the caring communities program at Walbridge Elementary School. Accord, N.Y.

Pinal County Human Services. 1990. Pinal County Prevention Partnership, Year End Report FY 1988–1989. Pinal County, Ariz.

Poehlman, B. 1992. Comprehensive School Health Programs Project, National School Boards Association. Alexandria, Va.: National School Boards Association.

Reynolds, G. Undated. Director of the School Based Youth Services Program, New Brunswick Public Schools. Visits to program and discussion with director.

Rienzo, B.A. 1994. Factors in the successful establishment of school-based clinics. *Clearinghouse* 67(6):356–362.

Rigden, D. 1992. *Business and the Schools: A Guide to Effective Programs.* 2nd ed. New York: Council for Aid to Education.

Santelli, J., Kouzis, A., and Newcomer, S. In press. Adolescent student attitudes toward school-based health centers. *Journal of Adolescent Health.*

Sizer, T. 1984. *Horace's Compromise.* Boston: Houghton-Mifflin.

Small, M.L., Majer, L.S., Allensworth, D.D., Farquahar, B.F., Kann, L., and Pateman, B.C. 1995. School health services. *Journal of School Health* 65(8):319–326.

State of Maryland. 1994. Report to the Subcabinet for Children, Youth, and Families from the School-Based/School-Linked Services Committee, May 12.

STC Partnership Center. 1994. Handout prepared for the Invitational Conference of the U.S. Department of Education and the American Educational Research Association: school-linked comprehensive services for children and families, Leesburg, Va., September 28 to October 2.

Stout, J. 1991. School-based health clinics: Are they addressing the needs of the students? Thesis for Master of Public Health, University of Washington.

Support Center for School-Based and School-Linked Health Care. 1995. *Assessing and Evaluating School Health Centers, Volume IV:.* Washington, D.C.: Advocates for Youth.

Taylor, L., and Adelman, H. In press. Mental health in the schools: Promising directions for practice. *Health Care in Schools, A Special Edition of Adolescent Medicine: State of the Art Reviews*, L. Juszak and M. Fisher, eds.

Teen Health Corps Project. Undated. Concept paper for National Cities in Schools, Inc. Washington, D.C.

Tyack, D. 1992. Health and social services in public schools: historical perspective. *The Future of Children: School Linked Services* . 2(1):107–117.

Wagner, M., Golan, S., Shaver, D., Newman, L., Wechsler, M., and Kelley, F. 1994. A healthy start for California's children and families: Early findings from a statewide evaluation of school-linked services. Menlo Park, Calif.: SRI International, June.

Wolk, L.I., and Kaplan, D.W. 1993. Frequent school-based clinic utilization: A comparative profile of problems and service needs. *Journal of Adolescent Health* 14:458–463.

E
Guidelines for Adolescent Preventive Services

INTRODUCTION

Changes in adolescent morbidity and mortality during the past several decades have created a health crisis for today's youth. Unintended pregnancy, STDs [sexually transmitted diseases] including HIV [human immunodeficiency virus], alcohol and drug abuse, and eating disorders are just some of the health problems faced by an increasing number of adolescents from all sectors of society. This health crisis requires a fundamental change in the emphasis of adolescent services—a change whereby a greater number of services are directed at the primary and secondary prevention of major health threats facing today's youth. School and community organizations have responded to the need for change by increasing health education programming. Primary care physicians and other health providers must respond by making preventive services a greater component of their clinical practice.

Guidelines for Adolescent Preventive Services (GAPS) can direct providers in how to deliver these services.

GAPS is a comprehensive set of recommendations that provides a framework for the organization and content of preventive health services.

Reprinted with permission from the American Medical Association, copyright, 1995, 2nd Edition.

GAPS recommendations are organized into four types of services that address 14 separate topics or health conditions.

- Three recommendations pertain to the delivery of health care services.
- Seven recommendations pertain to the use of health guidance to promote the health and well-being of adolescents and their parents or guardians.
- Thirteen recommendations describe the need to screen for specific conditions that are relatively common to adolescents and that cause significant suffering either during adolescence or later in life.
- One recommendation pertains to the use of immunizations for the primary prevention of selected infectious diseases.

The topics or health conditions addressed by GAPS are:

- promoting parents' ability to respond to the health needs of their adolescents;
- promoting adjustment to puberty and adolescence;
- promoting safety and injury prevention;
- promoting physical fitness;
- promoting healthy dietary habits and preventing eating disorders and obesity;
- promoting healthy psychosocial adjustment and preventing the negative health consequences of sexual behaviors;
- preventing hypertension;
- preventing hyperlipidemia;
- preventing the use of tobacco products;
- preventing the use and abuse of alcohol and other drugs;
- preventing severe or recurrent depression and suicide;
- preventing physical, sexual, and emotional abuse;
- preventing learning problems; and
- preventing infectious diseases.

A complete description of how GAPS recommendations were developed, the clinical approach to a comprehensive preventive services visit, and the scientific justification for each recommendation are contained in *Guidelines for Adolescent Preventive Services,* by Arthur B. Elster, M.D., and Naomi J. Kuznets, Ph.D. (1994), William and Wilkins: Baltimore.

GAPS recommendations are designed to be delivered ideally as a preventive service package during a series of annual health visits between the ages of 11 and 21. The recommended frequency of specific GAPS preventive services are presented in Table E-1. Annual visits offer

TABLE E-1 Preventive Health Services by Age and Procedure

Adolescents and young adults have a unique set of health care needs. The recommendations for *Guidelines for Adolescent Preventive Services (GAPS)* emphasize annual clinical preventive services visits that address both the developmental and psychosocial aspects of health, in addition to traditional biomedical conditions. These recommendations were developed by the American Medical Association with contributions from a Scientific Advisory Panel, comprised of national experts as well as representatives of primary care medical organizations and the health insurance industry. The body of scientific evidence indicated that the periodicity and content of preventive services can be important in promoting the health and well-being of adolescents.

Age of adolescent

Procedure	Early				Middle			Late			
	11	12	13	14	15	16	17	18	19	20	21
Health guidance											
Parenting*		•———			— • —						
Development	■	■	■	■	■	■	■	■	■	■	■
Diet & physical activity	■	■	■	■	■	■	■	■	■	■	■
Healthy lifestyles**	■	■	■	■	■	■	■	■	■	■	■
Injury prevention	■	■	■	■	■	■	■	■	■	■	■
Screening history											
Eating disorders	■	■	■	■	■	■	■	■	■	■	■
Sexual activity***	■	■	■	■	■	■	■	■	■	■	■
Alcohol & other drug use	■	■	■	■	■	■	■	■	■	■	■
Tobacco use	■	■	■	■	■	■	■	■	■	■	■
Abuse	■	■	■	■	■	■	■	■	■	■	■
School performance	■	■	■	■	■	■	■	■	■	■	■
Depression	■	■	■	■	■	■	■	■	■	■	■
Risk for suicide	■	■	■	■	■	■	■	■	■	■	■
Physical assessment											
Blood pressure	■	■	■	■	■	■	■	■	■	■	■
BMI	■	■	■	■	■	■	■	■	■	■	■
Comprehensive exam	———	•	———		— • —			———		•	———
Tests											
Cholesterol	———	1	———		—1—			———	1	———	
TB	———	2	———		—2—			———	2	———	
GC, Chlamydia, Syphilis & HPV	———	3	———		—3—			———	3	———	
HIV	———	4	———		—4—			———	4	———	
Pap smear	———	5	———		—5—			———	5	———	
Immunizations											
MMR	—•—										
Td	—•—										
Hep B	—•—				—6—			——6——			
Hep A	———	7	———		—7—			——7——			
Varicella	———	8	———		—8—			——8——			

1. Screening test performed once if family history is positive for early cardiovascular disease or hyperlipidemia.
2. Screen if positive for exposure to active TB or lives/works in high-risk situation, eg, homeless shelter, health care facility.
3. Screen at least annually if sexually active.
4. Screen if high-risk for infection.
5. Screen annually if sexually active or if 18 years or older.
6. Vaccinate if high risk for hepatitis B infection.
7. Vaccinate if at risk for hepatitis A infection.
8. Vaccinate if no reliable history of chicken pox.
* A parent health guidance visit is recommended during early and middle adolescence.
** Includes counseling regarding sexual behavior and avoidance of tobacco, alcohol, and other drug use.
*** Includes history of unintended pregnancy and STD.

SOURCE: *Guidelines for Adolescent Preventive Services* (GAPS), American Medical Association, 1995.

the opportunity to reinforce health promotion messages for both adolescents and their parents, identify adolescents who have initiated health risk behaviors or who are at early stages of physical or emotional disorders, provide immunizations, and develop relationships with the adolescents that will foster an open disclosure of future health information.

RECOMMENDATIONS FOR DELIVERY OF HEALTH SERVICES

The periodicity and manner in which services are delivered to adolescents can be important determinants of the effectiveness of preventive services. The rapid behavioral changes that occur during adolescence require frequent visits to screen for health risk behaviors and to provide health guidance. To ensure that providers obtain accurate information and deliver health guidance appropriate for each adolescent, GAPS recommends that services be tailored to the individual and that information shared by the adolescent during the medical visit remain confidential.

Recommendation 1: From ages 11 to 21, all adolescents should have an annual preventive services visit.

• These visits should address both the biomedical and psychosocial aspects of health, and should focus on preventive services.
• Adolescents should have a complete physical examination during three of these preventive services visits. One should be performed during early adolescence (age 11 to 14), one during middle adolescence (age 15 to 17), and one during late adolescence (age 18 to 21), unless more frequent exams are warranted by clinical signs or symptoms.

Recommendation 2: Preventive services should be age and developmentally appropriate, and should be sensitive to individual and sociocultural differences.

Recommendation 3: Physicians should establish office policies regarding confidential care for adolescents and how parents will be involved in that care. These policies should be made clear to adolescents and their parents.

RECOMMENDATIONS FOR HEALTH GUIDANCE

Adolescence is a time of experimentation and risk taking. Developmentally, adolescents are at a crossroads of health. Emerging cognitive abilities and social experiences lead adolescents to question adult values and experiment with health risk behaviors. Some behaviors threaten cur-

rent health, while other behaviors may have long-term health consequences. The changes in cognitive abilities, however, also offer an opportunity to develop attitudes and lifestyles that enhance health and well-
being. GAPS recommends that adolescents receive health guidance
annually to help them cope with developmental challenges, develop and
maintain healthy lifestyles, improve diet and fitness, and prevent injury.
In addition, GAPS recommends health guidance be given to parents and
guardians of adolescents to help them respond appropriately to the health
needs of their adolescent.

**Recommendation 4: Parents or other adult caregivers should receive
health guidance at least once during their child's early adolescence,
once during middle adolescence and, preferably, once during late adolescence.**

This includes providing information about:

• normative adolescent development, including information about
physical, sexual, and emotional development;
   • signs and symptoms of disease and emotional distress;
   • parenting behaviors that promote healthy adolescent adjustment;
• why parents should discuss health-related behaviors with their
adolescents, plan family activities, and act as role models for health-related behaviors;
• methods for helping their adolescent avoid potentially harmful
behaviors, such as:

   — monitoring and managing the adolescent's use of motor vehicles, especially for new drivers;
   — avoiding having weapons in the home. Parents who have
weapons in the home should be advised to make them inaccessible to
adolescents. If adolescents have weapons, parents and other adult
caregivers should ensure that adolescents follow weapon safety procedures.
   — removing weapons and potentially lethal medications from the
homes of adolescents who have suicidal intent;
   — monitoring their adolescent's social and recreational activities
for the use of tobacco, alcohol and other drugs, and sexual behavior.

**Recommendation 5: All adolescents should receive health guidance
annually to promote a better understanding of their physical growth,
psychosocial and psychosexual development, and the importance of
becoming actively involved in decisions regarding their health care.**

Recommendation 6: All adolescents should receive health guidance annually to promote reduction of injuries.

Health guidance for injury prevention includes the following:

- counseling to avoid the use of alcohol or other substances while using motor or recreational vehicles, or where impaired judgment may lead to injury;
- counseling to use safety devices, including seat belts, motorcycle and bicycle helmets, and appropriate athletic protective devices;
- counseling to resolve interpersonal conflicts without violence;
- counseling to avoid the use of weapons and/or promote weapon safety;
- counseling to promote appropriate physical conditioning before exercise.

Recommendation 7: All adolescents should receive health guidance annually about dietary habits, including the benefits of a healthy diet, and ways to achieve a healthy diet and safe weight management.

Recommendation 8: All adolescents should receive health guidance annually about the benefits of physical activity and should be encouraged to engage in safe physical activities on a regular basis.

Recommendation 9: All adolescents should receive health guidance annually regarding responsible sexual behaviors, including abstinence. Latex condoms to prevent STDs, including HIV infection, and appropriate methods of birth control should be made available, as should instructions on how to use them effectively.

Health guidance for sexual responsibility includes the following:

- counseling that abstinence from sexual intercourse is the most effective way to prevent pregnancy and sexually transmissible diseases (STDs), including HIV infection;
- counseling on how HIV infection is transmitted, the dangers of the disease, and the fact that latex condoms are effective in preventing STDs, including HIV infection;
- reinforcement of responsible sexual behavior for adolescents who are not currently sexually active and for those who are using birth control and condoms appropriately;
- counseling on the need to protect themselves and their partners from pregnancy; STDs, including HIV infection; and sexual exploitation.

Recommendation 10: All adolescents should receive health guidance annually to promote avoidance of tobacco, alcohol, and other abusable substances, and anabolic steroids.

RECOMMENDATIONS FOR SCREENING

GAPS includes recommendations for the screening of biomedical, behavioral, and emotional conditions. Some GAPS recommendations lead to a definitive diagnosis (e.g., cervical culture in females to diagnose gonorrhea). Other recommendations lead to a presumptive diagnosis (e.g., urine test for leukocyte esterase in males to screen for gonorrhea or asking about use of alcohol or other drugs during the past six months to screen for substance use) that must be confirmed with additional assessment. Physicians can use information from the initial screening to decide whether to continue the assessment themselves or to refer the adolescent elsewhere. Health risk behaviors may, in some adolescents, be interrelated and co-occur. Adolescents who are found to engage in one health risk behavior, therefore, should be asked about involvement in others.

Recommendation 11: All adolescents should be screened annually for hypertension according to the protocol developed by the National Heart, Lung, and Blood Institute Second Task Force on Blood Pressure Control in Children.

• Adolescents with either systolic or diastolic pressures at or above the 90th percentile for gender and age should have blood pressure (BP) measurements repeated at three different times within one month, under similar physical conditions, to confirm baseline values.
• Adolescents with baseline BP values greater than the 95th percentile for gender and age should have a complete biomedical evaluation to establish treatment options. Adolescents with BP values between the 90th and 95th percentiles should be assessed for obesity and their blood pressure monitored every six months.

Recommendation 12: Selected adolescents should be screened to determine their risk of developing hyperlipidemia and adult coronary heart disease, following the protocol developed by the Expert Panel on Blood Cholesterol Levels in Children and Adolescents.

• Adolescents whose parents have a serum cholesterol level greater than 240 mg/dl and adolescents who are over 19 years of age should be screened for total blood cholesterol level (nonfasting) at least once.
• Adolescents with an unknown family history or who have mul-

tiple risk factors for future cardiovascular disease (e.g., smoking, hypertension, obesity, diabetes mellitus, excessive consumption of dietary saturated fats and cholesterol) may be screened for total serum cholesterol level (nonfasting) at least once at the discretion of the physician.

• Adolescents with blood cholesterol values less than 170 mg/dl should have the test repeated within five years. Those with values between 170 and 199 mg/dl should have a repeated test. If the average of the two tests is below 170 mg/dl, total blood cholesterol level should be reassessed within five years. A lipoprotein analysis should be done if the average cholesterol value of the two tests if 170 mg/dl or higher, or if the result of the initial test was 200 mg/dl or greater.

• Adolescents who have a parent or grandparent with coronary artery disease, peripheral vascular disease, cerebrovascular disease, or sudden cardiac death at age 55 or younger should be screened with a fasting lipoprotein analysis.

• Treatment options are based on the average of two assessments of low-density lipoprotein cholesterol. Values below 110 mg/dl are acceptable; values between 110 and 129 mg/dl are borderline, and the lipoprotein status should be reevaluated in one year. Adolescents with values of 130 mg/dl or greater should be referred for medical evaluation and treatment.

Recommendation 13: All adolescents should be screened annually for eating disorders and obesity by determining weight and stature, asking about body image and dieting patterns.

• Adolescents should be assessed for organic disease, anorexia nervosa, or bulimia if any of the following are found: weight loss greater than 10 percent of the previous weight; recurrent dieting when not overweight, use of self-induced emesis, laxatives, starvation, or diuretics to lose weight; distorted body image; or body mass index (weight/height 2) below the fifth percentile.

• Adolescents with a body mass index (BMI) equal to or greater than the 95th percentile for age and gender are overweight and should have an in-depth dietary and health assessment to determine psychosocial morbidity and risk for future cardiovascular disease.

• Adolescents with a BMI between the 85th and 94th percentiles are at risk for becoming overweight. A dietary and health assessment to determine psychosocial morbidity and risk for future cardiovascular disease should be performed on these youth if:

— their BMI has increased by two or more units during the previous 12 months;

— there is a family history of premature heart disease, obesity, hypertension, or diabetes mellitus;
    — they express concern about their weight;
    — they have elevated serum cholesterol levels or blood pressure.

If this assessment is negative, these adolescents should be provided general dietary and exercise counseling and should be monitored annually.

Recommendation 14: All adolescents should be asked annually about their use of tobacco products, including cigarettes and smokeless tobacco.

• Adolescents who use tobacco products should be assessed further to determine their patterns of use.
• A cessation plan should be provided for adolescents who use tobacco products.

Recommendation 15: All adolescents should be asked annually about their use of alcohol and other abusable substances and about their use of over-the-counter or prescription drugs for nonmedical purposes, including anabolic steroids.

• Adolescents who report any use of alcohol or other drugs or inappropriate use of medicines during the past year should be assessed further regarding family history; circumstances surrounding use; amount and frequency of use; attitudes and motivation about use; use of drugs; and the adequacy of physical, psychosocial, and school functioning.
• Adolescents whose substance use endangers their health should receive counseling and mental health treatment, as appropriate.
• Adolescents who use anabolic steroids should be counseled to stop.
• The use of urine toxicology for the routine screening of adolescents is not recommended.
• Adolescents who use alcohol and other drugs should also be asked about their sexual behavior and their use of birth control products.

Recommendation 16: All adolescents should be asked annually about involvement in sexual behaviors that may result in unintended pregnancy and STDs, including HIV infection.

• Sexually active adolescents should be asked about their use and motivation to use condoms and contraceptive methods, their sexual orientation, the number of sexual partners they have had in the past six months, if they have exchanged sex for money or drugs, and their history of prior pregnancy or STDs.

• Adolescents at risk for pregnancy, STDs (including HIV), or sexual exploitation should be counseled on how to reduce this risk.

• Sexually active adolescents should also be asked about their use of tobacco products, alcohol, and other drugs.

Recommendation 17: Sexually active adolescents should be screened for STDs.

STD screening includes the following:

— a cervical culture (females) or urine leukocyte esterase analysis (males) to screen for gonorrhea;

— an immunologic test of cervical fluid (female) or urine leukocyte esterase analysis (male) to screen for genital chlamydia;

— a serologic test for syphilis if they have lived in an area endemic for syphilis, have had other STDs, have had more than one sexual partner within the last six months, have exchanged sex for drugs or money, or are males who have engaged in sex with other males;

— evaluation for human papilloma virus by visual inspection (males and females) and by Pap test.

• If a presumptive test for STDs is positive, tests to make a definitive diagnosis should be performed, a treatment plan instituted according to guidelines developed by the Centers for Disease Control, and the use of condoms encouraged.

• The frequency of screening for STDs depends on the sexual practices of the individual and the history of previous STDs.

Recommendation 18: Adolescents at risk for HIV infection should be offered confidential HIV screening with the ELISA [enzyme-linked immunosorbent assay] or confirmatory test.

• Risk status includes having used intravenous drugs, having had other STD infections, having lived in an area with a high prevalence of STDs and HIV infection, having had more than one sexual partner in the last six months, having exchanged sex for drugs or money, being male and having engaged in sex with other males, or having had a sexual partner who is at risk for HIV infection.

• Testing should be performed only after informed consent is obtained from the adolescent.

• Testing should be performed only in conjunction with both pre-
and post-test counseling.
• The frequency of screening for HIV infection should be determined
by the risk factors of the individual.

**Recommendation 19: Female adolescents who are sexually active or
any female 18 or older should be screened annually for cervical cancer
by use of a Pap test.**

Adolescents with a positive Pap test should be referred for further
diagnostic assessment and management.

**Recommendation 20: All adolescents should be asked annually about
behaviors or emotions that indicate recurrent or severe depression or
risk of suicide.**

• Screening for depression or suicidal risk should be performed on
adolescents who exhibit cumulative risk as determined by declining
school grades, chronic melancholy, family dysfunction, homosexual orientation, physical or sexual abuse, alcohol or drug use, previous suicide
attempt, or suicidal plans.
• If suicidal risk is suspected, adolescents should be evaluated immediately and referred to a psychiatrist or other mental health professional, or else should be hospitalized.
• Nonsuicidal adolescents with symptoms of severe or recurring
depression should be evaluated and referred to a psychiatrist or other
mental health professional for treatment.

**Recommendation 21: All adolescents should be asked annually about a
history of emotional, physical, or sexual abuse.**

• If abuse is suspected, adolescents should be assessed to determine
the circumstances surrounding abuse and the presence of physical, emotional, and psychosocial consequences, including involvement in health
risk behavior.
• Health providers should be aware of local laws about the reporting
of abuse to appropriate state officials, in addition to ethical and legal
issues regarding how to protect the confidentiality of the adolescent patient.
• Adolescents who report emotional or psychosocial sequelae should
be referred to a psychiatrist or other mental health professional for evaluation and treatment.

Recommendation 22: All adolescents should be asked annually about learning or school problems.

• Adolescents with a history of truancy, repeated absences, or poor or declining performance should be assessed for the presence of conditions that could interfere with school success. These include learning disability, attention deficit hyperactivity disorder, medical problems, abuse, family dysfunction, mental disorder, or alcohol or other drug use.
• This assessment, and the subsequent management plan, should be coordinated with school personnel and with the adolescent's parents or caregivers.

Recommendation 23: Adolescents should receive a tuberculin skin test if they have been exposed to active tuberculosis, have lived in a homeless shelter, have been incarcerated, have lived in or come from an area with a high prevalence of tuberculosis, or currently work in a health care setting.

• Adolescents with a positive tuberculin skin test should be treated according to CDC [Centers for Disease Control and Prevention] treatment guidelines.
• The frequency of testing depends on risk factors of the individual adolescent.

RECOMMENDATIONS FOR IMMUNIZATIONS

The fourth set of recommendations involves the use of vaccinations to prevent infectious disease. National immunization policies have changed recently with the development of the vaccination against Hepatitis B virus and the resurgence of measles and rubella among adolescent and adult populations. Providers will need to determine the number and type of previous vaccinations to assess the immunization needs of the adolescent.

Recommendation 24: All adolescents should receive prophylactic immunizations according to the guidelines established by the federally convened Advisory Committee on Immunization Practices.

• Adolescents should receive a bivalent Td [tetanus and diphtheria toxoid] vaccine booster at the 11–12 year visit if not previously vaccinated within 5 years. With the exception of the Td booster at 11–12 years, routine boosters should be administered every 10 years.
• Adolescents should receive a second dose of MMR [measles–

mumps–rubella] at age 11–12 years, unless there is documentation of two vaccinations earlier during childhood. MMR should not be administered to pregnant adolescents.

• Adolescents 11–12 years of age who have not been immunized as part of a routine childhood schedule and who do not have a reliable history of chickenpox should be offered varicella vaccine.

• Hepatitis B immunizations should be initiated at 11–12 years of age. Older unvaccinated adolescents with identified risk factors for HBV [Hepatitis B virus] infection should also be vaccinated. Major risk factors for acquisition of HBV infection in adolescents include multiple sex partners, intravenous drug abuse, living in areas with increased rates of parenteral drug abuse, teenage pregnancy, and/or sexually transmitted diseases. Widespread use of Hepatitis B vaccination is encouraged because risk factors are not always easily identifiable among adolescents.

• Hepatitis A immunizations should be given to adolescents who are traveling or living in countries with high or intermediate endemicity of Hepatitis A virus (HAV), live in communities with high endemic rates of HAV, have chronic liver disease, are injecting drug users or are males who have sex with males.

• Ideally all vaccinations should be administered at the scheduled 11–12 year visit.

CLINICAL APPLICATIONS

GAPS provides a strategy to organize the content and delivery of care within a clinical setting to address the health issues of adolescents. Most primary care providers offer some preventive services to adolescents but GAPS suggests a comprehensive approach that includes screening and health guidance on an annual basis. All adolescents should be scheduled for an initial GAPS visit at the 11–12 year visit.

DIFFERENCES BETWEEN GAPS AND TRADITIONAL APPROACHES TO HEALTH CARE

The major differences between GAPS services and the traditional approaches to health care are the emphasis on comprehensive rather than categorical services for adolescents, visits for their parents or guardians, and the orientation to preventive care. These differences are summarized in the following table.

GAPS Recommendations Compared with Traditional Approaches to Adolescent Health Care

GAPS Recommendations	Traditional Health Care
Provider plays an important role in coordinating adolescent health promotion. This role complements health guidance that adolescents receive from their family, school, and community.	Provider role is considered to be independent of health education programs offered by schools, family, and the community.
Preventive interventions target social morbidities such as alcohol and other drug use, suicide, STDs, (including HIV), unintended pregnancy, and eating disorders.	Emphasis is on biomedical problems alone, such as the medical consequences of health risk behaviors (e.g., STDs, unintended pregnancy).
Provider emphasizes screening of comorbidities; i.e., adolescent participation in clusters of specific health risk behaviors.	Emphasis is on the diagnosis and treatment of categorical health conditions.
Annual visits permit early detection of health problems and offer an opportunity to provide health education and develop a therapeutic relationship.	Visits are scheduled only as needed for acute care episodes or for other specific purposes (e.g., immunizations or an examination prior to participating in sports).
Provider performs three comprehensive physical examinations: one during early, middle, and late adolescence.	Current standards vary from as necessary to examinations every two years during adolescence.
It is recommended that all parents receive education about adolescent health care at least twice during the child's adolescence.	Parents are included in the health care of the adolescent solely at the discretion of the provider, who also serves as the sole decision maker of what health education topics should be addressed with parents.

Federal Funding Streams for Comprehensive School Health Programs

Provided by Kristine McCoy
Interagency Committee on School Health, Office of Disease
Prevention and Health Promotion, U.S. Public Health Service,
December 1995

Federal Programs Providing Funds Available to School Health Programs
Compiled by the Health Services Subcommittee of the Interagency Committee on School Health

This table offers basic descriptive information on federal programs providing funds for school-based or school-linked health programs. Available funding sources for training of school health professionals are also listed on this chart. In general, information on the dollar amount specifically targeted for school health programs was not available. The fixed year (FY) 1993 budget reported is for the entire program and not exclusively for the school health component.

NATIONAL COORDINATING COMMITTEE ON SCHOOL HEALTH

Member Organizations

American Academy of Family Physicians
American Academy of Pediatrics
American Alliance for Health, Physical Education, Recreation and Dance
American Association of Colleges for Teacher Education
American Association of School Administrators

American Cancer Society
American College Health Association
American Dental Association
American Federation of School Administrators
American Federation of Teachers
American Heart Association
American Indian Health Care Association
American Lung Association
American Medical Association
American Nurses Association
American Psychological Association
American Public Health Association
American Public Welfare Association
American School Counselor Association
American School Food Service Association
American School Health Association
Association of Maternal and Child Health Programs
Association of State and Territorial Health Officials
Council of Chief State School Officers
The Council of the Great City Schools
National Alliance of Black School Educators
National Association for Asian and Pacific American Education
National Association of City and County Health Officials
National Association of Community Health Centers
National Association of Elementary School Principals
National Association of School Nurses
National Association of Secondary School Principals
National Association of School Psychologists
National Association of Social Workers
National Association of State Boards of Education
National Coalition of Hispanic Health and Human Services Organizations
National Conference of State Legislators
National Education Association
National Governors Association
National Mental Health Association
National Parents/Teachers Association
National School Boards Association
National School Health Education Coalition
Society for Nutrition Education

Title of Program	Lead Agency
Medicaid (Title XIX), including Early and Periodic Screening, Diagnostic, and Treatment Program (EPSDT)	DHHS, HCFA, MB
Family Planning Program (Title X)	DHHS, OASH, OPA
Adolescent Family Life (Title XX)	DHHS, OASH, OPA
Indian Health Service Clinical Services	DHHS, IHS
Critical Populations Program Adolescent Track	DHHS, SAMHSA, CSAT
Community Partnership Demonstration Grant Program	DHHS, SAMHSA, CSAP
High Risk Youth Demonstration Grant Program	DHHS, SAMHSA, CSAP

Brief Description

Medicaid pays for health services provided to low-income individuals who meet eligibility criteria. There is a defined list of clinical services provided, including general health screenings, vision, dental, and hearing services and other medically necessary health services

EPSDT is a comprehensive preventive health program for Medicaid-eligible children under age 21. Through EPSDT, Medicaid-eligible children receive periodic health screenings, as well as medically necessary diagnostic and treatment services for conditions found through the screenings

FY 1994 expenditures: $979,836,854 (total Medicaid state and federal spending for children under age 21) (FY 1995 expenditures expected in May 1996)

Family planning services, personnel training, and service delivery research are all supported by this program. The health services include health education, some clinical services, and family planning counseling

FY 1995 Budget: $193,000,000

Provides communities with useful models of pregnancy prevention programs that promote abstinence for unmarried adolescents and deliver comprehensive care for pregnant adolescents to reduce negative outcomes. Counseling, health education, and clinical services are provided

FY 1995 Budget: $6,700,000

Comprehensive health services for Native Americans in areas serviced by the Indian Health Service. Services include counseling, health education, and clinical services

FY 1995 Budget: $1,800,000,000

Services for youth that use drugs. Services include counseling, health education, and limited clinical services

FY 1995 Budget: $23,600,000 (for all critical populations)

This program encourages the formation of community-based, public and private sector partnerships involving schools, business, industry, professional organizations, and others who will jointly sponsor long-term, comprehensive substance abuse prevention programs

FY 1995 Budget: $105,000,000

Demonstration grants for innovative and effective models to prevent substance abuse. The program targets most age groups as well as parents, health education is the major health service provided

FY 1995 Budget: $49,000,000

continued on next page

Title of Program	Lead Agency
Youth Violence Prevention Demonstration Grant Program	DHHS, SAMHSA, CSAP
Adolescent Females	DHHS, SAMHSA, CSAP
Child/Adolescent Planning and System Development Program (formerly the Child and Adolescent Service System Program [CASSP])	DHHS, SAMHSA, CMHS
Center for Mental Health Services Research Project	DHHS, SAMHSA, CMHS
Community and Migrant Health Centers	DHHS, HRSA, BPHC
Healthy Schools Healthy Communities	DHHS, HRSA, BPHC and MCHB
Maternal and Child Health State Block Grants	DHHS, HRSA, MCHB

Demonstration grants for innovative and effective models to prevent youth violence. The program targets most age groups as well as parents, health education is the major health service provided

FY 1995 Budget: $2,000,000

Demonstration grants for innovative and effective models to prevent alcohol, tobacco, and other drug use and gang activity among adolescent females. The program targets most age groups as well as parents, health education is the major health service provided

FY 1995 Budget: $8,200,000

Helps states and communities develop the infrastructure to provide comprehensive addressing physical, emotional, social, and educational needs), coordinated, (community-based services to children and adolescents with serious emotional disturbances

FY 1995 Budget: $12,100,000

Funds treatment services for children with serious emotional disturbances where there is an infrastructure to support coordinated and comprehensive service delivery for them and their families

FY 1995 Budget: $60,000,000

Comprehensive health services are provided to low-income children through community-based primary care providers. Many programs have a school-based or school-linked component. Services include counseling, health education, and clinical services

FY 1995 Budget: Section 329 $65,000,000
                  Section 330 $616,555,000
                  Section 340 $5,272,000

Funds school-based health services programs, health education or promotion programs, and school health staff development programs for extremely disadvantaged communities

FY 1995 Budget: $6,166,293

Ensures access to health care services for children, promotes the health of children by providing preventive and primary care services, and facilitates the development of community-based systems of services for children with special health care needs

FY 1995 Budget: $572,000,000

continued on next page

Title of Program	Lead Agency
Advanced Nurse Education	DHHS, HRSA, BHP
Nurse Practitioner/Nurse-Midwifery	DHHS, HRSA, BHP
Nursing Special Projects Grant Program	DHHS, HRSA, BHP
HIV Education Program	DHHS, CDC, DASH
Comprehensive School Health Program	DHHS, CDC, DASH
Food Labeling Education Program	DHHS, FDA, FSIS
Drug-Free Schools and Communities Act	DOEd, OESE
Elementary and Secondary Education Act (Chapter 1)	DOEd, OESE
Individuals with Disabilities Education Act	DOEd, OSERS

Supports the development and expansion of graduate programs in nursing. Programs that have a school health focus are eligible

FY 1995 Budget: $12,253,000

Provides support for educational programs that prepare nurse practitioners and nurse-midwives

FY 1995 Budget: $16,943,000

Supports continuing education for nursing, including nurses that work in school health. This program also provides funds for nurse managed clinics. These funds may be used for salary, support staff, equipment, and facilities

FY 1995 Budget: $10,410,000

Provides funding for all state departments of education, as well as for 18 large city departments of education, 25 national organizations, 4 city health departments, and 5 universities to help improve HIV education programs

FY 1995 Budget: $38,000,000

Funds demonstration programs in 10 states to implement comprehensive school health programs

FY 1995 Budget: $10,500,000

A major education campaign to help consumers use the new food label in planning a healthy diet. The federal government and public and private sector groups are producing educational materials and conducting research to help consumers understand the new food label

FY 1995 Budget: school health portion not reported

Provides state, local, and discretionary grants for drug abuse prevention, education, counseling, and referral services

FY 1995 Budget: $502,000,000

Provides formula grants to states for compensatory education programs. Many programs support integrated service delivery, including health education and services

FY 1995 Budget: $7,200,000,000

Provides health and education services at school to children with disabilities

FY 1995 Budget: $3,300,000,000

continued on next page

Title of Program	Lead Agency
Nutrition Education and Training	USDA, FNS, NTSD
Special Supplemental Food Program for Women, Infants and Children (WIC)	USDA, FNS
School Breakfast Program	USDA, FNS
National School Lunch Program	USDA, FNS

NOTE: BHP = Board of Health Promotion; BPHC = Board of Primary Health Care; CDC = Centers for Disease Control and Prevention; CMHS = Center for Mental Health Services; CSAT = Center for Substance Abuse Treatment; DASH = Division of Adolescent and School Health; DHHS = U.S. Department of U.S. Health and Human Services; DOEd = U.S. Department of Education; FDA = Food and Drug Administration; FNS = Food and Nutrition Services; FSIS = Food Safety and Inspection Service; HCFA = Health Care Financing Administration; HIV = human immunodeficiency virus; HRSA = Health Resources and Ser-

Brief Description

Promotes healthy eating habits for children in schools and child care facilities. Projects include in-service training and development of nutrition curricula guides

FY 1995 Budget: $10,200,000

Provides supplemental foods, nutrition education, and health care referrals at no cost to low-income pregnant women, non-breastfeeding postpartum women, infants and children up to 5 years old

FY 1995 Budget: $3,600,000,000

Provides low-cost and free breakfast to children in grades K–12

FY 1995 Budget: $1,000,000,000

Provides low-cost and free lunches to children in grades K–12

FY 1995 Budget: 4,500,000,000

vices Administration; IHS = Indian Health Service; MCHB = Maternal and Child Health Bureau; NTSD = Nutrition Technical Services Division; OASH = Office of the Assistant Secretary for Health; OESE = Office of Elementary and Secondary Education; OPA = Office of Population Affairs; OSERS = Office of Special Education and Rehabilitative Services; SAMHSA = Substance Abuse and Mental Health Services Administration; USDA = U.S. Department of Agriculture.

TABLE F-1 Target Population, Provided Services, and FY 1995 Budget Data of Federal Programs Providing Funds Available to School Health Programs

Program Title / Agency	Title XIX HCFA/MB	Title X OASH/OPA	Title XX OASH/OPA	Clinical Svcs IHS/OHP	Critical Popins SAMHSA/CSAT	Cmnty Ptnsp SAMHSA/CSAP	Hi-Risk Yth SAMHSA/CSAP	Yth Violence SAMHSA/CSAP	Adlst Female SAMHSA/CSAP	CASSP SAMHSA/CMHS	CMHS Svcs SAMHSA/CMHS	C/MHC HRSA/BPHC
Target Pop.												
preschool	X			X		X	X			X		X
elem. schl	X			X		X	X			X	X	X
junior high	X		X	X	X	X	X	X		X		X
high schl	X	X	X	X	X	X	X	X	X	X		X
college stud.	X	X		X		X	X			X		
stud.w/ sp.nds	X	X		X								X
high risk yth	X	X	X	X	X	X	X	X	X	X	X	X
out of schl yth	X	X	X	X	X		X					X
faculty/staff		X			X							X
parents		X		X	X							X
community		X	X	X	X							X
other	X	X			X			X	X	X	X	
Hlth Svcs.												
Counseling	X	X	X	X	X	X	X	X	X	X	X	X
Hlth Guidance	X	X	X	X	X	X	X	X	X	X	X	X
Screening	X			X								X
Immunizations	X			X								X
First Aid	X			X								X
Physical Exam	X	X	X	X								X
Diag and Refer	X	X	X	X	X	X	X	X	X	X	X	X
Diag.Trfmnt.F/u	X	X	X	X	X	X	X	X	X	X	X	X
Dental	X			X								X
Other	X	X						X	X	X		X
Health Ed.												
small group		X	X		X							X
classroom		X	X	X	X							X
Training												
faculty/staff				X								X
Funding												
FY 95 Budget in dollars ($)	980 M*	193 M	6.7 M	1.8 B	23 M	105.0 M	49.0 M	2.0 M	8.2 M	12.1 M	60.0M	N/A

*Denotes FY 94 expenditures; FY 95 expenditures expected May 1996.

TABLE F-1 Continued

Program Title	HSHC	MCH Blk Grts	Adv. Nurse Ed.	NP/Mid-wifery	Nursing Proj.	HIV Ed.	CSHP	Food Label	Drug-Free Schls	Chap 1	IDEA
Agency	HRSA	HRSA/MCHB	HRSA/BHP	HRSA/BHP	HRSA/BHP	CDC/DASH	CDC/DASH	FDA/FSIS	DOEd/OESE	DOEd/OESE	DOEd/OSERS
Target Pop											
preschool		X								X	
elem. schl	X	X				X	X	X	X	X	X
junior high	X	X				X	X	X	X	X	X
high schl	X	X				X	X	X	X	X	X
college stud.						X					
stud.w/ sp.nds	X	X				X	X			X	
high risk yth		X				X	X		X	X	
out of schl yth		X				X	X		X		
faculty/staff						X	X				
parents						X	X	X			
community						X	X				
other	X										
Hlth Svcs											
Counseling		X									
Hlth Guidance		X							X		
Screening		X								X	
Immunizations		X									
First Aid		X									
Physical Exam		X									
Diag./Ref.		X									
Diag/Trt/FU		X							X		
Dental		X									
other		X									
Health Ed.											
small group	X					X					
classroom	X					X	X				
Training											
faculty/staff	X		X	X	X	X	X		X	X	
Funding											
FY 95 Budget in dollars ($)	6.2 M	572 M	12.3 M	16.9 M	10.4 M	38 M	10.5 M	N/A	502.0 M	7.2 B	3.3 B

442

TABLE F-1 *Continued*

Program Title	NET	WIC	Schl Break	Schl Lunch
Agency	USDA/FNS	USDA/FNS	USDA/FNS	USDA/FNS
Target Pop				
preschool	x	x		
elem. schl	x	x	x	x
junior high	x	x	x	x
high schl	x	x	x	x
college stud.		x		
stud.w/ sp.nds	x	x	x	x
high risk yth				
out of schl yth				
faculty/staff	x	x		
parents		x		
community				
other				
Hlth Svcs				
Counseling				
Hlth Guidance		x		
Screening				
Immunizations				
First Aid				
Physical Exam				
Diag./Ref.				
Diag/Trt/FU				
Dental				
other				
Health Ed.				
small group		x		
classroom	x			
Training				
faculty/staff				
Funding				
FY 95 Budget in dollars ($)	10.2 M	3.6 B	1.0 B	4.5B

G-1

A Vision of Integrated Services for Children and Families

Maine Goals 2000 Study Group
Jacqueline Ellis, Facilitator
Spring 1995

Our vision includes the following elements:

• Communities provide all families and children from birth through school completion with the educational, social, and health services needed to enable children to grow and learn to their full potential. Children are ready to learn when they enter preschool or school, as well as being ready to learn every day throughout their school years and beyond.

• The integration of services involves attitudinal changes about and structural changes in the ways that the needs of children and families are met.

• Service providers work as partners with each other and with families and schools.

• The focus of these services is on prevention.

• Services are integrated to maximize access to and make efficient use of resources.

RECOMMENDATIONS ON INTEGRATED SERVICES FOR CHILDREN AND FAMILIES

Introduction

The Study Group on Integrated Services developed the following recommendations during the spring of 1995. We applaud the Task Force's recognition of the significance of integrated services in helping to give children an equal opportunity to learn, and we appreciate the opportunity to share our knowledge and experience about this topic.

Rationale for Integrated Services

1. The human services needs of children and their families are urgent and growing. Many children do not receive the services they need in order to learn and to reach their full potential. The National Commission on the Role of the School and the Community in Improving Adolescent Health issued a "Code Blue" alert:

> For the first time in the history of this country young people are *less* healthy and *less* prepared to take their places in society than were their parents and this is happening at a time when our society is more complex, more challenging, and more competitive than ever before (National Commission, 1989).

2. The current system is not working. Services are often fragmented, duplicative, or underused. They are more frequently driven by funding sources and program guidelines than by the needs of children and families.

3. Meeting the needs of the whole child would enhance the ability of children and teachers to focus on learning.

4. Integrated services make more efficient use of limited funds.

5. Coalitions are more capable of addressing multifaceted problems effectively and can accomplish more toward reaching common goals than organizations can when working independently.

The following statistics exemplify problems in Maine that interfere with learning and that can be addressed more effectively by integrated services:

• Thirty-seven thousand (12 percent) juveniles live in households with incomes far enough below the federal poverty line that they qualify for Aid to Families with Dependent Children (AFDC). The proportion of youth living in poverty has been steadily increasing.

• Nearly 30 percent of teenagers say they have seriously considered killing themselves, and 10 percent have tried to commit suicide at least once.

• Ten percent of all births are to unmarried teens who have not completed 12 years of school.

• More than one-fifth (21 percent) of youth report having carried a weapon such as a gun, knife, or club during the past month. This figure is for in-school youth in the safest state in the nation!

• One-half of teenagers use alcohol, with 25 percent of the girls and 32 percent of the boys drinking five or more drinks in a row.

Guiding Principles for Study Group Recommendations

• Support services, instruction, and administration or management are equally important components of successful school improvement and the development of healthy children.
• Support services are only one aspect of the increased family and community involvement in education necessary to improve children's learning. Indeed, it takes a village to raise a child.
• Effective prevention programs set high expectations for children and families, focusing on their strengths and the gains that they can make when given adequate support and appropriate services.
• School staff, such as guidance counselors, health educators, and school nurses, are potential facilitators of integrated services and provide critical links between other school staff, students, and community service providers.

Support for School Role in Integrating Services

Numerous organizations—such as the National Association of State Boards of Education, the National Education Association, the National School Boards Association, the National Association of Towns and Townships, the American Association of School Administrators, and the Carnegie Council on Adolescent Development—stress the interrelatedness of child health and learning and the pivotal role of schools in helping address these issues. Strong national support is reflected in Maine by position statements from such organizations as the Maine School Boards Association, the Maine Coalition on Excellence in Education, and the Maine Principals Association.

A 1992 national Gallup poll indicates strong public support for the school's involvement in service delivery. More than three-fourths (77 percent) of respondents favored using public school buildings to provide health and social services to students.

Recommendations

Study group recommendations are based on the following:

• a panel discussion of innovative Maine efforts to integrate services;
• a brief review of effective national programs;
• the results of a small survey of stakeholders in Maine;

• feedback from local focus groups on integrated services convened by the Maine Leadership Consortium in 1993;

• the comments on draft recommendations distributed to more than 40 reviewers (see list of reviewers at end of this appendix);

• the professional experiences of study group members who represent diverse perspectives and stakeholder groups (see list of members at end of this appendix).

Our recommendations were limited in depth and scope by the time available. The study group could offer more information later that would be more appropriate and useful for local schools and communities as they attempt to integrate services.

The following recommendations are organized by the issue areas or strands that emerged during our research. They attempt to address the barriers as well as to incorporate the effective strategies discussed. The strands in Part I describe *what type* of services are recommended and *how* services would be designed and delivered at the local level. Part II describes state and federal support for local efforts. All these strands need to be woven together to provide a seamless web of services for children and families.

I. LOCAL DESIGN AND DELIVERY OF SERVICES

The recommendations in this section are directed toward local communities. Local communities would decide on the exact type of services to meet the needs of their children and families (see Section A) and would select a convener for this effort (see Sections C and D).

A. Description of Services

Recommendations

1. Provide integrated services that are

a. **comprehensive:** a full range of basic social and health services to support educational services (see list of integrated services in Part II);

b. **child-centered:** services that focus on children, from birth through school completion;

c. **family focused:** services that address the needs of children within the context of the family;

d. **flexible and equitable**: services that meet the changing physical, emotional, social, and educational needs of children and families;

e. **preventive**: emphasize primary prevention as well as providing intervention and treatment.

Note: Other definitions related to the recommendations appear at the end of this appendix.

B. Access to Services

Recommendations

1. Establish contact between service providers and families of children **before or at birth**. A positive relationship would be initiated by hospitals through existing prenatal, sibling, and/or family classes or by providing visits from community health nurses. Maintain **continuity of care** from birth to school completion through collaboration by service providers, childcare providers, and preschool and public school staffs. Examples are: Healthy Families, Even Start, High Scope, Parents as Teachers, Headstart, Success by Six, Child Development Services, Division of Public Health Nursing, and Bureau of Children with Special Needs.

2. Provide low-barrier services for *all* children. Practices that increase accessibility include providing **childcare and transportation**, locating services in a **central location(s)** ("one-stop shopping"), reducing or eliminating **eligibility** requirements, and providing **affordable** care.

Schools represent an excellent potential location or conduit for services because of their regular contact with children. Research indicates that most successful collaborative services are located **in or near school buildings**. Administration of services seems to work best when done by service providers who are accountable to their agencies and who work as partners with school administrators or their designees. Consider using school space after class hours, utilizing space or facilities near a school, and planning space for service delivery in the design of any new school or community center.

3. Develop a single, straightforward form or method of gathering information from families and children; this is known as **"universal intake."** Agree upon a **common entry point** for those receiving services (e.g., a school, health clinic, or town office). Other institutions, such as employers or hospitals, would refer families with children to this entry point.

C. Communication and Positive Climate

Note: The following recommendations are essential for addressing the significant attitudinal barriers to fundamental changes in service delivery.

Recommendation

1. Develop a shared **vision** for integrated services among diverse families, students, providers, school staff and boards, community leaders, and other community members. This is an important early step of program development.

2. Build and maintain **trust and commitment** among schools, families, service providers, students, and other community members during the preplanning and planning phases. This takes a lot of time and patience but is essential to making lasting changes in service delivery.

One way to build trust and commitment is to hold neighborhood meetings, study circles, or community forums. These sessions could be used to provide input to the steering committee (see Section D).

3. Create a **safe physical and emotional setting** for those giving and receiving services. This can be achieved by respecting individual differences (including educational and economic level, gender, and disability), developing interagency partnership agreements, establishing clear policies and procedures regarding confidentiality, and providing opportunities for ongoing public dialogue about services.

4. Address **potential concerns** about loss of control and authority, uncertainty about new roles, differences in approach, and other sources of conflict early in the process. Set up a mechanism with written procedures to address these directly and regularly.

5. Provide opportunities for **ongoing, two-way communication** with the general public about available services, the purpose of integrating services, and the vision for integrating services in their community. Examples are: newsletters, open houses, the Internet, media coverage, and surveys.

6. Set **high expectations** for the health of children and the quality of services that are similar to those set for student achievement.

D. Governance and Management

Recommendations

1. Select a neutral and respected **leader** to convene a community-wide effort to integrate services. Examples are a: town manager or planner, school superintendent, businessperson, United Way, family or children's advocate, librarian, or service provider.

2. Create a steering committee with appropriate staff resources that is representatives of **all stakeholder groups**. Involve these groups in decisionmaking during all parts of the effort to improve services (i.e., from assessment, to development, implementation, and evaluation). These stakeholder groups should include but not be limited to parents and other primary caregivers, youth, senior citizens, service providers, churches, school administrators, and other community leaders.

3. Give specific individuals within service delivery and other stakeholder groups **responsibility** for assisting with integrated services, including participation on the steering committee. These responsibilities become part of their job description and evaluation.

4. Inventory and reassess **existing structures** and processes for service delivery. Build on effective processes such as that used by school Student Assistance Teams (SATs).

5. Identify and provide resources to support **case coordinators for multidisciplinary** teams. These teams would share information and plan strategies with families and children to address areas of concern.

E. Resources

Recommendations on Training

1. Restructure the **preservice training** of health, education, special education, and social service professionals to better meet the needs of the whole child. Without adding more courses, arrange for preservice education to include training on the roles and responsibilities of different professionals and on effective strategies for collaborating to deliver integrated services. Examples are: shared course work, skills training, field placement, job mentoring, and panel discussions. Adjust certification requirements to reflect these changes.

2. Provide **ongoing professional development** for those delivering and making decisions about services. Providers need training on such topics as communication, collaboration, team building, the roles and responsibilities of professionals from different disciplines, conflict resolution, grant writing, and confidentiality. Use a training-of-trainers model,

with experts providing professional development and technical assistance to enable local leadership teams to do their own training and work.

Recommendation on Time

1. Build in **time on the job** for individuals responsible for integrating services to complete relevant organizational activities. Examples are: case coordination, training, and evaluation.

Recommendations on Funding

1. Change the ways in which **existing public funds** and other resources are used; much can be done with existing funds.

Shift the balance of funding more toward primary prevention services, especially for young children. United Way estimates that every dollar spent in early childhood development saves society 6 dollars in remedial education, welfare payments, and court and prison expenses.

2. Search for **additional funding** from businesses or respond to requests for grant proposals (RFPs) only *after* developing community ownership and trust and *after* examining existing public resources and practices.

3. Take advantage of all available resources, including the skills, time, and energy of **volunteers**. People are our greatest resource.

4. Maximize the use of public and private **insurance options** for funding services. An example would be: Medicaid.

5. Use any **savings** resulting from the integration of services to increase services, provide services at less cost, or enhance the system's ability to collaborate.

F. Evaluation

Recommendations

1. Set **clear and manageable goals** for service delivery based on the vision developed by a steering committee. Evaluate and **document progress** toward goals. Involve key players in periodic reflection on and documentation of successes and failures, as well as on the factors affecting progress. Use this process to guide and adjust objectives, activities, and use of resources.

2. Use multiple **qualitative and quantative** strategies to evaluate the impact of integrated services. Qualitative evaluation strategies could in-

clude: case studies, interviews, observations in class and in the home, and feedback from family members. Establish a centralized database and track youth-related statistics to provide information for quantitative evaluation components.

3. **Recognize and celebrate** the efforts of those who collaborate to deliver more relevant and efficient services to children and families.

II. STATE OR FEDERAL ASSISTANCE FOR LOCAL EFFORTS

Recommendations

1. Increase cooperation and collaboration among the commissioners and the Departments of Education, Human Services, Corrections, and Mental Health and Retardation, and the Office of Substance Abuse. Governor King's attempt to rejuvenate the **Interdepartmental Council ("Children's Cabinet")** could lead to the types of changes in state government that are critical to fundamental and sustainable change at the local level. Related recommendations follow:

a. Make the **structural changes** that may be needed to facilitate interdepartmental collaboration.

b. Develop public **policies and legislation** that enhance the flexibility of local providers and state agencies in meeting children's needs. Eliminate policies and regulations that act as barriers to the integration of services.

c. **Standardize the regions** that state government and relevant statewide nongovernmental organizations use to organize funding, personnel, and services.

d. Combine **categorical sources of funding** from the state and federal government into one pool, the use of which is decided upon by local communities.

2. Plan a **Blaine House Conference** on integrated services for key stakeholder groups at the state and local levels. This would be an excellent catalyst for local communities to reexamine and begin to plan improvements in service delivery. It would also provide an opportunity to recognize and learn from communities that are currently collaborating. Organize a follow-up session to check on progress toward integration of services.

Integrated Services for Children and Their Families

The Maine Education Goals 2000 Study Group envisions a full range of basic social and health services being integrated with educational services to help ensure that children and adolescents have an equal opportunity to learn. These services include *but are not limited to* the following list. Note that many could be listed in more than one category.

Educational Services
Health education
Guidance
Student assistance teams (SATs)
Alternative education
Special education
Speech and language
Physical therapy
Occupational therapy
School psychology

Basic Services
Housing, food, clothing
Family welfare
Childcare
Transportation
Graduate Education Degree
(GED) adult education
Job training
Crisis intervention (all areas)
Legal services

Social Services
Support groups
Mentoring
Peer leadership and mediation
Recreation, culture, clubs, sports
School-to-work preparation
Parenting education and support

Health Services
Health screenings
Routine medical services
Dental services
Mental health services
Nutrition and weight management
Family planning
Child abuse and neglect prevention
Sexual abuse prevention
Policing and violence prevention
Substance abuse treatment

DEFINITIONS

Case coordination	Multidisciplinary teams of professionals and support staff share information and plan strategies with families and children to address areas of need
Categorical funding	Funding to be used for a specific purpose or activity
Collaboration	Partners establish common goals, they share leadership, pool resources, and accept public responsibility for what the collaborative does or does not accomplish

Cooperation	Partners help each other meet their respective goals, but without making any major changes in their basic services, policies, or administrative regulations
Coordinated services	Providers of separate services communicate and share resources
Developmentally appropriate services	Services that are responsive to changes in age, maturity, and other conditions
Family	The primary caregiver in a child's daily life, including but not limited to parents
Integrated services	Separate services that are connected by common intake, eligibility determination, and individual family service planning so that each family's entire range of needs is addressed; integrated services require collaboration
Local community	Town or a group of towns with a shared center
Parent	A person who is a biological parent or appointed as a legal guardian of a child
Prevention	Includes primary, secondary, and tertiary phases (see below)
Primary prevention	Promotion of health and prevention of problems or disease (e.g., health education, immunizations)
Secondary prevention	Intervention
Stakeholders	People who are affected by actions or policies
Tertiary prevention	Treatment of a problem or disease

Study Group on Integrated Services Membership

Candace Crane, Director of School Services (Millinocket)
Ruth Davison, Reading Coordinator, Chapter One Director (Boothbay)
Debora Duncan, Guidance Counselor (Randolph)
Jacqueline Ellis, Educational Consultant, Study Group Facilitator
Barbara Estes, Bureau of Children with Special Needs (Bath region)
Denison Gallaudet, Task Force on Learning Results, businessperson
DeEtte Hall, Division of Maternal and Child Health (U.S. Department of
    Health and Human Services [DHHS])
Thomas Hood, Principal, Montello School (Auburn), Task Force on
    Learning Results
Debra Houston, Director of Special Services, SAD #53, (Pittsfield)
Orene Nesin, Maine School Boards Association, Task Force on Learning
    Results
Arlene Nicholson, Guidance Counselor, School Board member, Task
    Force on Learning Results
William Primmerman, Maine Department of Education (Augusta)
Wendy Pullen, Director of School Health Center (Dover-Foxcroft)
Christine Snook, Special Needs Parent Information Network (Hallowell)
Cheri Stacy, Partnerships for a Healthy Community (Bangor area)
Meredith Tipton, Director of Public Health Division (City of Portland)
Patti Wooley, Director of Headstart (Waterville)
Gail Werrbach, School of Social Work (University of Maine at Orono)

Panelists

Myrt Collins, Principal, Jack Elementary School (Portland)
Donna Finley, Family Development Specialist, Western Maine
    Community Action Program (Auburn)
Roger Merchant, Piscataquis County Cooperative Extension (Dover-
    Foxcroft)
Kenneth Schmidt, Director, Regional Medical Center at Lubec (Lubec)

Recommendations on Integrated Services for Children and Families

Reviewers

Michael Brennan, Maine House of Representatives (Portland)
Paul Brunelle, Executive Director, Maine School Management
    Association
Michael Clifford, Substance Abuse Counselor, Portland Schools
Myrt Collins, Principal, Jack Elementary School (Portland)

Dale Douglass, Executive Director, Maine Superintendents Association (Augusta)

Donna Finley, Family Development Specialist, Western Maine Community Action Program (Auburn)

Thomas Godfrey, Juvenile Justice Advisory Group, Maine Department of Corrections

Judy Kany, Project Director for Health Professions Regulation Task Force, Medical Care Development (Augusta)

Joseph Lehman, Commissioner, Maine Department of Corrections

Susan Lieberman, Case Management for Youth, United Way of Greater Portland (Portland)

Sylvia Lund, Maine Office of Substance Abuse (Augusta)

Bette Manchester, Principal, Mt. Ararat Middle School, SAD #75 (Topsham)

Frank McDermott, Associate Superintendent, SAD #6 (Bar Mills)

Joanne Medwid, Elementary Education Specialist, Office of Substance Abuse (Hallowell)

Roger Merchant, Piscataquis County Cooperative Extension (Dover-Foxcroft)

James Moll, Acting Associate Commissioner for Programs, Maine Department of Mental Health and Retardation (Augusta)

Irving Ouellette, incoming Executive Director, Maine Association for Supervision and Development (Brunswick)

John Rosser, Senior Administrator, Spurwink School (Portland)

Charlene Rydell, Maine Health Care Finance Commission Advisory Board, former Maine legislator (Brunswick)

Stanley Sawyer, Superintendent, SAD #52 (Turner)

Roger Spugnardi, Superintendent, Biddeford Schools (Biddeford)

Mark Steege, Department of Human Resource Development, University of Southern Maine (Portland)

Richard Tyler, Executive Director, Maine Principals Association (Augusta)

Nelson Walls, Maine Leadership Consortium (Augusta)

Carol Wishcamper, Organizational Consultant (Freeport)

REFERENCE

National Commission on the Role of the School and the Community in Improving Adolescent Health. 1989. *Code Blue: Uniting for Healthier Youth.* Alexandria, Va.: National Association of State Boards of Education.

G-2
The West Virginia Experience: An Infrastructure Model

West Virginia Department of Education and
West Virginia Bureau for Public Health, 1993–1995

Lenore Zedosky, M.N.
Director, Office of Healthy Schools

West Virginia began to build an infrastructure for comprehensive school health programs (CSHPs) in the mid-1980s, when business leader C. E. "Jim" Compton urged Governor Gaston Caperton to appoint a blue-ribbon School Health Task Force. The Task Force's report became the framework for the development of a multicomponent program with multiagency program implementation responsibility.

Ten demonstration school districts received training and technical assistance to begin to design and implement programs at the local level, while state and private agency individuals continued to develop law, policy, and other necessary support for effective program delivery. In 1992, West Virginia was selected as an "Infrastructure Demonstration State" by the Division of Adolescent and School Health at the Centers for Disease Control and Prevention, which provided funds to place senior-level staff responsible for CSHP coordination in the state Departments of Education and Health. These individuals have been responsible for assessing policy and fiscal and manpower resources in their respective agencies, and for planning program expansion into additional school districts. CSHP training was jointly designed and funded by several offices in each agency and was delivered to "infrastructure" teams from 90 percent of the state's school districts.

FUNDING, PLANNING, AND TRAINING RESOURCES

Department of Education

Office of Healthy Schools
  (CSHP office)
Drug-Free Schools Project
Office of Child Nutrition
Office of Evaluation and Research

Department of Health

Office of Health Promotion
AIDS/HIV Division
Office of Primary Care and
  Recruitment
Office of Maternal and Child Health
Office of Local Health

The local teams had the following configuration:

- Local education agency administrator
- Local health agency administrator
- Local school board member
- Local primary care center director
- Education agency health coordinator (health educator, school
nurse)
- Parent
- Community business representative
- One or two others as determined by the community

Each team developed an action plan with priority objectives for beginning program implementation. School reform legislation in West Virginia, which emphasized increased local planning and decisionmaking, created School Senates in each school and set aside specific time during the instructional calendar (one-half to one day per month) for school-based groups to meet for curricular planning and teacher staff development. In addition, each school must have a school improvement team with both school and community representation. These provisions have been most helpful in promoting school and community communication about CSHP and providing time for health team members to meet.

Examples of infrastructure accomplishments in an eight-component comprehensive school health program are described as follows.

COMPREHENSIVE SCHOOL HEALTH PROGRAM INFRASTRUCTURE ACCOMPLISHMENTS

Health Education

During the spring and summer of 1994, the West Virginia Department of Education and the West Virginia Bureau for Public Health jointly planned and delivered infrastructure training for 10-member teams from 50 of the 55 school districts in the state. A total of 500 school and health department administrators, primary care center directors, local board of education members, business representatives, social service agency staff, and parents participated in the training sessions. Each team began the development of an action plan for implementing a comprehensive school health program in their local school district. Grants of $5,000 were given to each district for further planning and teacher training based on an assessment of needs identified during the training. During the 1994–1995 school year, approximately 1,000 teachers participated in training to strengthen classroom delivery of health education.

Additional training has been provided by the State AIDS Task Force, comprised of representatives from the Department of Education, the Bureau for Public Health, community health providers, and others. This Task Force sponsors an annual AIDS conference and develops strategies for implementing AIDS prevention education in schools and communities throughout the state.

An HIV/AIDS Higher Education Consortia was formed following training conducted at Rutgers University. One goal of the consortia is to determine preservice and inservice teacher training needs so that appropriate staff development programs and educational programs can be developed.

Training needs are identified and delivered in a coordinated fashion by these groups.

Health Services

The West Virginia Department of Education (Office of Healthy Schools) and the Bureau for Public Health (Office of Primary Care and Recruitment) recently received funding from the Claude Worthington Benedum Foundation for development of school-based health centers and Healthy Schools initiatives. The foundation provided $950,000 to be used over a period of two years to plan and implement school-based health centers in 14 new sites across the state. In three of the sites, a comprehensive school health program is also in place that will be closely aligned with the health centers. One aspect of the grant is to evaluate the effectiveness of the health centers and compare results in schools that have a traditional health education program with those that have the expanded Healthy Schools program model.

The Office of Maternal and Child Health at the Bureau for Public Health and the Office of Healthy Schools at the Department of Education have collaborated on the development of a manual entitled *Guidelines for Developing and Implementing School-Based Early Periodic Screening, Detection and Treatment (EPSDT) Services.* The Superintendent of Schools, the Commissioner of Health and Human Services, and the Director of Public Health have approved the distribution of this document.

The Department of Education (Office of Child Nutrition), in collaboration with the Department of Human Resources, received permission from the U.S. Department of Agriculture to place an affirmative checkoff section on the free and reduced meal application form that allows parents to indicate their interest in being reviewed for Medicaid eligibility. This has resulted in a significant number of additional children being identified as eligible and being provided with primary care health services.

The State Maternal and Child Health Program, in collaboration with the West Virginia Healthy Schools Program, has entered into a written agreement to provide for the development of a dental health initiative in a Regional Education Service Agency. The Office of Maternal and Child Health provides funds to employ a dental hygienist, who develops teaching modules and other educational materials that promote prevention practices and the use of oral health care services. The curriculum and services developed through this venture may be used as a model for other regions in the state.

Physical Education

The Physical Education Program of Study Instructional Goals have been revised to reflect a focus on lifetime fitness activities. The goals were jointly reviewed by physical educators in the field and by members of the staff at the Bureau for Public Health who have expertise in the area. A statewide physical education summit was held in the summer of 1995 to introduce the new program to physical educators and to assess future training needs. The summit was a collaborative effort of the Department of Education, the Institutions of Higher Education, and the Bureau for Public Health. More than 300 physical educators participated in the summit.

In 1990, the West Virginia Legislature passed a law requiring that all children in grades K–9 be given the President's Physical Fitness Test. Many teachers in the elementary grades indicated that they were not familiar with this test. The Department of Education, in collaboration with the Office of the Governor, has developed a videotape that demonstrates the correct administration of this test. The children in the video are students from three school districts in the state who all qualified for the Physical Fitness Award. This renewed emphasis on the importance of physical fitness has resulted in a significant increase in the number of students who pass the fitness test.

School Counseling, Psychological, and Social Services

A new program entitled the "Responsible Students Program" was initiated in middle schools within the past two years. The program emphasizes personal responsibility for students, and it has resulted in a significant decrease in student discipline problems and a significant increase in student preparedness for class. In addition, students receive one lesson weekly related to the importance of taking personal responsibility for behaviors and performance. The Office of Student Services and Assessment has been primarily responsible for helping to spread this program to schools throughout the state. Because of the strong relationship between responsible behavior and good health outcomes, a student assignment book and accompanying video that correlate good study habits and good health and physical fitness habits were jointly developed by the two offices and distributed to more than 1,000 students.

School Environment

The West Virginia Board of Education has adopted two very significant policies that reflect the importance of sending the correct messages about the importance of good health habits. The Child Nutrition Policy requires that all meals served as part of the school foodservice program meet the new national Dietary Guidelines in 1995. In addition, the policy requires that snack foods sold in vending machines must have limited fat and sugar content. No soft drinks may be sold to students during the school day. The Tobacco Control Policy prohibits the use of any tobacco products, by any individual, at any time on school property. The West Virginia Tobacco Control Coalition has offered assistance in developing educational programs to encourage compliance with this policy.

Recently enacted legislation is providing for the construction of many new school facilities and has also provided an opportunity to ensure that these facilities provide space for school-based health centers and/or full-service facilities for community members.

Staff from the Adolescent Health Initiative Program is working with numerous school systems across the state in conducting Teen Issue Forums, which address such issues as stress, conflict resolution, teenage pregnancy, and other topics selected by the students in participating schools.

Child Nutrition Services

The Child Nutrition Policy is one of the first in the nation to require that foods served in school meet the national Dietary Guidelines. The original policy was developed by a committee comprised of members of the West Virginia University School of Medicine, the West Virginia School Health Committee, the Dairy and Nutrition Council, the Nutrition and Education Trainees Program Cadre, and agency staff. Training for policy implementation is taking place throughout the state.

Teacher and Staff Wellness

The West Virginia School Health Committee is one of five member organizations of the Healthy West Virginia Coalition. The goal of the coalition is to increase the capacity of participating groups and organizations to sustain and enhance their roles in promoting health and preventing disease in the state. The five member organizations and the groups they represent are as follows:

Organization	Representing
West Virginia School Health Committee	All education employees
West Virginia Bureau for Public Health	All other state employees
West Virginia State Medical Society	All health care providers
Wellness Council of West Virginia	Private industry wellness programs
West Virginia State Health Education Coalition	All other state residents

Numerous school districts have initiated staff wellness programs and are reporting significant improvements in physical activity, dietary habits, and other health-promoting activities.

Community Involvement

During the local infrastructure training held in 1994, representatives from the community attended as members of each team. They represented parents, health care providers, Chambers of Commerce, and other interested or influential groups. Action planning has resulted in involvement of community members in the development and implementation of Healthy Schools programs.

In addition, a resource manual was prepared for each participant that listed all of the regional specialists and training opportunities that were available to schools. The lists included adolescent health specialists, community development specialists for substance abuse prevention, regional health educators, and others who have expertise in a variety of areas that are useful to schools.

West Virginia is the only state with a statewide Education Fund that assists in the development of school–business partnerships. Recently, members of the staff of the Office of Healthy Schools and the West Virginia Education Fund received funding from the Public Education Funds Network to help local school improvement councils develop Healthy Schools programs.

The previously mentioned Benedum Foundation initiative is linking primary care centers and federally qualified health centers with school-based health centers. The foundation is supporting this initiative as one of a series of activities that bring better health care to rural communities.

The West Virginia Tobacco Control Coalition staff has worked with local community leaders in successfully passing clean indoor air policies for public facilities in numerous counties.

The Adolescent Health Initiative is working with approximately 30 community groups in improving parenting education skills. The training is modeled after the How to Live with 10–15 Year Olds curriculum, developed in North Carolina.

APPENDIX
G-3
Connecticut School
Health Services Models

State of Connecticut,
Department of Public Health and Addiction Services

STANDARD MODEL FOR INCREASED BASIC SERVICES
SCHOOL AND ADOLESCENT HEALTH SERVICES—LEVEL II

I. The scope of services at this level does not require an outpatient clinic license.

II. The Increased Basic School Health Services Model must enhance existing basic school health services. These services should be available on a regular basis during the academic year. Extended hours beyond the regular school day are encouraged, when possible.

III. Staff should be efficient and appropriate to carry out the services of the project. Project activities must complement the school's responsibilities and programs but not substitute for or replace them. Staff may include but is not limited to social worker (MSW); bachelor's-prepared registered nurse (BSN); certified health educator; allied health professional (medical assistant, community educator, outreach worker, parent aide, clerical staff, etc.).

IV. Health and mental health services

    A. Health services must be provided in accordance with nationally recognized and accepted standards, such as the American Acad-

463

emy of Pediatrics school health manual, *School Health: Policy and Practice* (American Academy of Pediatrics Committee on School Health, 1993), or those of the National Association of School Nurses. The standards to be used must be clearly identified in the project application.

B. Mental health services must be provided in accordance with a nationally recognized and accepted standard, such as the National Association of Social Workers *Guidelines for School Settings.* The standards to be used must be clearly identified in the project application.

C. Examples of possible increased or additional services include the following:

1. Health maintenance and promotion
2. Nursing assessments, nursing diagnosis, and EPSDT screenings
3. Support or educational groups for students with chronic conditions (e.g., asthma, diabetes)
4. Consultation with school staff and parents
5. Referral and follow-up for specialty services that are beyond the scope of mandated school health services
6. Crisis intervention
7. Individual, family, and group counseling and referral
8. Outreach to students at risk, including those in jeopardy of dropping out or who have recently dropped out
9. Support and/or psychoeducational groups focusing on topics of importance to the target population (pregnancy prevention, grief, conflict resolution skills, etc.)
10. Training for school health services staff (through regular consultation, clinical supervision, or additional education)
11. Individual and group health education
12. Home visits or early intervention

V. Linkages with the community; Establishing linkages with medical, mental health, social service providers, and other relevant groups is encouraged. These may include the local health department, community health center, medical schools and hospitals, and schools of public health, mental health and family service agencies, youth service bureaus, and recreational agencies.

VI. The administration of these increased services must be integrated with the current administration (i.e., additional nursing services should be supplied by the same agency that currently supplies nursing services to the school). Should subcontractors with community agencies be utilized, a plan for project and administrative integration with existing school-based services must be clearly outlined.

STANDARD MODEL FOR ENHANCED CLINICAL SERVICES
SCHOOL AND ADOLESCENT HEALTH PROGRAM—LEVEL III

I. A project at this level *may* be required to hold a State of Connecticut license for outpatient clinics as outlined in the Public Health Code, Sections 19-13-D45 through 19-13-D53. The scope of services offered will dictate whether or not a license would be required.

II. The enhanced clinical services should be available on a regular basis during the academic year. Extended hours beyond the regular school day are encouraged, when possible. Specific plans for the provision of services and continuity of care during nonoperational times must be clearly outlined.

III. Staff should be appropriate to carry out the services of the project.

   A. A project coordinator or manager must be identified.

   B. Staffing may include health and/or allied health professionals as needed (e.g., pediatric, family or psychiatric nurse practitioner, pediatric or family physician assistant, social worker, nutritionist, substance abuse prevention specialist, certified health educator, outreach worker, parent aide, clinical psychologist, M.D., dentist, dental hygienist, clerical support.

IV. Certain services may require written parental permission. Services may include but not be limited to the following:

   A. Health or physical services, must be provided in accordance with nationally recognized and accepted standards, such as the American Academy of Pediatrics school health manual, *School Health: Policy and Practice* (American Academy of Pediatrics Committee on School Health, 1993), or those of the National Association of School Nurses. The standards to be used must be clearly identified in the project application.

    1.   Primary health care, including the following:

       a. Physical exams, health assessments, and screening for health problems
       b. Diagnosis and treatment of acute illness and injury
       c. Diagnosis and management of chronic illness
       d. Immunizations
       e. Health promotion and risk reduction
       f. Nutrition and weight management
       g. Reproductive health care
       h. Laboratory tests
       i. Prescription and/or dispensing of medication for treatment
       j. Prenatal and postpartum referral and follow-up
       k. Adolescent pregnancy prevention and parenting services

    2. Referral and follow-up for specialty services that are beyond the scope of services provided by this project

   B. Mental health or social services must be provided in accordance with nationally recognized and accepted standards, such as the National Association of Social Workers *Standards for Social Work in Health Care Settings*. The standards to be used must be clearly identified in the project application.

    1.   Assessment and treatment of psychological, social, and emotional problems
    2.   Crisis intervention
    3.   Individual, family, and group counseling or referral for same, if indicated
    4.   Substance abuse and HIV/AIDS (human immunodeficiency virus/acquired immunodeficiency syndrome) prevention, risk reduction, and early intervention services
    5.   Support and/or psychoeducational groups focusing on topics of importance to the target population
    6.   Advocacy and referral for such services as day care, housing, employment, and job training
    7.   Referral for students requiring long-term or residential treatment
    8.   Consultation with school staff and parents on issues of child and adolescent development

   C. Health education services (complementary to the curriculum provided by local education agencies)

1. Consultation with school staff regarding issues of growth and development
2. School staff and parent training regarding issues of importance to target population
3. Individual and group health education

D. Dental services, including the following:

1. Screenings and cleanings
2. Sealant applications
3. Treatment for caries or extractions
4. Referral and follow-up for services beyond the scope of the project

V. Linkages with the community: Establishing linkages with medical, mental health, social service providers, and other relevant groups is encouraged. These may include the local health department, community health center, medical schools and hospitals, schools of public health, mental health and family service agencies, youth services bureaus, and recreational agencies.

VI. The administration of these clinical services *may* need to be distinct from the administration that currently exists, depending on the scope of services provided. The rationale and design of the administrative structure must be clearly outlined in the proposal. A plan for how these new services will integrate with existing school-based services must be described.

STANDARD MODEL FOR PART-TIME COMPREHENSIVE SCHOOL-BASED HEALTH CENTER—LEVEL IV

I. A part-time school-based health center (SBHC) is similar to a full-time SBHC and closely follows the Level V Standard Model for a comprehensive SBHC. A school would be eligible for a part-time SBHC if the student body is less than 500. The administration and coordination of the part-time SBHC must emanate from a full-time SBHC.

II. The part-time SBHC must hold a State of Connecticut license for outpatient clinics as outlined in the Public Health Code, Sections 19-13-D45 through 19-13-D53.

III. The part-time SBHC should operate regularly at specified times during the academic year:

    A. It should be open September through June (excepting weekends, holidays, and school vacations).

    B. It should be open specific hours during school operation. Extended hours may be appropriate to increase access.

IV. Solid plans for the provision of services during nonoperational times must be clearly identified.

    A. Medical and social services "backup" must be clearly defined (with letters of agreement) to cover medical and psychiatric emergencies and other needed services during times the center is not open (i.e., after school hours, weekends, holidays, vacations).

    B. *Ideally*, the center staff would have privileges at the backup site(s) in order to enhance continuity of care for the target population.

    C. Administration and coordination must be under the direction of the full-time SBHC with which it is affiliated.

V. Staff should be sufficient to provide services for the number of hours the SBHC is to be open and should include the following:

    A. A center coordinator or manager responsible for the full-time SBHC with which the part-time SBHC will be affiliated

    B. A nurse practitioner who must have experience serving the target population (including age and ethnicity), with clinical supervision or consultant backup

    C. A social worker (MSW) who must have experience in working with the target population (including age and ethnicity), with clinical supervision or consultant backup

    D. Additional health and/or allied health professionals as needed (e.g., nutritionist, substance prevention specialist, health educator, outreach worker, parent aid, psychologist, dentist, dental hygienist

    E. Clerical support

VI. Utilization of center services requires written parental permission.

A. Physical health or medical services must be provided in accordance with such standards as the American Academy of Pediatrics *Guidelines for Health Supervision*. Other nationally recognized and accepted standards may be used as a framework for professional practice with prior department approval.

   1. Primary health care, including the following:

      a. Physical exams, health assessments or screening for health problems
      b. Diagnosis and treatment of acute illness and injury
      c. Diagnosis and management of chronic illness
      d. Immunizations
      e. Health promotion and risk reduction
      f. Nutrition and weight management
      g. Reproductive health care
      h. Laboratory tests
      i. Prescription and/or dispensing of medication for treatment
      j. Prenatal and postpartum referral and follow-up

   2. Referral and follow-up for specialty services that are beyond the scope of services provided by this project

B. Mental health or social services must be provided in accordance with nationally recognized and accepted standards, such as the National Association of Social Workers *Standards for Social Work in Health Care Settings*. Other nationally recognized and accepted standards may be utilized as a framework for professional practice with prior department approval.

   1. Assessment and treatment of psychological, social, and emotional problems
   2. Crisis intervention
   3. Individual, family, and group counseling or referral for same, if indicated
   4. Substance abuse and HIV/AIDS prevention, risk reduction, and early intervention services
   5. Outreach to students at risk
   6. Support and/or psychoeducational groups focusing on topics of importance to the target population
   7. Advocacy and referral for such services as day care, housing, employment, and job training

8. Referral for students requiring long-term or residential treatment
9. Consultation with school staff and parents on issues of child and adolescent development

C. Health education services should be supportive of existing health education activities of local education agencies.

1. Consultation with school staff regarding issues of growth and development
2. School staff and parent training regarding issues of importance to target population
3. Individual and group health education
4. Classroom presentations

VII. Linkages with the community: Establishing linkages with medical, mental health, social service providers, and other relevant groups is encouraged. These may include the local health department, community health center, medical schools and hospitals, schools of public health, mental health and family service agencies, youth services bureaus, and recreational agencies.

STANDARD MODEL FOR A FULL-TIME COMPREHENSIVE SCHOOL-BASED HEALTH CENTER—LEVEL V

I. The school-based health center must hold a State of Connecticut license for outpatient clinics as outlined in the Public Health Code, Sections 19-13-D45 through 19-13-D53.

II. The SBHC should operate full-time during the academic year, according to the following schedule:

A. It should be open September through June (excepting weekends, holidays, and school vacations).

B. It should be open specific hours during school operation. Extended hours are encouraged when possible.

III. Solid plans for the provision of services during nonoperational times must be clearly identified.

A. Medical and social services back-up must be clearly defined (with letters of agreement) to cover medical and psychiatric emergencies and other needed services during times the center is not open (i.e., after school hours, weekends, holidays, vacations).

B. *Ideally*, the center staff would have privileges at the backup site(s) in order to enhance continuity of care for the target population.

IV. Staff should be sufficient to operate a full-time SBHC (as defined in part I of this section) and should include the following:

A. A center coordinator or manager with training and experience in health or mental health systems management, supervision, and administration

B. At least one nurse practitioner who must have experience serving the target population (including age and ethnicity), with M.D. backup

C. At least one social worker (MSW) with expertise in working with the target population (including age and ethnicity), with clinical supervision or consultant backup

D. Additional health and/or allied health professionals as needed (e.g., nutritionist, substance prevention specialist, health educator, outreach worker, parent aide, psychologist, dentist, dental hygienist)

E. Clerical support

V. Utilization of center services requires written parental permission. Minimum services to be provided include the following:

A. Physical health services must be provided in accordance with nationally recognized standards, such as the American Academy of Pediatrics school health manual *School Health: Policy and Practice* (American Academy of Pediatrics Committee on School Health, 1993), or those of the National Association of School Nurses. The standards to be used must be clearly identified in the project application.

1. Primary health care, including:

a. Physical exams, health assessments or screening for health problems

    b. Diagnosis and treatment of acute illness and injury
    c. Diagnosis and management of chronic illness
    d. Immunizations
    e. Health promotion and risk reduction
    f. Nutrition and weight management
    g. Reproductive health care
    h. Laboratory tests
    i. Prescription and/or dispensing of medication for treatment
    j. Prenatal and postpartum referral and follow-up
    k. Adolescent pregnancy prevention and parenting services

2. Referral and follow-up for specialty services that are beyond the scope of services provided by the SBHC

B. Mental health services must be provided in accordance with a nationally recognized and accepted standard such as the National Association of Social Workers (NASW) *Standards for Social Work in Health Care Settings*. The standards to be used must be clearly identified in the project application.

1. Assessment and treatment of psychological, social, and emotional problems
2. Crisis intervention
3. Individual, family, and group counseling or referral for same, if indicated
4. Substance abuse and HIV/AIDS prevention, risk reduction, and early intervention services
5. Outreach to students at risk
6. Support and/or psychoeducational groups focusing on topics of importance to the target population
7. Advocacy and referral for such services as day care, housing, employment, and job training
8. Referral for students requiring long-term or residential treatment
9. Consultation with school staff and parents on issues of child and adolescent development.

C. Health education services (complementary to the curriculum provided by the local education agencies)

1. Consultation with school staff regarding issues of growth and development

2. School staff and parent training regarding issues of importance to target population.
3. Individual and group health education

D. Dental services, including the following:

1. Screenings and cleanings
2. Sealant applications
3. Treatment for caries or extractions
4. Referral and follow-up for services beyond the scope of the project

VI. Linkages with the community: Establishing linkages with medical, mental health, social service providers, and other relevant groups is encouraged. These may include the local health department, community health center, medical schools and hospitals, schools of public health, mental health and family service agencies, youth services bureaus, and recreational agencies.

REFERENCE

American Academy of Pediatrics Committee on School Health, 1993. *School Health: Policy and Practice*, Nader, P.R. (ed), American Academy of Pediatrics, Elk Grove Village, IL.

Acronyms and Abbreviations

AAHE	Association for the Advancement of Health Education
AAP	American Academy of Pediatrics
ACCESS	Administration, Community, Curricula, Environment, School, Services
ACS	American Cancer Society
ADA	Americans with Disabilities Act
AFDC	Aid to Families with Dependent Children
AFY	Advocates for Youth
AIDS	acquired immunodeficiency syndrome
AMA	American Medical Association
ASFSA	American School Food Service Association
ASHA	American School Health Association
BOCES	Boards of Cooperative Educational Services
CAS	Children's Aid Society
CATCH	Child and Adolescent Trial for Cardiovascular Health (National Heart, Lung and Blood Institute)
CCSSO	Council of Chief State School Officers
CDC	Centers for Disease Control and Prevention
CIS	Cities in Schools
CPR	cardiopulmonary resuscitation
CSHP	comprehensive school health program

DASH	Division of Adolescent and School Health (Centers for Disease Control and Prevention)
DHHS	U.S. Department of Health and Human Services
DOEd	U.S. Department of Education
EDC	Education Development Center
EPSDT	Early Periodic Screening, Detection, and Treatment
ESA	Educational Service Agency
ESEA	Elementary and Secondary Education Act
ETR	Education, Training, and Research Associates
FRC	Family Resource Center
FY	fiscal year
FPL	federal poverty level
GAO	U.S. General Accounting Office
GAPS	Guidelines for Adolescent Preventive Services
Goals 2000	Educate America Act, 1994
Healthy People 2000	National Health Promotion and Disease Prevention Objectives, U.S. Public Health Service, DHHS, 1991
HDL	high-density lipoprotein
HIV	human immunodeficiency virus
HMO	health maintenance organization
HRSA	Health Resources and Services Administration (U.S. Public Health Service)
ICSH	Interagency Committee on School Health (federal)
IDEA	Individuals with Disabilities Education Act
IEP(s)	Individualized Education Plan
IHP	Individualized Health Plan
IOM	Institute of Medicine
K–12	kindergarten through grade 12
LEAs	local education agency
LST	Life Skills Training
MCH	Maternal and Child Health Bureau (U.S. Public Health Service)

MCO	managed care organization
Met Life	Metropolitan Life Insurance Foundation
NAEP	National Assessment of Educational Progress
NAPSO	National Alliance of Pupil Services Organizations
NASN	National Association of School Nurses
NASP	National Association of School Psychologists
NASPE	National Association for Sport and Physical Education
NASW	National Association of Social Workers
NCATE	National Council for Accreditation of Teacher Education
NCCSH	National Coordinating Committee on School Health
NEA	National Education Association
NET	Nutrition Education and Training (Program)
NIAAA	National Institute on Alcohol Abuse and Alcoholism
NIH	National Institutes of Health
NIMH	National Institute of Mental Health
NRC	National Research Council
NSBA	National School Boards Association
NSLA	National School Lunch Act
NSLP	National School Lunch Program
OBRA	Omnibus Reconciliation Act
OSHA	Occupational Safety and Health Administration,U.S. Department of Labor
OT	occupational therapy
OTA	Office of Technology Assessment, U.S. Congress
PHS	U.S. Public Health Service
P.L.	Public Law
PTA	Parent Teachers Association
RDA	recommended daily allowance
RQES	Research Quarterly on Excercise and Sport
RWJ	Robert Wood Johnson Foundation
SAP	Student Assistant Program
SBHC	school-based health center

SBP	School Breakfast Program
SCASS	State Collaborative on Assessment and Student Standards
SEA	state education agency
SEBHI	School Enrollment-Based Health Insurance
SHA	state health agency
SHEE	School Health Education Evaluation (Project)
SHES	School Health Education Study
SHPPS	School Health Policies and Programs Study (Centers for Disease Control and Prevention)
SREB	Southern Regional Education Board
STD	sexually transmitted disease
Title I	of the Elementary and Secondary Education Act
Title IV, Title IV-B	of the Elementary and Secondary Education Act
Title V	Maternal and Child Health block grants
Title XI	of the Elementary and Secondary Education Act
Title XIX	Medicaid program
Title XX	social services grants
USDA	U.S. Department of Agriculture
USPHS	U.S. Public Health Service, Department of Health and Human Services
YRBS	Youth Risk Behavior Surveillance (Centers for Disease Control and Prevention)

Index

Abortion counseling and birth control, 257, 398, 409-410. *See also* Teen pregnancy prevention

Absenteeism and tardiness, 24, 35, 67, 73, 160, 174, 189, 193, 397-398

Academic performance
grade retention/repeated grades, 24
health services and, 193, 396-398
health status and, 19, 51
parental involvement and, 25
physical activity/education and, 68, 85, 90-91
poverty and, 24
psychosocial environment and, 65-66

Accelerated schools, 385

ACCESS model of CSHP, 56, 57

Access to health care
health insurance and, 27-28
professional training in adolescent health care and, 28
psychosocial interventions and, 67
school health services and, 7, 15, 158, 196, 217-218, 226, 298, 365-366, 394
transportation, convenience, and cultural issues, 28

Adolescent and School Health Initiative, 242

Adolescent females, 434-435

Adolescent Parenting Program, 378

Advanced Nurse Education, 436-437

Advisory Committee on Immunization Practices, 427

Advocates for Youth, 190-191, 389-390

After-school programs, 37-38, 121

AIDS/HIV prevention, 16, 49, 69, 100, 106-107, 112-115, 119, 207, 242, 248, 403, 436-437, 458

AIDS Prevention Education Curricula, 106-107

Alcohol and drug abuse, 20, 21, 23, 72

Alcohol and drug abuse prevention, 16, 157
access to care for, 28
cost-effectiveness, 122
funding for, 250
health education and guidance, 46, 47, 69, 100, 101, 112-115, 122, 129, 130, 283-284, 314-317, 320-323, 422, 424
model programs, 378
outcomes of interventions, 103, 393-394
physical activity/education and, 68, 85
professional development/training, 118
Student Assistance Programs, 174, 372-373, 394
temperance movement and, 336-337

Alternative schools, 396

American Academy of Pediatrics, 59, 64 n.6, 154, 161-162 n.3, 163, 166, 216, 217 n.7, 219, 221, 241, 463-464, 469, 471

American Alliance for Health, Physical
    Education, Recreation and Dance, 59
    n.5
American Association for the Advance-
    ment of Science, 70 n.9, 129, 130-131
American Association of School
    Administrators, 40, 245
American Cancer Society, 124, 136, 207, 246
American Child Health Association, 43
American College Health Association, 59 n.5
American Dental Association, 241
American Heart Association, 86-87
American Medical Association, 18, 39, 44,
    47, 222-223, 241, 245, 298
American Nurses Association, 44-45, 48,
    163, 241
American Occupational Therapy
    Association, 168
American Physical Therapy Association, 168
American Public Health Association, 44-45,
    48, 59 n.5
American Red Cross, 207
American School Counselor Association,
    154, 162 n.3, 171
American School Food Service Association,
    154, 162 n.3
American School Health Association, 44,
    45, 48, 59 n.5, 63 n.6, 154, 222-223
American Speech, Language, and Hearing
    Association, 168-169
Americans with Disabilities Act, 64
ASSIST grant program, 251
Association for the Advancement of Health
    Education, 44, 59, 108, 109
Association of State and Territorial
    Directors of Public Health Education,
    59 n.5
Astoria Plan, 41, 43-44
Audiologists, 169

Baltimore, Maryland, 43, 182-183, 191, 298,
    386, 390, 394, 397
Beacons program, 185, 382
Behaviors, problem. *See also* Health
    behavior change
    and adolescent mortality and morbidity,
        1, 4, 20-21, 22, 139
    CDC priority areas, 20, 101, 132, 141
    clusters of, 13, 21, 120, 286-287, 290, 310
    and dropout rates, 21

environmental factors in, 5, 117, 120, 127,
    140, 272, 279, 357
    expectancy values and, 310
    family structure and, 26-27
    perceived norms and, 260, 310, 359-361
    poverty and, 24
    survey, 20-21
    theory, 286-287, 290, 309-310
Beyond Rhetoric, 46
Big Brother/Big Sister organization, 385
Blacks
    family structure, 26
    poverty, 23
Boards of Cooperative Educational
    Services, 251-252
Boys Clubs of America, 184, 381
*Bright Futures: Guidelines for Health
    Supervision of Infants, Children, and
    Adolescents*, 18, 299-300
Brookline Project, 189
Brown University, 387
Bureau of Education, 38-39
Bureau of the Census, 20

California, 398
    comprehensive multicomponent
        programs, 383-384
    Family Resource Centers, 185, 379, 405-
        406
    full-service schools, 387
    Healthy Start program, 193, 207, 298,
        393-394, 395, 396, 397, 404
    school-based health centers, 161, 191,
        196, 242 n.3, 374, 400, 403, 406
    School-Community Health Project, 43
*Cardinal Principles of Secondary Education,
    The*, 39
Cardiopulmonary resuscitation, 112, 114,
    118, 218-219
Cardiovascular Heart Healthy Eating and
    Exercise, 104-105
Carnegie Corporation, 47, 404
Carnegie Council on Adolescent
    Development, 67, 245
Carnegie Task Force on Meeting the Needs
    of Young Children, 23
Case management, 165, 174, 184, 380-381,
    398
Cattaragus County Studies, 43
Causes of death, 22-23

Center for Mental Health Services Research Project, 434
Center for Reproductive Health Policy Research, 395
Center for School Mental Health Assistance, 184
Centers for Disease Control and Prevention, 1
 Chronic Disease and Health Promotion, 250
 definition of health education, 99
 Division of Adolescent and School Health, 46, 54, 64 n.6, 75 n.11, 103, 108, 155, 242, 244, 247-248, 251, 403, 456
 funding for school health services, 207, 250
 Guidelines for School and Community Health Programs to Promote Physical Activity Among Youth, 4, 64 n.6, 97-98, 139
 health education evaluation guidelines, 280
 physical education recommendations, 97-98
 SHPPS study, 4, 5, 69, 71, 85, 92, 110-116, 132, 135, 138-139, 140, 141, 153, 155, 163, 182, 297, 373
 social morbidity findings, 20, 101, 139, 141
 Youth Risk Behavior Survey, 20-21
Child abuse evaluations and follow-up, 155, 156, 378
Child/Adolescent Planning and System Development Program, 434-435
Child and Adolescent Health Policy Centers, 243 n.4
Child and Adolescent Trial for Cardio-vascular Health (CATCH), 89, 179
Child Health Organization, 38
Child Nutrition Act, 45, 176
Children's Aid Society, 387, 397
Children's Defense Fund, 245
Children's Health Charter, 299, 300
Christmas Seal drive, 36
Cities in Schools, 184, 380-381
Claude Worthington Benedum Foundation, 458, 462
Clearinghouses, for family support programs, 380
Clinics, *see* School-based health centers
Closer Look, A, 71, 155, 157, 163, 218 n.8

Coalition of Essential Schools, 386-387
Coalition of National Health Organizations, 59
Collaborative Study of Children with Special Needs, 187, 189
Colorado, 191-192, 243 n.4, 374, 391, 393
Comer School Development Program, 383, 404
Commission of the European Communities, 58
COMMIT trial, 324-325
Committee for Economic Development, 181
Committee on War Time Problems of Children, 38
Communicable disease control, 34, 35, 127
Communities in Schools, 195
Community
 definition, 313
 health instruction, 112, 114, 118
 programs, 14, 51, 316-318, 323-324
Community and Migrant Health Centers, 243, 434-435
Community Health Center Program, 45
Community participation in CSHPs
 components, 63, 313, 318-322, 324-326, 353-354
 coordinating council, 10-11, 63, 165, 173-174, 240
 effectiveness, 74, 121, 313, 318-322, 324-326, 328-329
 extended services, 181, 184, 185, 225, 369
 goals and objectives, 51, 63, 353
 health education, 7, 51, 74, 75, 121, 137, 223-224, 306-311, 313, 316-326
 health services, 165, 172, 173, 187, 217, 225-226, 464, 467
 historical examples, 37-38, 40, 41, 42, 43
 importance of, 41
 infrastructure building, 252-253, 259-260, 264-265, 266, 461-462
 issues, 326-328
 mental health services, 71
 mobilization of, 252, 259-260
 models, 55-56, 307-308
 physical education, 98
 policy and administration, 63, 353
 practical considerations, 308-309
 rationale for, 308-311
 research and evaluation, 63, 74, 329
 school linkages for, 67, 165, 172, 173, 187, 217, 225-226, 464, 467

strategic prevention concept, 311-313
theoretical considerations, 309-311
and turf wars, 259, 406-407
Community Partnership Demonstration
Grant Program, 432-433
Competitive sports, 4, 88, 94, 139
Comprehensive School Health Program,
436-437
Comprehensive school health programs
(CSHPs). *See also individual*
components
ACCESS model, 56, 57
Allensworth model, 56-57
charge to the committee, 2, 17
community participation in, 15, 55-56,
63, 74, 297-298
components, 14-15
DASH models, 46, 54, 247-248
deficiencies, 15, 297-298
definitions, 2, 28, 51-60, 301, 355
effects of, 121, 273, 281, 284-285
eight-component model, 3, 52-54, 64 n.6
family–school–community (Nader)
model, 55-56
feasibility, 15, 280
full-service schools, 3, 59
goals and desired outcomes, 2, 16-17, 50-
51, 242, 271, 338-339
governance, 405-406, 449
guidelines, 337-355
implementation, 17, 273-274
infrastructure, *see* Infrastructure building
for CSHP
integration of elements of, 60, 74-76, 165,
310-311
international models, 58-59
issues and questions, 29, 402-411
key elements, 2-3, 63-76, 446-447
models, 56, 58, 443-455
organization, 382-384
origin, 1-2, 16
principles, 445
rationale for, 271, 296-297, 308-311, 444-
445
school-based versus community-based,
407-408
status, 14-15, 17, 297-298
three-component model, 3, 52, 53
types of services, 452
Conferences, 44-45, 47, 246, 261. *See also*
specific conferences

Confidentiality of student records, 8-9, 191,
204-206, 227, 256, 390, 419
Conflict resolution, nonviolent, 100, 112,
114, 118, 250, 378, 393-394
Connecticut
dental services, 375-376
Family Resource Centers, 185, 379
school-based health centers, 374, 407
School Development Plan, 386
school health services model, 199, 202-
203, 463-473
vision screening, 35
Consumer health instruction, 112, 114, 118
Controversies
birth control and abortion counseling,
257, 398, 409-410
funding, 207
in health education, 69, 257
historical, 49
management of, 11, 257-259, 409-411
in school health services, 7, 11, 158, 398,
409-410
Cooperative learning, 67
Coordinated Services Project, 242
Coordination of health programs. *See also*
Community participation in CSHPs
advisory and coordinating councils, 66,
138-139, 241, 252-254, 263, 297-298, 386
family services, 73
federal interagency, 238-241, 242
funding for, 73 n.10, 374
historical efforts, 39
psychosocial environment, 67
research, 240
school-based health centers, 398
Cost-effectiveness
health education, 5, 122-123, 140, 327
health services, 400
Council of Chief State School Officers, 47,
108, 240, 245
Council of Europe, 58
Council of Great City Schools, 241
Counseling. *See also* School guidance
counselors; Vocational counseling
mental health, 3, 49, 155, 156, 157, 169,
171-172, 184, 192, 391
nutrition, 155, 156, 158, 176
Creating an Agenda for School-Based Health
Promotion: A Review of Selected
Reports, 245
Crisis medical situations, 218-219

Critical Populations Program, Adolescent Track, 432-433
Curriculum
    AIDS/HIV instruction, 49
    "back to the basics" movement, 46
    crowding issue, 141
    dissemination of effective programs, 103, 108, 242, 244
    health education, 4, 40, 41, 45, 49, 52, 53, 58, 69, 72, 100-101, 103-108, 110-115, 132-133, 139, 258, 284, 288, 342
    How to Live with 10–15 Year Olds, 462
    implementation of effective programs, 132-133
    nutrition, 72
    physical education, 37, 52, 68, 84, 85, 88-92, 95, 98, 139, 347-348
    social skills, 66, 122
    substance abuse prevention, 101

Dallas, Texas, 375, 383
Danforth Foundation, 382
Databases, 242, 243 n.4
Day care centers, 375, 385
Death and dying, instruction, 112, 114, 118
Definitions and terminology, 452-453
    Committee's definition, 2, 60-62
    community, 313
    comprehensive school health program, 355
    extended services, 181
    health, 1 n.1, 354
    health education, 99
    need for definition, 51-52
    previous definitions, 52-60
    primary care and primary health care, 154 n.1
    school-based health centers, 373
    School Health Coordinating Council, 355
    school health services, 153
Delaware, 191, 374, 390-391, 395
Delivery of health services
    funding for, 248
    models/guidelines, 202-203, 417, 419, 447
    primary care in schools, 45, 187
    regional approaches, 186, 188
Dentists and dental services
    controversies, 49
    demand for, 365-366
    funding, 168, 376
    health education, 112, 114, 118
    history, 37, 42, 49

    models, 376, 459, 467
    poverty and, 24
    in school-based health centers, 473
    standards, 467
    types of services, 71, 167-168, 375-376
Denver, Colorado, 191-192, 391, 393
Depression, 16, 28
Dietary behaviors, 112-115, 119
Dietary Guidelines for Americans, 177-178, 243, 460
Diffusion of innovation theory, 310
Disease prevention, 112, 114, 119
District school health advisory councils, 252-253, 297-296
Driver training, 41
Drop-Out Prevention Initiative, 195
Drug abuse, *see* Alcohol and drug abuse
Dummer Grammar School, 33

Eagle Forum, 409
Early and Periodic Screening, Diagnostic, and Treatment Program, 24, 207, 209, 219, 221, 243-244, 402-403, 432-433
Early Intervention Group, 378
Eat Smart School Nutrition Program, 179
Education. *See also* Health education; Physical education
    elements of, 3
    importance of, 18-20
Education Audiology Association, 169
Education for All Handicapped Children Act, 45, 214
Education of the Handicapped Act, 168, 187
Educational Service Agencies, 188
Elementary and Secondary Education Act, 45, 48 n.4, 73 n.10, 170, 172, 173, 207, 241-242, 248, 250, 436-437
Elementary school
    dental services, 167, 376
    extended services, 386
    health education in, 5-6, 7, 110-112, 115, 140, 141-142
    nutrition, 179
    physical education, 93
    professional development and qualifications, 141
    pupil personnel teams, 371
Emergency Medical Services for Children, 218-219
Employee Assistance Programs, 174
Employment, *see* Youth employment
Environment, *see* School environment

Environmental health, 112, 114, 119
European Network of Health Promoting
    Schools, 58
Evaluation of programs, *see* Research and
    evaluation
Even Start, 172, 380
Extended services. *See also* Dentists and
    dental services; School-based health
    centers
  basis for, 181
  case management, 165, 174, 184, 380-381,
    398
  Cities in Schools, 184, 380-381
  community role, 7, 181, 184, 185, 225,
    369, 381
  components, 367, 370
  comprehensive multicomponent
    programs, 382-384
  coordination of, 374
  definition, 181
  effectiveness, 366
  Family Resource Centers, 185, 379-380,
    398
  full-service schools, 3, 59, 185-186, 204,
    365, 380, 387-389
  funding, 181, 185, 371, 378, 379, 380, 382,
    389
  goals, 367
  issues, 225, 366
  mental health centers, 184, 376-379, 391,
    394, 395
  models, 202-203, 464, 465-467
  organization of, 366-389
  parental permission for services, 465-467
  personnel/staffing, 173-174, 367, 368,
    370-372, 377-378, 465
  pupil personnel teams, 173-174, 370-372
  recommendations, 8, 227
  regional approaches, 186, 188, 203
  research and evaluation, 227
  school reorganization, 66, 385-387
  standards, 465-466
  student assistance programs, 174, 372-
    373, 378, 394
  success factors, 399-400
  target groups, 367, 395
  teen parent programs, 384-385
  user characteristics, 365-366
  youth service centers, school-based, 184-
    185, 382, 393, 395
Extracurricular activities, 98, 121

Family and Community Endeavors, 382
Family Educational Rights and Privacy Act
    of 1974, 205
Family Planning Program (Title X), 183,
    374, 432-433
Family Preservation Act, 48 n.4
Family Resource Centers, 185, 379-380, 388,
    398, 403-404, 405
Family Resources Coalition, 380
Family services, elements of, 73-74
Family structure. *See also* Single-parent
    households
  and health and welfare of children, 18
  and school health programs, 16, 25-27
  traditional, 26
  wages and earnings and, 26
Family support teams, 66-67, 386, 397
Federal Interagency Committee on School
    Health, 238-240
Federal programs, infrastructure building,
    241-245
First aid, 71, 112, 114, 119, 155
Florida
  Family Resource Centers, 185, 379, 380
  full-service schools, 207, 403-404
  Funding for School Services Act, 199,
    203-204, 251
  school-based health centers, 242 n.3, 374,
    391, 392-393, 397, 398-399, 403, 406, 408
  School Enrollment-Based Health
    Insurance concept, 210-211, 298-299
  Supplemental School Health Program,
    371-372, 392-393
Focus on Youth, 194
Food Labeling Education Program, 436-437
Framingham, Massachusetts, 43
Full-service schools, 3, 59, 185-186, 204, 207,
    380, 387-389, 403-404, 406, 407
Funding of school health services
  categorical, 203-204, 244-245, 264, 406
  controversial, 207
  coordination of, 10, 188, 239, 248-251
  for coordination of services, 73 n.10
  dental services, 168, 376
  by excise taxes and penalties, 9, 216, 251
  extended services, 181, 185, 203-204, 378-
    379, 380, 382, 389
  federal, 179, 207, 213, 239, 430-442
  Great Society and, 46
  health care services, 168, 203-204
  health education, 248, 250

health insurance, school-based, 9, 210-212
infrastructure building, 241-245, 248-251, 262-264
Medicaid, 9, 208-209, 212, 213, 214, 219, 221, 402-403
mental health or pupil services, 169, 170, 173, 378, 379
multisource, 188
nonprofit intermediary for contracting services, 213-215
nutrition and foodservice, 175, 177, 179-180, 243
overview, 206-208
personnel/staffing, 248, 250
pooled-fund approach, 213, 263
private foundations, 208
recommendations, 9, 10, 227, 450
research and evaluation, 262-263
school-based health centers, 46, 183, 212-213, 243, 250, 374, 398, 402-405
screening, 209, 219, 221
sources, 9, 183, 207-208, 249, 250, 264, 298-299, 402-405
in standard benefit packages, 9, 216
state and local, 179-180, 207-208, 213, 239, 248, 249
surcharge on health care payers, 215
training and professional development, 248, 250

Gallup Organization, 124
Girls Clubs of America, 381
Go for Health, 104-105
Goals 2000: Educate America Act, 48 n.4, 73 n.10, 238
Golden Anniversary Conference on Children and Youth, 44
Great Society programs, 45, 46
Growing Healthy, 104-105, 132
Guidelines
  health education, 64 n.6
  mental health center, 377
  nutrition, 64 n.6
  physical activity, 4, 64 n.6, 97
  professional training and education, 44-45
  tobacco prevention programs, 64 n.6
Guidelines for Adolescent Preventive Services (GAPS)
  abuse (emotional, physical, sexual), 426
  alcohol and drug abuse, 422, 424
  barriers to implementation, 222

clinical applications, 47, 428
confidentiality of adolescent care, 419
delivery of health services, 417, 419
depression/suicide risk, 426
frequency of preventive services, 417-419
health guidance, 47, 417, 418, 419-422
immunizations, 417, 418, 427-428
injury prevention, 421
learning or school problems, 427
nutrition/diet-related, 421, 422-424
overview, 416-419
parental involvement, 419, 420
physical activity, 421
physical assessment, 418, 423-424
primary care providers, 222-223, 298
recommendations, 222
screening, 417, 418, 422-427
sexual behavior and responsibility, 421-422, 424-426
sociocultural sensitivity, 419
tests, 418
tobacco use, 424
topics/health conditions addressed by, 417
traditional approaches contrasted with, 428-429
Guidelines for Comprehensive School Health Programs, 63-64 n.6
Guidelines for Developing and Implementing School-Based Early Periodic Screening, Detection and Treatment Services, 458-459
Guidelines for Health Supervision, 469
Guidelines for School and Community Health Programs to Promote Physical Activity Among Youth, 4, 64 n.6, 97, 139
Guidelines for School Settings, 464

Head Start, 45, 48 n.4, 170, 175, 380
Health
  aides, 163
  centers, *see* School-based health centers
  defined, 1 n.1, 16 n.1, 45, 354
  examination surveys, 167-168
  guidance, 419-422
  information, access to, 16
  insurance, 27-28, 67, 160, 161, 165, 210-211, 214, 216, 241, 247, 298, 365
  literacy, 4, 102, 137, 138, 139-140
  records and medical information, 155, 156
  services, *see* School health services
Health Appraisal of School Children, 40

Health behavior change. *See also* Social
    learning theory
  expectations and, 359-361, 362-363
  goals and, 361-363
  health education and, 5, 103-107, 109-
    110, 116, 117, 120-121, 122-123, 140,
    281, 313-322, 341-342, 356-363
  hours of instruction and, 103, 109-110,
    115, 135, 140
  individual characteristics and, 117, 120
  measuring, 271-272
  models used in health education
    programs, 356-363
  as outcome measure, 278-279
  parental involvement and, 120
  peer involvement in prevention and, 120
  relapse prevention, 117, 120
  school-based health centers and, 7, 190,
    191-192, 226, 366, 390-391
  self-efficacy and, 120, 357-359, 362-363
  skills and, 13, 117, 120, 362-363
  social support and, 117, 120
  teacher/professional qualifications and,
    103, 118-119, 140
Health Care Financing Administration, 208
Health care services, *see* Access to Health
    care; Extended services; School-based
    health centers; School health services
Health education
  alternative approaches, 6, 103, 110, 141
  barriers to, 309
  and behavior change, 5, 103-107, 109-
    110, 116, 117, 120-121, 122-123, 140,
    281, 283-284, 286-287, 341-342, 356-
    363
  booster sessions, 103, 110, 141, 283-284,
    285, 287, 309
  cardiovascular, 316-317, 320-321
  community role, 121, 137, 223-224, 306-
    311, 313, 316-326
  controversies, 69
  cost-effectiveness, 5, 122-123, 140, 327
  current practice, 110-116, 140, 141
  curriculum, 4, 40, 41, 45, 49, 52, 53, 58,
    69, 72, 99, 100-101, 103-108, 110-115,
    132-133, 139, 258, 284, 288, 309, 342
  effectiveness, 116-124, 136, 140, 284-285,
    316-323
  environment for, 135
  exemptions from, 112
  funding for, 248

GAPS recommendations, 47, 417, 418,
    419-422
goals and objectives, 3, 4, 39-40, 47, 52,
    69, 81, 99-100, 101-110, 112, 136, 140,
    341
grade level and, 5-6, 7, 110-112, 115-116,
    140-141
health services and, 166, 182, 215, 218-
    219, 223-224, 373, 417, 418, 419-422
hours of instruction, 103, 109-110, 115,
    140, 141, 281-282, 283-284
infrastructure, 457-458
infusion/integration approach, 13, 40,
    68, 69-70, 74-75, 98, 111, 112-116, 125-
    131, 136-137, 138, 176, 180-181
instructional elements, 45, 46, 99, 100-
    101, 117, 120, 121-122, 126, 127, 132-
    133, 141, 285-286, 342
interagency collaboration, 247
issues, 326-328
legislation, 41
literature review, 306
local education agency role, 137
media role, 121, 309, 318-323, 325
models, 307-308
national action plan, 135, 136, 140
national organizations' role, 138
National Science Education Standards
    and, 129-130
needs, 132-135
outcomes, 103, 116-117, 287-288, 341-342
parental involvement, 101, 117, 120, 318-
    323, 325, 420
peer-based, 286
performance assessment, 102-103, 108,
    141, 240
physical fitness, 98, 112-115, 125, 126,
    128, 134, 320-321, 421
policy and administrative support, 135,
    239-240, 325, 341
priorities, 4, 101, 138, 139, 140, 141
professional development and
    qualifications, 5, 6-7, 103, 108-109,
    115-116, 117, 118-119, 121, 133-134,
    137, 138, 140, 141-142, 343, 457-458
public perceptions of, 123-124, 140
recommendations, 5-7, 135-142
requirements for graduation, 5, 6, 110-
    112, 140, 141
research and evaluation, 5, 103-107, 116-
    124, 132, 135, 280-288, 312

risk-factor specific vs. problem behavior intervention, 286-287
role in CSHPs, 99-139
in school-based health centers, 182, 373, 470, 472-473
Science for All Americans standards, 130-131
sexuality and reproductive, 49, 69, 100, 112-115, 119, 130, 166, 286, 314-315, 318-319, 421
SHPPS findings and recommendations, 110-116, 135, 138-139, 140, 141
sociocultural issues, 117, 121
standards, 4, 5-6, 48, 101-103, 108, 109, 129-131, 132, 135, 136-138, 139-140, 141, 238-239, 466-467
state education and health agencies, 137
strategic prevention concept, 311-313
teaching/learning materials, 342-343
theoretical framework, 116, 117, 120, 309-310, 356-363
trends, 104-107, 117, 121
Health Insurance Association of America, 67-68
Health promotion
effectiveness of programs, 314-315, 320-321
objectives, 46-47
movement, 38, 117, 121
for staff, 3, 53, 67-68, 352-353, 461
Health status
and academic achievement, 19, 51
nutrition and, 72-73
physical education and, 4, 68-69, 81-82, 83, 84, 139
school-based health centers and, 7
Health Supervision and Medical Inspection of Schools, 39
Health: You've Got to Be Taught, 123
Healthy Caring, 183, 258-259
Healthy Kids Corporation, 299
Healthy Kids: Nutrition Objectives for School Meals, 175
Healthy People 2000 initiative, 22, 39-40, 46-47, 67-68, 83-84, 85, 99, 102, 112-115, 177-178, 215 n.6, 271
Healthy Schools, Healthy Communities, 48, 243, 280, 434-435
Healthy Start program, 193, 207, 298, 393-394, 395, 396, 397
Hearty Heart, 104-105

High Risk Youth Demonstration Grant Program, 432-433
High schools, *see* Secondary schools
Hillsdale County Elementary Success Program, 195
Hispanics
family structure, 26
poverty, 23
History of school health programs, 1
lessons learned from, 48-50
1960s to present, 45-48
1700s through early 1900s, 33-38, 82
World War I to 1960s, 38-45
HIV/AIDS Higher Education Consortia, 458
HIV Education Program, 100, 436-437
Hogg Foundation for Mental Health, 383, 404
Home economics, 69, 70, 72, 125, 126, 128, 129
Honeywell Corporation, 384-385
How to Fund Public Health Activities, 215
How to Live with 10–15 Year Olds, 462
Human Genome Project, 127
Human growth and development, 69, 112, 114, 119
Human Services Reauthorization Act, 48 n.4
Human sexuality, 49, 69, 100, 112-115, 119, 130, 166, 409, 421

Illinois, 35, 56, 58, 194, 374, 380
Immunizations, 34, 155, 157, 160, 396, 398, 427-428
Improving America's Schools Act, 48 n.4, 73 n.10
Indian Health Service Clinical Services, 432-433
Individualized Education Plans, 50, 155, 156, 168, 177
Individuals with Disabilities Education Act, 168, 170, 172, 173, 187, 207, 210, 242, 244, 248, 436-437
Infant mortality rates, 18
Infrastructure building for CSHPs
advisory and coordinating councils, 247, 252-254, 259-260, 263, 264-265, 297-298
barriers to, 11, 256-259, 298-299, 448
CDC/DASH models, 247-248
collaboration in, 256, 259, 260-261, 298
communications, 250, 263, 298, 448
community or district level, 10-11, 252-253, 259-260, 264-265, 266, 461-462

community support mobilization, 252, 259-260

controversy management, 11, 257-259

district school health coordinator, 253

extension service, 10, 251-252, 263, 264

federal programs, 241-245, 451

funding streams, 10, 241-245, 248-251, 262-264, 298-299, 450

health education, 457-458

health services, 247, 253-254, 265-268, 458-459

interagency collaboration, 9-11, 247, 256, 263

Interagency Committee on School Health, 9-10, 47, 238-240, 262

interdisciplinary teams, 254-256, 257, 265, 267-268, 298, 457

leadership, 9, 247

local level, 252-261

mental health and pupil services, 460

models, 456-462

National Coordinating Committee on School Health, 9, 10, 240-241, 262

national level, 9-10, 238-246, 262-263, 266

objectives, 246

nutrition and foodservices, 460-461

personnel training needs, 11, 249, 256-257, 265, 267-268, 449-450

physical education, 459

recommendations, 9-11, 261-268

research and evaluation, 262-263

resources, 249, 259, 449-450

school environment, 460

school level, 11, 253-254, 265-268, 460

state level, 10, 239, 246-252, 263-264, 266, 451

teacher and staff wellness, 461

technical assistance, 251-252, 263, 264

and turf battles, 259, 406-407

Injury prevention and control, 100, 112-115, 119, 218-219, 320-321, 421

Institute of Medicine

Committee on Comprehensive School Health Programs in Grades K–12, 154 n.1

Committee on the Future of Primary Care, 154 n.1

Instruction

duration, sequence, and timing of, 103, 109-110, 115, 135, 140, 141, 283-284

health education, 45, 46, 52, 98, 99, 100-101, 103, 109-110, 115, 117, 120, 121-122, 126, 127, 132-133, 135, 140, 141, 283-284, 342

physical education, 98, 348

social skills, 132-133

Instructional materials, 342-343

Interagency Committee on School Health, 9-10, 47, 238-240, 262

Interdisciplinary teams, 171, 254-256

International models of CSHPs, 58-59

Inwood House, 372-373

Jackson-Hinds Comprehensive Health Center (Mississippi), 374

Johns Hopkins University, 66, 196, 243 n.4, 386

Joint Committee on Health Education Terminology, 59-60

Joint Committee on National Health Education Standards, 101-102, 129, 131

Jump Rope for Heart, 94

Junior high, *see* Middle school

Junior League, 184, 381

Just Say No clubs, 378

Kentucky, 185, 379, 382, 403, 406, 408

Kiwanis Club, 376

Know Your Body, 104-105, 132, 281, 282

Language arts, 69, 70, 125, 126, 127, 128-129

Latchkey children, 26-27

Leadership, 9, 247

Legislation, 41, 45, 48 n.4, 73 n.10, 100-101, 157, 179, 379. *See also specific statutes*

Lehigh University College of Education, 381

Life Skills Training, 284-285

Local community

extended service providers, 369

funding sources, 207-208

health education role, 137

infrastructure building, 252-261

process evaluation, 12

Locust Point Demonstration, 43

Los Angeles, 191, 377, 390

Louisiana, 175, 374

Low-income families. *See also* Poverty

children in, 23

health problems in, 160-161

utilization of extended services, 365-266

Maine, 248, 443-455
Making the Grade, 183, 212, 213, 246, 404
Managed care, 10, 207-208, 211, 213, 214-215, 241, 247, 298-299, 374, 403, 404-405
March of Dimes, 207
Maryland, 43, 182-183, 191, 368, 386, 390, 394
Massachusetts, 34, 35, 82, 251, 374, 376
Maternal and child health agencies, 40, 207, 458, 459
Maternal and Child Health Bureau, 47, 48, 217 n.7, 243
Maternal and Child Health State Block Grants, 183, 213, 243, 244, 250, 374, 402, 434-435
Mathematics, 69, 70, 75, 126, 127, 128-129
Media role, 55, 121
Medicaid, 45, 244
    and access to health care, 160
    Early and Periodic Screening, Diagnostic, and Treatment Program, 24, 207, 209, 219, 221, 243-244, 402-403, 432-433
    eligibility screening, 459
    nutrition-related funding, 177
    for school health services, 160, 183, 207, 208-209, 212, 213, 214, 243-244, 374, 389, 402-403, 459
Memphis City Schools Mental Health Center, 377-378
Mental health and pupil services. See also Mental health centers
    community health linkages, 71, 172, 173-174
    counseling, 3, 49, 155, 156, 157, 169, 171-172, 184, 192, 248, 297, 391, 460
    demand for, 365-366
    direct services to students, 349-350
    education, 112, 114, 119, 125
    funding, 169, 170, 172, 173
    goals, objectives and outcomes, 3, 71, 349
    guidelines, 349-350
    infrastructure building, 460
    issues, 170-172, 173
    mechanisms for providing, 173-174
    models, 464, 469-470
    need for, 71-72, 297
    outcomes, 394
    policy and administrative support, 349
    poverty and, 160

    problem identification and resolution, 222
    professional development, 119, 170, 171, 173, 350
    psychological, 3, 8, 155, 156, 169-171, 297, 460
    recommendations, 8, 226
    in school-based clinics, 464, 469-470, 472
    social morbidities and, 71-72
    social services, 3, 71, 169, 172-173, 222, 460, 472
    staffing, 170, 171, 172-173
    standards, 170, 173, 464, 469-470, 472
    student assistance programs, 174, 372-373
    team approach, 66, 67, 171, 173-174, 370-372, 386
    utilization, 191, 395
Mental health centers, 184, 376-379
Metropolitan Life Foundation, 123
Metropolitan Life Insurance Company, 43, 283
Michigan, 242 n.3, 374, 395, 407
Mid-Century White House Conference on Children and Youth, 44
Middle school
    health education, 5-6, 110-112, 140, 283-284
    physical education, 85, 88
    psychosocial interventions, 67, 460
    school health services programs, 201
    substance abuse prevention, 283-284
Milbank Memorial Fund, 43
Minimum Health Requirements for Rural Schools, 39
Minnesota, 192-193, 242 n.3, 384-385
Missouri, 195, 199, 201, 382, 396, 397
Modern Health Crusaders, 36
Motor vehicles
    driver training, 41
    and mortality, 23
    and risky behaviors, 20

Nashville, Tennessee, 380, 398
Nation at Risk, A, 46
National Action Plan for Comprehensive School Health Education, 5, 135, 136, 140, 246, 262
National Adolescent Health Information Center, 243 n.4
National Adolescent Health Resource Center, 217 n.7, 243 n.4

National Alliance of Pupil Services Organizations, 173, 370
National Assembly for School-Based Health Care, 48, 374
National Assessment for Educational Progress, 240
National Association of:
Community Health Centers, 242
Elementary School Principals, 241
School Nurses, 48, 153-154, 161 n.3, 162, 163, 241, 464, 465, 471
School Psychologists, 154, 162 n.3, 170
Secondary School Principals, 241
Social Workers, 154, 162 n.3, 172-173, 464, 469-470, 472
State Boards of Education, 47, 245
National Cancer Institute, 251
National Center for:
Education in Maternal and Child Health, 243 n.4
Health Statistics, 168
Leadership Enhancement of Adolescent Programs, 243 n.4
Partnership Development, 381
National Cholesterol Education program, 158
National Commission on Children, 46, 245
National Commission on the Role of the School and the Community in Improving Adolescent Health, 444
National Committee on School Health Policies, 40
National Conference for Cooperation in Health Education, 40
National Congress of Parents and Teachers, 36
National Coordinating Committee on School Health, 9, 10, 47, 238, 240-241, 262, 430-431
National Council for the Accreditation of Teacher Education, 44, 108, 109
National Education Association (NEA), 36, 39, 40, 241
National Education Goals, 4, 19-20, 47, 89-90, 101, 102, 139, 238
National Food Service Management Institute, 177
National Health and Education Consortium, 183
National Health Education Standards, 4, 5-6, 48, 101-103, 108, 109, 129-131, 132,

135, 136-138, 139-140, 141, 176, 240, 246, 262
National Heart, Lung, and Blood Institute, 179, 422
National Institute of Alcohol Abuse and Alcoholism, 372
National Institute of Dental Research, 168
National Nursing Coalition for School Health, 48, 163
National organizations. *See also individual organizations*
extended services from, 369
health education role, 138
infrastructure building, 238-246, 262-263, 266
National Parent Teachers Association, 241
National School-Based Oral Health/Dental Sealant Resource Center, 243 n.4
National School Boards Association, 47, 109-110, 167, 241, 245-246, 253, 376
National School Health Bill, 42
National School Health Leadership Conference, 244
National School Health Project, School-Based Adolescent Health Care, 246
National School Lunch Act, 41, 175, 177, 179
National School Lunch Program, 25, 175, 211, 438-439
National Science Education Standards, 129-130
National Standards for Physical Education, 4, 48, 83, 85, 97, 139
National State School Nurse Consultants Association, 48
National Tuberculosis Association, 36, 43
NEA–AMA Joint Committee on Health Problems in Schools, 39, 40, 166
New Beginnings (San Diego), 383-384, 405-406
New Futures School, Inc. (Albuquerque), 384
New Jersey, 175, 378-379, 403, 404
New Mexico, 54, 242 n.3, 384
New Vistas High School (Minneapolis), 384-385
New York City
Astoria Plan, 41, 43-44
Beacons program, 185, 382
Drop-Out Prevention Initiative, 195
full-service schools, 387-388, 408
Health Day, 41

lunch program, 49, 179
medical inspection of schools, 34-36, 41
school health services, 37, 396
Teen Choice program, 372-373
New York State, 36, 193, 242 n.3, 372, 374, 396, 400
North Carolina, 185, 371, 379, 410, 462
Nurse Practitioner/Nurse-Midwifery, 436-437
Nurses and nurse practitioners
    burdens and responsibilities, 165, 407
    evaluation of activities, 189, 400
    historical role in schools, 35, 42, 45, 366
    issues related to, 164-165, 222-223, 406
    as primary care providers, 222-223
    qualifications and professional training, 153-154, 163, 164, 345-346
    services provided by, 45, 71, 75, 153, 162-163, 386, 388, 400, 406
    staffing patterns, 163-164
    standards, 48, 153, 163
Nursing Special Projects Grant Program, 438-439
Nutrition and foodservice. See also Dietary behaviors
    breakfast program, 41, 45, 73, 175, 243, 438-439
    counseling, 155, 156, 158, 176-177
    education, 69, 72, 74-75, 112-115, 119, 129, 130, 176, 180-181, 243, 421
    funding, 175, 177, 179-180, 243
    goals and objectives, 3, 52-53, 351
    guidelines, 350-352
    and health status, 72
    infrastructure building, 460-461
    integrated approach, 74-75, 129, 247
    issues related to, 20, 23, 177-181
    legislation, 175, 176, 179
    lunch programs, 25, 37, 41, 49, 175, 178, 179, 211, 243, 244, 438-439
    perceptions of nutrition, 180
    personnel, 177
    policy and administrative support, 179, 350-351
    professional development/training, 119, 177, 181, 352
    profit-making, 180
    recommendations, 8, 226
    research, 73
    and risky behaviors, 21
    screening related to, 158, 176-177

services provided, 174-177, 351-352
Snack Program, 243
Special Milk Program, 243
for special-needs children, 177
standards, 48, 154, 177, 178, 180, 239
and student performance, 73, 178
vending machines, special events, and fundraisers, 73, 75, 176, 178, 460
Nutrition Education and Training Program, 45, 176, 243, 248, 436-437
Nutrition for Life, 106-107
Nutrition in a Changing World, 106-107

Obese children, 86-87
Obsessive-compulsive disorder, 24
Occupational Safety and Health Administration, 64
Occupational therapists, 168
Office of Technology Assessment of the U.S. Congress, 47, 64-65
Ohio Research Study, 43
One-Stop-Shopping in a Northeast Nashville Community, 380, 398
Open-air classrooms, 36
Opportunity-to-Learn Standards, 136-138
Oregon, 191, 258, 390
Outcomes
    behavioral change as, 278-279, 313-322
    community, 51
    desired, 50-51
    dose-response relationship, 282-283
    effectiveness trials, 187, 273, 276
    efficacy testing, 273, 276, 277
    evaluation, 11-12, 13, 14, 50-51, 271-272, 273, 275, 276, 287-288
    of health education curricula, 103-107, 116, 282-283, 287-288, 313-322
    health-services-related, 14, 189, 394-396
    implementation effectiveness trials, 273-274
    measures of, 7-8, 12-13, 277, 278-279, 289
    mental health, 14, 394
    null or negative, interpretation of, 12-13
    positive, protective factors for, 23
    poverty and, 159-161
    pregnancy-related, 192-193, 392-393
    programmatic and organizational, 51
    realistic, 287-288
    school-based health centers and, 7-8, 190, 191-193, 366, 392-398
    school-related, 14, 396-398

of standards development, 102-103
student, 50
substance abuse-related, 393-394

Parental consent for health services, 190, 205, 206, 389, 399, 465-467, 468-470, 471-473
Parental involvement. *See also* Teen parent programs
   and academic achievement, 25
   and confidentiality of student records, 205, 206, 419
   disadvantaged students, 66
   funding for programs, 248
   goals for, 47, 54
   and health and welfare of children, 18
   in health education, 101, 117
   in health services, 185-186, 190
   historical examples, 44
   importance of, 41, 398
   in infrastructure building, 258-259
   interventions involving, 66, 386, 387
   in physical education, 98
Parent to Parent training, 378
Partnership for Prevention, 215
Pawtucket Heart Health Program, 106-107
Peer cluster theory, 310
Peer Mediation Training, 250
Peer Power and ADAM, 106-107
Pennsylvania, 35, 37, 386, 387
Personal health, 112, 114, 119
Philadelphia, 35, 37, 386
Physical education
   and academic achievement, 68, 85, 90-91
   academic rigor and, 90-92
   attendance, 21
   CDC recommendations, 97-98, 139
   community-based programs and facilities, 98
   contributions of, 3, 94, 97-98, 139
   current practice, 85, 88-92
   curriculum, 37, 52, 68, 84, 85, 88-92, 95, 98, 139, 347-348
   evaluation, 88-89, 98
   exemptions from, 85
   extracurricular activities, 98
   goals and objectives, 4, 47, 52, 68, 81, 82, 83-84, 92-93, 97, 101, 346-347
   grade level and, 68, 85, 88, 93-94, 95
   guidelines, 139, 346-349

health education and, 98, 112-115, 125, 126, 128, 134, 421
   and health services, 98
   and health status, 4, 68-69, 81-82, 83, 84, 90-91, 94, 97, 139
   history of movement, 37, 41, 82
   infrastructure building, 459
   instruction methods, 98, 348
   intensity of activity, 89, 92-93
   legislation, 41
   motor skill development, 84, 90-91
   nutrition education in, 72
   parental involvement, 98
   personnel/teachers, 92-94, 96, 98
   policy and administrative support, 97-98, 346
   professional development/training, 84, 90-91, 93-94, 96, 98, 119, 134, 348
   and public health, 82, 92-93
   quality of, 83-84, 85, 88-89
   recommendations, 97-98, 139
   requirements, 68, 85, 88, 94, 95
   research evidence on, 81-82, 84-85, 86-91, 139
   research needs, 85
   role in CSHPs, 81-98
   scheduling and environmental factors, 89-90
   school-based programs and facilities, 98
   standards, 4, 83, 139, 239
   strategies to promote physical activity, 94
   student outcomes, 68-69, 84, 347
   and substance abuse, 85
   testing of students, 94, 459
Physical environment of schools, 340-341
   hazards, 65
   legislation, 64-65
   program elements of, 2, 64-65
   structural condition of schools, 24-25
Physical examinations, 36, 43-44, 419
Physical fitness, health-related, 20, 84
Physical therapists, 168
Physicians
   historical role in schools, 37-38, 42, 166
   issues related to, 166-167
   qualifications and professional training, 166, 345
   services provided by, 71, 165-166
   "snip doctors," 37
   social contract, 167
   staffing patterns, 164

Pinal County Prevention Partnership
  (Arizona), 381
Pinkston High School (Dallas) , 375
Policy and administrative support, 349, 352
  elements of, 2
  environment, 2, 65, 135, 339
  health education, 135, 341
  health services, 225-226, 343-344
  nutrition and foodservice, 179, 350-351
  physical education, 97-98, 346
Population-based prevention, 157-158
Portland, Oregon, 258
Postponing Sexual Involvement, 106-107
Poverty
  and academic achievement, 24
  and health care, 24
  and health outcomes, 22-25, 159-161,
    167-168
  measure of students in, 25
  and nutrition, 180
  rates, 18
  and school environment, 24-25
  and school health services, 16, 38, 158-
    161, 167-168
  and social morbidities, 24
Pregnancy, *see* Teen pregnancy
Preschool programs, 66
President's Physical Fitness Test, 459
Primary care
  defined, 154
  nurses as providers, 222-223
  regional approaches to delivery, 186, 188
  in school-based health centers, 15, 42, 45,
    58, 154, 158, 160-161, 182, 187, 201, 217-
    218, 222-223, 373, 466, 469, 471-472
Principles and Practices of Student Health, 64
  n.6, 219
Principles to Link By, 47 n.3, 261
Professional development, training, and
    certification
  computer network discussion groups, 109
  demand for, 5, 116, 118-119, 140
  elementary school teachers, 141
  funding for, 248, 250
  health care services, 153-154, 163, 164,
    166, 169, 345-346
  health education, 5, 6-7, 103, 108-109,
    115-116, 117, 118-119, 121, 133-134,
    137, 138, 140, 141-142, 343
  infrastructure building, 11, 256-257, 265,
    267-268, 449-450, 457-458

  interdisciplinary approach, 11, 257, 265,
    267-268
  issues, 408-409
  mental health and pupil services, 66,
    170, 171, 184, 350
  nurses, 153-154, 163, 164, 345-346
  nutrition and foodservice, 119, 177, 181,
    352
  and outcomes, 103
  peer coaching, 109
  physical education, 84, 90-91, 93-94, 96,
    98, 348
  physicians, 166
  recommendations, 6-7, 11, 137, 138, 265,
    267-268, 449-450
  research on, 44
  for special-needs services, 169
  standards, 108-109
  transfer of training, 109
Program facilitators and coordinators, 66
Programs That Work project, 108
Project Pride, 194
Project School Care, 189
Psychologists
  issues related to, 170-171
  personnel, 170
  services provided by, 169-170, 371
Psychosocial environment
  and academic achievement, 65-66
  elements of, 2-3, 65-67, 339-340
  School Development Program, 66
  Success for All, 66-67
  Turning Points, 67
Public education, compulsory, 33-34
Public health, physical education and, 82,
    92-93
Public perceptions
  of health education, 36, 123-124, 140
  of nutrition, 180
  of school health services, 410
  of school role in integrating services, 445
Pupil personnel teams, 173-174, 370-372

Quality
  physical education, 83-84, 85, 88-89
  school-based health centers, 190, 196,
    389, 391
  school health services, 8, 14, 154
Quincy, Florida, 398-399

Race/ethnicity
   and poverty, 23
Ranier Beach High School (Seattle), 396
Reading, 66, 90-91
Recommendations
   CDC, 97-98
   confidentiality of health records, 227
   data collection, 227
   extended services, 227
   funding, 227
   health education, 5-7, 135-142
   infrastructure building, 9-11, 261-268
   physical education, 97-98, 139
   research, 13-14, 289-291
   school health services, 8-9, 226-227
   SHPPS, 138-139
Recommended Dietary Allowances, 178
Reducing the Risk, 106-107
Regional approaches, 186, 251-252
Reports and publications, influential/
      landmark, 34, 38-41, 245
Requirements for graduation
   health education, 5, 6, 110-112, 140, 141
   physical education, 68, 85, 88, 94, 95
Research and evaluation. *See also individual
      projects and studies*
   basic, 11-12, 13, 272-273, 288, 290
   challenges, 12, 75-76, 240, 271-272, 275, 289
   components of programs, 12, 14, 285-
      286, 291
   coordination of, 240
   data collection, 198-199, 280
   dependent variables, defining, 278-279
   diffusion-related, 13
   dose-response relationship, 275, 281-284
   effects of comprehensive programs, 281,
      284-285
   ethical issues, 277
   feasibility, 280, 289, 327
   funding for, 262-263
   goals, 51
   guidelines/manuals on, 280
   Hawthorne effect, 279
   health education, 5, 103-107, 108, 110,
      116-124, 132, 135, 138, 281-288, 312
   historical context, 43-44
   independent variables, defining, 277-278
   infrastructure building, 262-263
   on integration of program components,
      75-76
   linking outcome and process
      evaluations, 275
   methodological challenges, 190, 274, 276-
      280, 389
   organization, governance, and financing,
      186, 187, 398-400
   outcome evaluation, 7-8, 11-12, 50-51, 63,
      170, 189, 271-272, 273, 275, 276, 287-
      288, 290, 392-398
   overview, 271-276
   physical education, 81-82, 84-85, 86-91,
      98, 116-124
   process evaluation, 11-12, 247-248, 274,
      275, 276, 288, 289, 312
   professional education and training, 44
   recommendations, 13-14, 289-291, 450-451
   reporting bias, 280
   researchers, 275-276
   school-based health centers, 7-8, 226,
      190-199
   school health services, basic, 8, 40-41,
      186-189
   self-reporting biases, 279
   student health needs, 186-187
   Type III error, 279
   types of, 272-276
   uses for, 276
   utilization studies, 389-392
   validity assessment, 277-280
   workforce issues, 186, 187
Resource Coordinating Team, 173-174, 370-
      371
Responsible Students Program, 460
Rhode Island, 34, 242 n.3
Risks to Students in Schools, 64-65
Robert Wood Johnson Foundation, 45, 46,
      183, 187, 190, 192, 193, 212, 246, 258,
      374, 390, 391, 395, 399, 404
Rules of the Health Game, The, 39

Safe and Drug-Free Schools and
      Communities, 172, 174, 183, 207, 242,
      244, 250, 374, 377, 436-437
Safety programs, 41, 165, 218-219
San Antonio, Texas, 383
San Diego, California, 383-384, 405-406
San Fernando, California, 394-395, 396
San Francisco, California, 106-107, 394
San Jose, California, 394
School advisory councils and committees,
      66, 138-139, 253-254, 386
School-Based Adolescent Health Care
      Program, 46, 183, 193

School-Based Clinics That Work, 183
School-based health centers. *See also* Mental
    health centers
  and academic performance/graduation
      rates, 396-398
  and access to care, 7, 196, 226, 298, 366,
      394, 403
  administration, 467
  and behavior change, 7, 190, 191-192,
      226, 366, 390-391
  case studies, 183
  client characteristics, 161, 190-192, 390-392
  community health linkages with, 7, 374,
      470, 473
  confidentiality issue, 191, 390
  controversies, 398
  cost-benefit studies, 193-196, 389, 400
  data collection and management, 198-200
  definition, 373
  dental services, 473
  education role, 182, 373, 470, 472-473
  enrollment, 389-390
  funding and expenditures for, 46, 183,
      212-213, 243, 374, 398, 403
  and hospital/emergency room
      utilization, 193, 196, 366, 394, 400
  measures of effectiveness, 7-8, 226, 366
  mental health services, 464, 469-470, 472
  mobile vans, 182-183, 373-374, 375
  models, 203, 374, 467-473
  number of, 182, 373
  organization of, 373-375, 470-471
  outcome data, 7-8, 190, 192-195, 392-398,
      400
  parental consent, 190, 389, 399, 468-470,
      471-473
  part-time, 467-470
  personnel/staffing, 182, 312, 398, 468, 471
  primary care in, 15, 42, 45, 58, 154, 158,
      160-161, 182, 187, 217-218, 373, 466,
      469, 471-472
  quality of care, 190, 196, 389, 391
  referral and follow-up, 466, 469
  research and evaluation, 190-199, 226
  research needs, 7, 196, 199
  services, 71, 167, 182, 183, 203, 374-375
  standards of care, 239, 469-470, 471-473
  strengths and weaknesses, 196, 197-198
  utilization, 161, 190-192, 389-392, 393,
      394-396

School Breakfast Program, 45, 175-176, 438-
    439
School–Community Health Project, 43
School Development Program, 66, 385-386
School Enrollment-Based Health Insurance
    concept, 210-211
School environment
  CSHP, 64-68, 339-341
  eight-component program, 53
  goals, 51, 53, 101
  guidelines, 339-341
  infrastructure building, 460
  issues, 224
  physical, 2, 24-25, 34-35, 64-65, 340-341
  policy and administrative, 2, 65, 135,
      224, 339
  poverty and, 24-25
  psychosocial, 2-3, 65-67, 339-340
  sanitary inspections, 34-35
  three-component program, 52, 53
School guidance counselors. *See also*
    Vocational counseling
  issues related to, 171-172
  personnel, 171
  services provided by, 75, 169, 171
  visiting teachers, 38
School Health Care Online!!!, 199, 200
School Health Challenge, 64 n.6
School Health Coordinating Council, 11, 355
School Health Education Evaluation, 282,
    313, 322-323
School Health Education Study (SHES), 4,
    45, 100-101, 117
*School Health Education Study: A Summary
    Report*, 45
School health extension service, 10, 251-
    252, 263, 264
School Health Policies and Programs Study
    (SHPPS), 4, 5, 69, 71, 85, 92, 110-116,
    132, 135, 138-139, 140, 141, 153, 155,
    163, 182, 247, 252, 297, 373
School Health: Policy and Practice, 64 n.6, 154,
    163, 217 n.7, 219, 464, 465, 471
School health programs. *See also*
    Community participation in CSHPs;
    Comprehensive school health
    programs; History of school health
    programs
  access to health care and, 27-28
  components, 313-316

conferences and collaborative efforts, 44-45

context for, 16, 18-28

effectiveness, 313-316, 322-323

family structure changes and, 25-27

importance of education and, 15, 18-20

models, 167

nature of, 41-43

poverty and, 22-25

reports and publications influencing, 38-41

research and experimentation, 43-44

social morbidities and, 16, 20-22

School Health Resource Services, 243 n.4

School health services. *See also* Extended services; School-based health centers; Screening programs

barriers to utilization, 212

basic, 14-15, 161-181, 186-189, 201, 202, 463-465

community linkages, 165, 172, 173, 187, 217, 225-226, 403-404, 464, 467

components, 7, 71, 153-157, 225, 367

confidentiality of records, 8-9, 204-206, 227

coordination of, 345

crisis medical situations, 218-219

data collection, 8-9, 198-199, 227

definition, 153

delivery of, 15, 45, 186, 187, 188, 202-203, 419

evaluation of programs, 8-9, 187, 224-225

financing, *see* Funding of school health services

first aid and administration of medicines, 71, 155, 156, 218

goals and objectives, 3, 42, 51, 52, 53, 71, 154, 216-217, 344, 367

guidelines, 343-346, 458-459

health education, 166, 182, 215, 218-219, 223-224, 373

history, 37, 42

implementation steps, 216-225

infrastructure building, 247, 253-254, 265-268, 458-459

issues of concern, 70-71, 164-165, 166-167, 169

legislation affecting, 157

levels matched with needs, 199, 201-204

medical inspections of schools, 35-36, 41-42

mental health, *see* Mental health and pupil services

need for, 157-159, 186-187, 225

needs assessment, 217, 245

nurses and nurse practitioners, 162-165, 189, 345-346, 366

nutrition, *see* Nutrition and Foodservice

organization and governance, 186, 187, 188, 464

outcomes, 189, 192-193

parental consent for, 190, 205, 206, 389, 399, 465-467, 468-470, 471-473

personnel/staffing, 40, 71, 186, 187

physical education and, 98

physicians, 165-167, 345

policy and administrative support, 225-226, 343-344

poverty and, 158-161

primary care, 15, 42, 45, 58, 154, 158, 160-161, 163, 182, 201, 217-218

problem identification and resolution for students, 221-223

professional development/training, 163, 166, 169, 346

quality, 8, 14, 154, 226

rationale for, 401-402

recommendations, 8-9, 226-227

referral and follow-up of students, 40-41, 42, 174, 218 n.8, 221-222

research on, 40-41, 186-199

and school environment, 224

SHPPS survey, 155, 157

for special-needs students, 155, 156, 157, 165, 168-169, 170, 177, 187-188, 189, 209, 210, 214

standards, 162, 463-464, 466

status of, 401

student services, 344-345

team approach, 43, 121, 165, 188, 221, 247, 254-256

School Health Study, 43

School Mental Health Centers, 243 n.4

School Mental Health Project, 184, 377

School Nutrition Dietary Assessment Study, 73, 178

School-to-Work Opportunities Act, 48 n.4

Schools for the Future Project, 383, 404

Science

assessment measures, 108

health education in, 13, 69, 70, 125, 126, 127-128, 129-131, 134

national standards, 129-130
nutrition education in, 72, 75
profession qualifications and training, 134
Science for All Americans, 130-131
Screening programs
    alcohol and drug, 156, 422, 424
    anticipatory guidance, 209, 403
    cardiovascular, 156, 316-317, 422-423
    child abuse, 426
    cholesterol, 158, 422-423
    criteria for effective programs, 220
    dental, 167, 209
    Early and Periodic Screening, Diagnostic, and Treatment Program, 24, 207, 209, 219, 221, 243-244, 402-403, 432-433
    eating disorders and obesity, 165, 176-177, 423-424
    emotional/mental health, 426
    evaluation of, 187, 189
    follow-up and referral, 40-41, 42, 176-177, 221-222
    funding for, 209, 219, 221
    GAPS recommendations, 422-427
    height and weight, 71, 156, 165, 209, 423
    HIV, 425-426
    hypertension, 422
    implementation, 219-221
    issues, 221
    learning or school problems, 427
    Pap tests, 426
    physical fitness, 156
    rationale for, 157
    recommendations, 219
    responsibility for, 42
    scoliosis, 155, 166, 189
    sexual behavior, 424-425
    sexually transmitted diseases, 425
    tobacco use, 424
    tuberculin skin test, 427
    vision and hearing, 71, 155, 156, 165, 189, 209, 221-222
Search Institute, 27
Seattle, Washington, 396
Secondary schools
    completion rates, 20
    dropouts, 19-20, 21, 195, 380-381
    health education, 6, 110-112, 115-116, 182
    school-based health centers, 182
Self-efficacy, 68, 357-359, 362-363

Services. *See also* Nutrition and foodservice; School health services; *other specific services*
    elements of, 3
Settlement-house workers, 38
Sex education, *see* Human sexuality
Sexual behavior, 20
    cost-effectiveness of interventions, 122, 123
    health education and, 123, 132
    and mortality, 23
    trends, 20-21, 72
Sexually transmitted diseases, prevention, 16, 20, 46, 69, 100, 112-114, 119, 122, 123, 129, 196, 400
Single-parent households, 18, 26-27
Skills, *see* Social skills
Smallpox, 34
Smoking, *see* Tobacco use
Social learning theory
    goals, 116, 361-363
    and health education, 116, 117, 120, 310
    outcome expectations, 359-361, 362-363
    self-efficacy, 357-359, 362-363
    skills, 362-363
Social morbidities, new, 20-22, 46, 49-50, 72, 101, 139, 158-159, 245, 401-402, 416, 444-445
Social services. *See also* Social workers
    community linkages, 71, 222
    model programs, 38, 466
    standards, 466
    Title XX, 374
Social skills
    and behavior change, 13, 117, 120, 131, 285-286, 362-363
    communication and decision-making, 133
    conflict resolution, nonviolent, 100, 112, 114, 118, 133, 378
    curriculum, 66, 122, 132-133, 386
    goal-setting, 133
    measures of, 13
    practice by students, 132-133
    resisting social pressures, 133
    stress management, 133
Social studies, 69, 70, 75, 125, 126-127, 128-129
Social support theory, 310
Social workers
    issues related to, 173
    personnel, 172-173

services provided by, 169, 172, 371, 380-381

Society for Public Health Education, Inc., 59 n.5

Society of State Directors of Health, Physical Education, and Recreation, 59 n.5

Sociocultural perspectives
in delivery of health services, 419
in health care utilization, 212
in health education, 117, 121

South Tama County Partnership Center (Iowa), 379, 397

Southern Council on Collegiate Education for Nursing, 165

Southern Regional Education Board, 165

Solving School Health Problems, 44

Special-education and special-needs students, 37-38, 50, 71, 155, 156, 157, 165, 170, 177, 187-188, 189, 209, 210, 214, 248

Special Supplemental Food Program for Women, Infants, and Children (WIC), 438-439

Speech, language, and hearing therapists, 168-169

Spiral of silence theory, 310

Sports, *see* Competitive sports

Sports medicine programs, 166

Standards for Social Work in Health Care Settings, 469-470, 472

Stanford Adolescent Heart Health Program, 106-107

Stanford University, 385

St. Louis, Missouri, 195, 382

St. Paul, Minnesota, 192-193, 298

State agencies and organizations
advisory councils, 247
extended services from, 369
funding sources, 179-180, 207-208, 213
health education role, 137
infrastructure building, 10, 246-252, 263-264, 266
interagency coordinating council, 241, 247

State Collaborative on Assessment and Student Standards project, 108, 240

State Nurse Practice Act, 163

Strategic prevention concept, 311-313

Stress prevention, 314-315

Student Assistance Model, 372

Student assistance programs, 174, 250, 312-313, 372-373, 378, 394

Student Leadership Training, 378

Student outcomes
desired, 50
expectations, 359-361, 362-363
health centers and, 192-193
health education, 341-342
physical education, 347

Student services, 344-345

Substance abuse, *see* Alcohol and drug abuse

Substance Abuse and Mental Health Services Administration, 280

Success for All, 66-67, 386, 397

Suggested School Health Policies, 40

Suicide and suicide prevention, 20, 22, 72, 112, 114, 119, 322-332

Supplemental School Health Program, 371-372, 392-393

Teachers and personnel. *See also* Professional development, training, and certification
burden on, 44
health education, 5, 108-109, 115-116, 133-134, 138
health promotion for, 3, 53, 67-68, 224, 352-353, 461
health status of, 41
physical education, 84, 92-94, 96, 98
as role models, 68, 109
training/qualifications, 42, 84, 98

Teaching methods, *see* Instruction

Team Nutrition program, 243

Technical assistance, 184, 251-252, 263, 264

Teen Choice, 372-373, 393

Teen Health Centers, 214, 395, 407-408

Teen Health Corps, 381

Teen parent programs, 384-385

Teen pregnancy, 16, 20, 46
outcomes of interventions, 192-193, 196, 392-393, 400
prevention, 112, 114, 119, 122, 123, 192-193, 316-319, 322-323, 372-373, 375

Teenage Health Teaching Modules, 104-105, 132, 282

Television, 27

Temperance movement, 36-37

Tennessee, 377-378, 380

Texas, 129, 195, 371, 374, 375, 383

Tobacco use, 20, 21, 23
Tobacco use prevention, 69, 100, 112-115,
    119, 122-123, 251, 314-315, 318-321,
    460
Transportation, 37, 408
    safety, 64
Travis County Health Department (Texas),
    371
Trois Riveres study (Canada), 90-91
Tuberculosis, 36, 43
Turner School (Philadelphia), 387
Turning Point, 67, 404

United Way, 184, 185, 381
University of:
    Colorado Health Sciences Center, 155,
        162, 243 n.4
    Maryland at Baltimore, 184, 243 n.4
    Medicine and Dentistry of New Jersey,
        378-379
    Minnesota, 217 n.7, 243 n.4
    Texas Health Sciences Center at
        Galveston, 214
U.S. Children's Bureau, 43
U.S. Department of Agriculture, 175, 177,
    238, 243, 248, 459
U.S. Department of Education
    Comprehensive School Health
        Education Program, 117
    cooperation with the Department of
        Health and Human Services, 238
    funding for health services, 207, 241
    National Diffusion Network, 103, 108, 242
U.S. Department of Health and Human
    Services, 21, 207, 208, 217 n.7, 238,
    243, 280
U.S. Department of the Interior, 38-39
U.S. General Accounting Office, 19, 24, 175
U.S. Office of Education, 40
U.S. Public Health Service, 21
    Bureau of Primary Health Care, 48
    Healthy People 2000 initiative, 22, 39-40,
        46-47, 67-68, 83-84, 85, 99, 102, 112-
        115, 177-178
    Healthy Schools, Healthy Communities
        initiative, 48
    Maternal and Child Health Bureau, 47, 48

Vaccination, *see* Immunizations
*Values and Opinions of Comprehensive School
    Health Education in U.S. Public Schools*,
    124
Vanderbilt study, 189
Victorian attitudes, 36
Violence, 16, 72
Violent Crime Control and Law
    Enforcement Act of 1994, 48 n.4
Vision examinations, 35
VISTA, 184, 381
Visual and Performing arts, 69, 70, 126
Vocational counseling, 38, 172
Vocational education, 69
Volusia County, Florida, 210-211

Walbridge Caring Community (Missouri),
    195, 382, 396, 397
War on Poverty, 45
Washington Heights, New York, 387-388
Washington, D.C., 242 n.3
Washington State, 396
West Virginia, 242 n.3, 248, 251, 456-462
Westchester County Student Assistance
    Model, 372
White House Conference on:
    Child Health and Protection, 42, 44
    Child Welfare, 44
    Children and Youth, 44, 46
    Children in a Democracy, 44
    Food, Nutrition, and Health, 44
Wisconsin, 185, 242 n.3, 379
W.K. Kellogg Foundation, 43
Workforce 2000 report, 19
World Health Organization, 16 n.1, 58, 154

Yale University Child Study Center, 66,
    385-386
Youth employment, 46, 184
Youth Risk Behavior Survey, 20-21
Youth Service Centers, school-based, 184-
    185, 382, 393, 404
Youth Violence Prevention Demonstration
    Grant Program, 434-435

Zigler's Schools of the 21st Century, 383, 404